EVERY
SECOND
COUNTS

EVERY
SECOND
COUNTS

The Race to Transplant the First Human Heart

DONALD McRAE

G. P. PUTNAM'S SONS   *New York*

ılP

G. P. PUTNAM'S SONS
Publishers Since 1838
Published by the Penguin Group
Penguin Group (USA) Inc., 375 Hudson Street, New York, New York 10014, USA • Penguin Group
(Canada), 90 Eglinton Avenue East, Suite 700, Toronto, Ontario M4P 2Y3, Canada (a division of
Pearson Penguin Canada Inc.) • Penguin Books Ltd, 80 Strand, London WC2R 0RL, England •
Penguin Ireland, 25 St Stephen's Green, Dublin 2, Ireland (a division of Penguin Books Ltd) •
Penguin Group (Australia), 250 Camberwell Road, Camberwell, Victoria 3124, Australia (a division
of Pearson Australia Group Pty Ltd) • Penguin Books India Pvt Ltd, 11 Community Centre,
Panchsheel Park, New Delhi–110 017, India • Penguin Group (NZ), Cnr Airborne and Rosedale
Roads, Albany, Auckland 1310, New Zealand (a division of Pearson New Zealand Ltd) • Penguin
Books (South Africa) (Pty) Ltd, 24 Sturdee Avenue, Rosebank, Johannesburg 2196, South Africa

Penguin Books Ltd, Registered Offices: 80 Strand, London WC2R 0RL, England

Library of Congress Cataloging-in-Publication Data

McRae, Donald, date.
    Every second counts : the race to transplant the first human heart / Donald McRae.
        p.   cm.
    Includes bibliographical references and index.
    ISBN 0-399-15341-1
        1. Heart—Transplantation—History.   2. Transplant surgeons—Biography.
    3. Heart surgeons—Biography.   4. Kantrowitz, Adrian.   5. Shumway, N. E.
    (Norman Edward), 1923–2006.   6. Lower, Richard R.   7. Barnard, Christiaan, 1922–2001
    I. Title.
    RD598.35.T7M45   2006   2005056627
    617.9'54092—dc22
    [B]

Printed in the United States of America
10   9   8   7   6   5   4   3   2   1

This book is printed on acid-free paper. ∞

Book design by Meighan Cavanaugh

For Alison

CONTENTS

All these years later I can still see it clearly. It was an unforgettable sight. We had taken the old heart and we needed to move damn fast to fill that huge hole with a new heart. No wonder they were frightened of us then. No wonder they thought we were out of our minds.

—ADRIAN KANTROWITZ, DETROIT, MICHIGAN, OCTOBER 2003

What is it they always say about being the first? We all know the first guy to get to the North Pole or the South Pole—or to step across the moon. It's just that second or third guy's name that is a little more elusive. I understand the whole drama of being the first.

—NORMAN SHUMWAY, STANFORD UNIVERSITY SCHOOL OF MEDICINE, STANFORD, CALIFORNIA, JANUARY 2004

Prologue: Into the Void . . .

On a fevered and restless summer night, with the vast darkness of the un-known in front of him, Adrian Kantrowitz moved carefully, almost delicately, in the scrub room. He leaned forward and, gingerly dunking his right elbow into the hot stream pouring from the tap, set to work with the detergent. The huge and imposing forty-eight-year-old surgeon scrubbed as if, rather than being freshly showered, he were grimy with dirt. It was the last time he would be alone before he began the world's first human heart transplant, at Mai-monides Hospital in Brooklyn, New York, on June 29, 1966.

The lower half of Kantrowitz's face was covered in ribbed white gauze. Thin cotton strips held the mask against his mouth and nose, wrapping around the top of a surgical cap and the back of his powerful neck. A short-sleeved top, the same green as his trousers, pulled tightly at his shoulders as he bunched his muscled arms. He looked ready to lift a mighty load—one freighted with risk and history.

Moving into strange and dangerous territory, Kantrowitz was about to attempt a once unthinkable act. Even the idea of touching the human heart, let alone cutting it out and placing it inside another living body, had been considered impossible for all but the last twenty years. Kantrowitz knew the myths and warnings. Aristotle had established the belief that "the heart alone of all viscera cannot withstand serious injury." Ovid was equally emphatic that no man, no matter how gifted, could heal a damaged heart: "Although Aesculapius himself applies the sacred herbs, by no means can he cure a wound of the heart."

The heart was mysterious and sacrosanct.

Even Theodore Billroth, the Viennese master whom Kantrowitz regarded as the greatest of all surgeons, insisted it was the one organ in the human body that lay beyond reach. In 1883, Billroth claimed that "a surgeon who tries to suture a heart wound deserves to lose the esteem of his colleagues."

Kantrowitz wondered how much had really changed in eighty-three years. In his own hospital they called him a maverick. It was not just the fact that he roared through the streets of the hushed and black-robed Orthodox Jewish community surrounding Maimonides on a classic Indian motorcycle, the surgeon's heavy frame dwarfing his bike. They had also grown used to his image as a daredevil as he took to the skies to fly his own small plane. It was even part of his legend that when they were young and still dating in the Bronx, he and his future wife, Jeannie, used to hunt down stray cats for his innovative laboratory experiments.

The Maimonides board, and some of its leading doctors, thought Kantrowitz was crazy for a different reason. They called their director of surgery a force of nature, a man difficult to work with as he swept aside their orders to temper the breadth of his experimental animal research. Kantrowitz looked beyond them and focused instead on a far more formidable enemy.

Death hung over the two tiny bodies about to be packed in small tubs of ice in preparation for transplant surgery. Kantrowitz knew that he could bring back only one baby from the table. At least he did not have to choose between them.

They called the first, an eighteen-day-old boy, a "Gypsy prince." He was regarded as a future leader by the Gypsies who lived and wandered in and around Coney Island, and as far north as Boston. His new heart would be taken from a body born into oblivion. Kantrowitz found it incredible that in 1966, even in modern medical textbooks, the second baby was identified as an anencephalic "monster." He refused to use the term to describe a victim of anencephaly, a rare condition that, caused by some inexplicable genetic flaw, prevents the creation of a brain, or even the development of the upper skull in an otherwise normal fetus. Kantrowitz insisted on a more neutral expression. The smaller baby was the two-day-old "donor patient" who had been flown to Brooklyn from Portland, Oregon.

Earlier that night, Kantrowitz had made his last tour before scrubbing. He'd stood over the cot in which the anencephalic baby had been placed on its arrival. A white towel had been draped over the missing section of his head, as if to spare any passing nurses and orderlies a grotesque sight. Kantrowitz peeled back the towel and stared at the deformed skull. Instead of the soft and rounded curve of a newborn head, a leathery mass of reddened skin covered the top half of a face. A mouth and a nose were crudely visible, but it was hard for Kantrowitz to shift his gaze from the blankness above. Although the eyes protruded oddly, they were vacant. It was as if everything that made this body human had been cut away.

Kantrowitz thought of the remarkable parents. He wondered if he and Jeannie would have been willing to allow some doctor they had never met to fly their brainless baby across the country so that his heart could be taken to save another. He eased his gaze downward. The skin below the deformity was pale. Kantrowitz placed his giant hand over the baby's minuscule chest and stomach. His index finger rested on the fluttery heart beating inside.

Then he walked to the room where the Gypsy baby waited. A toy polar bear had been propped in the bottom right-hand corner of the hospital cot. The bear looked bigger than the baby he was guarding. The little prince was dressed in white and matched the furry coat of his arctic bear. He lay on his back, his short arms held high above his head in surrender, looking peaceful in the dim light.

Kantrowitz moved methodically through the last stages of preparation. He met his surgical teams, one assigned to the donor table and the other to the recipient's operating room, and announced his readiness to begin. The most vibrant doctors on his team—Jordan Haller, his first assistant, who was the head of thoracic surgery, and William Neches, a young pediatric intern—were inspired by his forceful presence. They saw the historic opportunity before them, not only to save an infant life but to shatter a surgical barrier with the world's first cardiac transplant.

There was unease and dissent, however, in the eyes of the older men. Harry Weiss, the silvery-haired anesthesiologist, and Howard Joos, the pedantic chief pediatrician at Maimonides, led the opposition. Kantrowitz sensed their thirst for battle but he was not about to reopen the debate as to when he might remove the donor heart. The Maimonides administrators had been emphatic. They had instructed him not to touch the organ to be transplanted until it stopped beating inside its original body. Kantrowitz thought differently. He wanted to take the living heart.

Kantrowitz was ready to risk everything in the next few hours. He was about to attempt a radical operation that he and his two main rivals— Norman Shumway and Richard Lower—had been racing toward for years. Close friends and research collaborators at the Stanford Medical Center from 1958 to 1965, Shumway and Lower were acknowledged as the leading pioneers in heart transplant research. Through rigorous exploration and surgical precision they had developed and refined the concept of switching a heart from one body to another. As they worked in isolation from other surgeons across America and around the world, Shumway and Lower's radical experiments had resulted in the first successful heart transplant between two dogs, six and a half years earlier, in December 1959.

Kantrowitz had followed them into the transplant field in 1962, but the Stanford pair still dominated the race to replicate their technique in man. In 1965, Lower succumbed to an irresistible offer to lead his own team, at the Medical College of Virginia, in Richmond, but even that departure from Stanford did not lessen his friendship with Shumway or their surgical pact to turn a revolutionary concept into a clinical reality.

Shumway and Lower were meticulous and cautious scientists. Kantrowitz came from a similar academic background—having trained under the renowned cardiovascular physiologist Carl Wiggers—but he was far more instinctive. He was willing to gamble in his bid to become a surgical leader.

Kantrowitz felt even more certain when he completed his scrubbing ritual in front of the gushing taps. Water glistened on his skin. His mind was clear and his hands were strong. The blunt sight of them rarely soothed any of those patients who believed in the romantic notion that a surgeon's hands should be elegant and slim with long, tapering fingers that might play the piano beautifully on a free evening away from the gore of the operating table. But Kantrowitz knew how many lives they had saved down the years—just as he never forgot how many patients he had lost.

Surgery was not just a brutal art; it was a bloody trade shrouded by death but seamed with great human attributes of hope and skill, courage and compassion. You could write about death, or sing about it, or paint it in streaks of black and red, but surgery went beyond artifice. Kantrowitz looked into the void every time his knife sliced through skin and muscle and exposed the heart. When he cut into the heart, he moved deep into another world. It was a world impossible to wholly conquer, but now Kantrowitz was about to try.

He would cut out a heart, lift it from the raw chasm, and then, holding it in a steel container filled with an icy saline solution, walk slowly to the room next door. He would place that same heart into the second baby's empty chest and, moving fast and sure, stitch and fasten it to a new home. He might imagine it as a kind of miracle had he not already proved that the technique worked in the hundreds of heart transplants he had carried out in puppies—the longest survivor was still alive more than two hundred days after surgery. And the human heart, he knew from twenty years in the OR and the laboratory, was far easier to handle than the bloodier and less pliant canine model.

Kantrowitz understood that the pressure about to bear down on him would be immense. It would make him sweat and swear, forcing him to holler with frustration when they hit trouble, or if one of his team moved too slowly. Yet the sheer enormity of his tilt at surgical history felt exhilarating.

Using his back to push open the door, he found his way into the room next door. Haller, Neches, and a few of the others were waiting for him. He took the pristine blue towel offered to him and dried his hands. He reached for his latex gloves and pulled them on with a snap, smoothing away the wrinkles as he flexed his fingers.

Kantrowitz turned and nodded to his surgical assistants. Haller, his eyes glinting behind operating glasses, winked in assent.

"Okay," Kantrowitz said, "let's go. . . ."

Adrian Kantrowitz was not alone. He was one of an exceptional quartet of heart surgeons who between 1958 and 1968 ventured deep into this uncharted terrain. All that Norman Shumway, Richard Lower, Christiaan Barnard, and Kantrowitz pursued now glitters before us in magnificent detail. But in those early years they were true explorers, and even icons. Some were friends, while others were medical rivals or plain old enemies from the 1950s, when two of them had worked together uncomfortably at the University of Minnesota in the thrilling early days of open-heart surgery. They were men who dared do the "impossible." They made the journey into the heart as compelling as the parallel race between the Americans and the Soviets to the moon.

If they were entranced by the work, and by the quest to be first, they had little notion that the winner of the race would become one of the world's most famous men—courted by the most powerful leaders on earth, from the American president to the pope, and trailed by breathless movie stars from Europe to Hollywood. The fallout from such a searing burst of celebrity would be tinged with tragedy and delusion. An even more deadly struggle against post-transplant rejection—when the patient's immune system acts instinctively to destroy the new heart, in the same way it attacks any "foreign" organism—preoccupied the men while they adjusted to the shock of public euphoria and antagonism toward the operation they had all helped pioneer.

In the midst of this surgical adventure and human drama, each of the four men recognized that, for all its ceaseless wonder, the pumping heart cannot match the calculating brain. Humanity resides in thought, or consciousness, rather than a beating heart. While that prosaic understanding may seem obvious today, U.S. law then accepted only the absence of a heartbeat as its definition of death. The concept of brain death did not exist then in American jurisprudence. Any attempt to remove a beating heart from a brain-dead body, even with permission from the donor's family, risked a charge of murder. Shumway ridiculed this antiquated "boy-scout definition of death" and, together with Lower and Kantrowitz, campaigned to overturn the law. Meanwhile, their rival, Chris Barnard, benefited dramatically from a far looser legal definition of death in apartheid South Africa.

After the race had been decided, in 1967, and the world had gone a little crazy with "transplant fever," one of the men suffered more than any other. He was finally put on trial four years later. There had been a time when it seemed as if he might even be accused of murder—for taking the heart from a brain-dead donor—but in the end he was charged with "causing wrongful death," in a million-dollar lawsuit. His career, his reputation, and the very future of cardiac transplantation were put on trial.

Such indestructible commitment—that readiness to face down risk and confront ruin—separates the transplant pioneers from the rest of us. If we read the details of the case again today, the magnitude of all they achieved and endured emerges again—from the very roots of their daring research in the animal laboratory, through accusations of medical "theft," as one surgeon stood accused of appropriating years of work done by others, to the seething aftermath of arguably the most famous operation in medical history. Yet they were united, too, in their surgical battle to overcome public fear of the unknown and even the antipathy of colleagues who engaged them in blazing confrontations over the bodies of both donor and recipient patients.

Such contrasting emotions shape this book, which is built around my own interviews with the American surgeons—and with the immediate family and members of the late Chris Barnard's unit, most notably his brother, Marius, who was a crucial member of his surgical team. Ambition and envy, compassion and resentment, dedication and despair, glory and infamy shadow this story. Most powerful of all, perhaps, remains the now virtually unknown fact that all four surgeons were on the brink of being the first to transplant a human heart.

More than a year before the famous first transplant, Kantrowitz and Lower were each poised on the verge of success—amid incredible scenes of acrimony over issues ranging from medical ethics to donor compatibility. Their stories became entwined still further in early December 1967, when three of the four were, separately and simultaneously, only hours from making medical history.

In Brooklyn, Cape Town, and Palo Alto, Kantrowitz, Barnard, and Shumway each stood alone at the abyss. They did not know exactly what would happen when, once they found an appropriate donor, they removed the diseased heart of their patient. They had so little time left to save a life—and to become the first. That astonishing collision of fates has, until now, barely been recorded.

Darkness came early that cold November afternoon as I pushed back the moment I would call her. Instead of drawing up a list of questions I might put to a woman I had never met, about the heart of her dead baby, I sat at my desk and watched the light fade from a wintry sky. It was not the first time I had felt adrift in the depths of this book. But this was different. Rhoda Senz was not a great heart surgeon, not a giant of medical research, nor a crucial member of a historic cardiac transplant team. The apprehension I had felt before approaching the revered but mysterious Shumway and Lower, the formidable Kantrowitz, or the notoriously irascible Marius Barnard was not the same as the disquiet that spread through that afternoon in late 2003.

Rhoda Senz's obscure place in history was of a more private nature. Even after thirty-seven years Senz seemed unlikely to discuss with a stranger the powerful distinction separating her from the rest of humanity. She was the first mother to have been asked if the heart of her living child could be taken from its chest and planted inside the body of another. Rhoda and her husband, Richard, were the first couple to face each other and consider such a stark request. She was the first woman to agree that someone in her family could be used as a donor in a cardiac transplant. And Richard Senz was the first man.

Kantrowitz, a surgeon accustomed to danger and risk, had told me about the "brave people" who had given him their son when he prepared himself to make history in June 1966. He remembered how the Senzes had allowed their anencephalic baby, whom they had just named Ralph, to be flown through the darkness from Portland to New York. It had taken immense courage, and he knew it.

Just before six p.m. in London, mid-morning in Oregon, I pressed the thirteen digits that might connect me to them. The number I had been given for the Senzes by Kantrowitz was almost ten years old. Richard and Rhoda had been living then, as they had back in the summer of 1966, in a small town in Oregon called Newbury. I had no idea what might have happened to them during the intervening years.

While I waited for a voice to answer, I watched a young woman on the rainy street below push a stroller through a small pile of leaves glistening beneath the yellow streetlights. She looked up at my window, almost accusingly, as I stood with the phone pressed to my ear. It was as if she sensed I was about to invade another mother's life. But she walked on, and the phone kept ringing.

I was still unsure what I would say to either Rhoda or Richard Senz if and when they picked up the phone. It was not the kind of call you could plan. This felt far more tangled. And then, at last, she answered.

Even as I bumbled around the subject, Rhoda Senz waited for me to get the words out. Calmly, almost serenely, she understood. The birth and death of her fourth son had happened many years before, but she still could not stop thinking of him every day. Only a few people outside their family knew what they had endured that fated summer, but she was proud rather than ashamed of their decision to help Kantrowitz and his dying patient. Yet this memory was not the kind you tossed lightly into an ordinary conversation. It remained a painful and fragile part of their lives.

We agreed that I would write to them in more detail in an attempt to explain the intentions of this book. "Do you have e-mail?" I asked tentatively of a sixty-seven-year-old woman who had stepped out into the unknown of medical science in the mid-1960s, a time when transplanting a human heart seemed a truly frightening and alien experiment.

Rhoda Senz laughed. Yes, she said, she and Dick had joined the modern world and mastered the Internet. She told me how they corresponded almost daily with their grandchildren in Tennessee. So an e-mailed letter would allow them to prepare themselves for my questions.

Later that night I began my letter to Rhoda and Richard by explaining that at the time of the first successful transplant I had been a six-year-old boy living in South Africa. Christiaan Barnard, the handsome and charismatic Afrikaner surgeon, had seemed like a magician to us in a country scarred and twisted by apartheid. We did not understand it then, but we lived in a warped and backward place. Even television was banned by the South African state, for until 1976 it was considered a tool of propaganda that Communist forces would use to deform our innocent minds. And so the very idea that South Africa could be at the center of heart transplantation in December 1967 thrilled us to the core. We might have been hated by the rest of the world, but the mystical Dr. Barnard, working alongside his brother, Marius, rose up as a heroic figure.

It was only years later, when I left South Africa, that I learned more about the other surgeons who for so long had led the race to transplant the first human heart. I explained that when I began this book Chris Barnard had just died. Both Marius Barnard and Norman Shumway had long been notorious for their refusal of any and all interview requests. So I sought out Kantrowitz first, and with him I was lucky.

In 2002, at the age of eighty-four, Kantrowitz had nodded sagely and folded his hands across his vast stomach when I told him that the extent of my scientific knowledge of the heart extended, then, to a few lonely facts—it comprised four chambers, of which those on the left were the more powerful, while, most miraculous of all, it would beat approximately three billion times in the life of a man as old and venerable as himself.

He nodded and smiled. Kantrowitz was equally patient while I mused on the philosophical and romantic myths of the heart—whether it was the ancient belief that the heart symbolized the very seat of the soul or any of the old rhetorical flourishes that insist wearily that "my heart goes out to them" or "I lost my heart that night" or "she's a heartbreaker." He grinned again. When it came to matters of love, Kantrowitz suggested, there are always more appropriate organs to use ahead of the heart.

He had now led me to the Senzes. It seemed invasive, but I wanted to know how they had felt when Kantrowitz asked if they would give up the heart of their son. Rhoda and Richard were ready to talk. And they wanted to hear about the surgeons and all that they had faced. They wanted to hear news from those epic days in which, however briefly, they had played a role. "Tell us more," she said, "tell us more . . ."

And so it became easy to talk. "Back then, in 1966," Rhoda said, "not everybody agreed with our decision. We tried to respond by saying that you must live by your beliefs and not try to influence ours—or be judgmental of us. We, in turn, won't judge your feelings. It was hard. We were doing something no one had ever done before. No one had ever tried to transplant a heart from one human to another. It just so happened that the heart being taken, or given, came from our baby."

Dick Senz was equally compassionate and thoughtful. But the more we spoke the harder it became for him. "The shock of it," he said, his voice cracking again after thirty-seven years, "was something terrible . . ." When he began to cry, his voice soft and muffled on the phone, it was time to set aside our interview. His openness and decency shone through the tears.

"Always feel free to call us," he said. "We appreciate your interest in our son."

I could still hear him crying quietly when, after I thanked him for talking to me, Dick Senz managed to say, "You bet." That simple and homely phrase stuck in my head. It reminded me of the amiable and magnanimous way that Shumway, Lower, Kantrowitz, and Marius Barnard eventually shared their recollections.

A few months later Rhoda wrote to tell me that "our media are keeping a close watch on the latest local heart transplant. Little four-month-old Baby Peyton is doing well and will be home with her family in time to begin the new year with a new heart. I pray that the donor baby's family will always carry their lost child close to their heart and feel they have done the right and best thing for both little ones."

Every year in America, around two and a half thousand heart transplants are carried out successfully. The number rises to four thousand when the annual global count is made. It represents a long line of lives that have been saved around the world after almost forty years and is testimony to Barnard, Kantrowitz, and, especially, Lower and Shumway. Following the progress of "Baby Peyton" made me remember yet again how incredibly close each of the surgeons had come to performing the first transplant.

I felt the power of this story all over again when I told Rhoda that Shumway, Kantrowitz, and Barnard had each been only hours away from making history.

"It might sound strange to you," Rhoda Senz said, "but this is all new to us. So what happened next?"

One

ON THE BRINK

Cape Town, South Africa, November 21, 1967

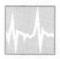Chris Barnard's old suit was black and frayed. It matched his mood as he rifled furiously through his pockets in search of a cigarette. He knew it was hopeless. He hadn't bought a pack in weeks. The surgeon usually stole a smoke at work from a sultry nurse he liked, or from one of the boys who sliced open his dogs in the dark and stinking Animal House. Alone in his wife's little red Toyota, Barnard was stuck at a set of broken-down lights on Main Road. The Tuesday-evening traffic was as thick as the frustration that overwhelmed him.

It had been a long and terrible day. His arthritic hands were raw and swollen as they gripped the steering wheel. Barnard's knuckles had turned red, as if in raging protest at the endless waiting. It seemed as if he did nothing but wait—whether for the light to change or for a human heart he might transplant into the chest of his dying patient. It sometimes felt as if he had even less time to make history than poor Louis Washkansky, a bloated and breathless wreck of a man, had days to live. The race closed in on them, tormenting Barnard with the thought that they might both be beaten before the month was out.

Black and colored workers ghosted past, heading for the crammed buses and trains that would rattle and clatter away from the city to the barren townships of Langa and Gugulutu, Athlone and Mannenberg. Cape Town was still "white by night." Only domestic servants were exempt from the racial curfew. They were allowed to stay in rooms at the bottom of suburban gardens so that they could clear tables and wash dishes before they rose early the next morning to polish shoes and prepare breakfast for their white masters and madams.

Barnard did not rail against apartheid. He just said that whenever he pulled on his surgical mask and the lights shone down on the table, it was the same old story. The color of skin, once he started cutting, was of no consequence. On the inside he always faced a field of red.

If he had been cruising along in a swanky American convertible, drifting through Sea Point and then past the golden beaches of Clifton and Camps Bay before climbing smoothly up Chapman's Peak, where the blue mountains and the glittering ocean stretched out majestically in front of him, perhaps he might have been able to dream of worldwide fame and medical immortality. Instead, on grimy old Main Road, he was just another middle-aged white commuter jammed to a standstill in a small and tinny car—a popular 1962 model called the Toyopet Crown.

The gaunt surgeon had to fold his six-foot-two-inch frame into the cramped front seat. His short black hair, slicked down with a morning dash of Brylcreem, sometimes left an oily stain on the low interior of the upholstered roof of the car. He was a good-looking man, even if his ears stuck out too much like jug handles for the comfort of his own vanity, but Barnard sometimes wondered if driving his wife's car made him look like a bank clerk. Who would guess, either by looking at his clothes or car, that he was the country's premier cardiac surgeon—a man accustomed to flipping open hearts? No one else trapped on Main Road that evening would have glanced over at him and imagined that he barely flinched when he encountered something as terrible as the tangled cluster of cardiac abnormalities known as a tetralogy of Fallot—the congenital heart defect that would have otherwise killed those hundreds of blue and tiny babies he had saved on the operating table.

Louwtjie, his wife, enjoyed the anonymity of driving the unremarkable little Toyota. Yet Christiaan Barnard had never been interested in obscurity.

Two weeks earlier he had turned forty-five—the same age as the unquestioned frontrunner in this race. Norman Shumway, based at Stanford University, in California, was already celebrated as a great American surgeon and a master of transplant research. Now, more than ever, Barnard craved recognition for his own brilliance. He knew this might be his last chance.

Washkansky's health had continued to deteriorate as speculation surrounding the world's first heart transplant intensified. Although Barnard had tried to keep his plans for the operation secret, that morning the *Cape Times,* quoting "a hospital source," revealed that surgeons were "on standby to perform a human heart transplant." The brief report suggested that the surgical team would "probably be led by Professor Chris Barnard."

It had been another day of grinding emptiness in which they seemed as far from finding a donor for Washkansky as they had ever been. Flicking on the car radio just after six, Barnard realized hazily that he had switched on the national evening news. The first few words slipped from the car's speakers in a senseless blur—but the final phase jumped out as if intent on wounding him: "*. . . a heart transplant at Stanford Medical Center.*"

The words hit him with shocking force. His hand reached out instinctively to crank up the volume, but the robotic newscaster had already moved on to another story, something about the high morale of the South African Defense Force. Barnard stared in anguish at the radio, as if he might force a miraculous replay of the report he had just missed. It was, of course, useless. And Barnard was suddenly sure of it. It was over. He had lost the race.

Shumway had done it. Jesus! Shumway won.

He had not even needed to hear Shumway's name. Stanford meant Shumway—the same coolly acerbic and grinning surgeon Barnard remembered from ten years earlier. In 1957 and the first six months of 1958 they had worked together under Owen Wangensteen and Walt Lillehei at the University of Minnesota. Barnard knew that Shumway had little regard for him. He didn't care, because he, sure as hell, had never cared much for Shumway.

Barnard's quest to become the first surgeon to transplant a human heart was driven in part by his desire for a measure of revenge. He wanted to prove that he was more than just some dumb Afrikaner from a despised country. He thought he was just as smart as Shumway. He was just as dedicated and just as inspired. He didn't know then how much the rest of the world might care about the winner of the race. His ambition was far more narrow in its focus. He thought of all those who had mocked or sneered at him in the past. Barnard pictured the surprise, perhaps the awe, in their faces when one day they might hear that he had made history.

His dream now lay in ruins. If Shumway had made the SABC (South African Broadcasting Corporation) news, that surely meant he had successfully transplanted a human heart. Barnard yearned for a twine of hope to which he might cling—but the sound of hooting and shouting made him look up instead. A cop in a brown uniform and white gloves gestured impatiently at him. Standing tall and grand on a wooden box, from which he directed the passing cars like an imperious conductor, he stared witheringly down at Barnard.

"Hey!" the traffic cop yelled above the noise of snarling traffic. "Are you *blerrie* [bloody] stupid?"

The surgeon drove home in a daze. When he got back after a typical day Barnard usually burst through the front door of The Moorings, the house he'd bought on the water's edge at Zeekooivlei (an Afrikaans name meaning Hippopotamus Lake), in an ordinary suburb on the edge of Cape Town. He would kick off his shoes and socks and head for the bedroom, leaving a trail of clothes for his wife to pick up while he soaked in a hot bath. Barnard would then dry himself, flop down on the bed and cover his face with a pillow while he recovered from the day.

But this evening was different. By the time he reached home he was deeply agitated—especially when Louwtjie shrugged and replied that she had not listened to the news and so could not tell him whether Shumway had already done a transplant. The weariness in her voice suggested she cared little either way. She was more interested in the unlikely dream of her husband getting home at a decent hour than in his pursuit of medical stardom.

An irate Barnard brushed past her and reached for the phone. He called Groote Schuur Hospital where he was finally put through to François Hitchcock, a young registrar who had been among those assisting him in transplanting the first kidney on the African continent in early October. Hitchcock had since been given a place on the cardiac team. He quietly explained to

Barnard that he had been working and had not had time to listen to his radio. He had no idea what Shumway might have done.

"You'd better go out and find a donor *now*!" Barnard snapped.

He slammed down the phone and scrambled for the telephone number of the state-run SABC. He was still convinced the race was over. Barnard felt it in his bones and aching hands. His rheumatoid arthritis had been diagnosed in the bitter Minnesota winter of 1956. He knew that it was an incurable disease. While a student doctor in Cape Town, his first patient had been an old woman crippled so badly by the illness that she could no longer wash or feed herself. When he was told that he suffered from the same ailment, his future threatened to collapse around him. How could he cut and heal when his own hands were so damaged?

It took him almost twenty minutes to locate the relevant editor on the news desk who could confirm that they had run the Stanford story. Barnard gripped the phone as tightly as his hands allowed.

And then, slowly, he let a long breath slide from him. The SABC, picking up on an American wire report, had merely reported Shumway's *readiness* to carry out a transplant. He had not, as yet, fulfilled his ambition. Shumway was frighteningly close. Yet, as long as they lacked a donor at Stanford, Barnard still had a chance. Relief swept through him.

Groote Schuur Hospital, Cape Town, South Africa, December 2, 1967

Eleven days later, on a sweltering Saturday afternoon, the hospital seemed desolate. Before his round of the wards, including A1, where Washkansky lay dying, not one nurse or resident seemed to share Barnard's craving for a cigarette. They all claimed to be nonsmokers. The surgeon was incredulous.

"What kind of people are you?" Barnard yelled.

The race again seemed to be slipping away from him. His American rivals— Shumway, Lower, and Kantrowitz—had already amassed a vast bank of transplant research that mocked his own limited experience. He knew that each surgeon in that esteemed trio was now preparing separately for the first clin-

ical trial. Shumway led a crack team at Stanford, while Lower, his former research partner, headed his own unit at the Medical College of Virginia in
Richmond, where the great kidney transplant pioneer, David Hume, was desperate that they should be the first to claim the heart. At Maimonides Hospital
in Brooklyn, Kantrowitz had at his command a $3 million grant and thirty-
five international researchers and surgeons.

Barnard relied instead upon his younger brother, Marius, who was just
making his way in cardiac surgery, and their lab's untrained "nonwhite" staff.
Chris and Marius argued bitterly and frequently—but they were bound together by love for their father, Adam, a Calvinist minister who had suffered in
the harsh desertlike region of the Karoo. Adam Barnard and his family had
been reviled by the local Afrikaans community in the small town of Beaufort
West because he preached in a colored church. Chris and Marius's sense of
isolation and insecurity had been forged amid such hostility.

They had still not endured the same hardship as the men they worked
alongside at the Animal House. Victor Pick was a colored man from the barren Cape Flats. Hamilton Naki, like the imprisoned Nelson Mandela, was
a Xhosa. Apartheid dictated that they could never officially claim to be anything more than a laboratory attendant and a former gardener turned cleaner.
But Victor ran the lab and opened and closed the dogs, removing and
transplanting kidneys and hearts alongside Marius. And Hamilton proved
himself a competent anesthetist and an even better experimental surgeon.
Chris taught them well, but they had both exhibited an instinctive aptitude
for the work.

By mid-November 1967, the unlikely Cape Town team had transplanted
forty-eight hearts in dogs—250 less than Shumway and 210 less than Kantrowitz
in New York. Unlike the Americans, who could restore their transplant-dogs
to full health for a year and more, the South Africans' longest survivor died
after ten days. Yet Barnard insisted that "in over ninety percent of [our] experiments the new heart had begun to beat regularly. It was a technique built on
that developed by Shumway and Lower, who had experimented on more than
300 dogs. The body of their work was formidable—especially in their studies
of rejection. With their findings joined to ours, there was little sense in continuing the further sacrifice of animals."

Barnard had, in his own words, "plagued [his chief cardiologist] Val Schrire day and night" for permission to transplant a human heart. Finally, despite also suffering from kidney and liver failure, Louis Washkansky was put forward by Schrire as a possible recipient. For once, the meticulous cardiologist set aside the empirical evidence and spoke of Washkansky as a fighter—a fifty-three-year-old former boxer who refused to give up until he was "knocked out for good."

While Washkansky believed utterly in the transplant, his wife, Ann, worried that he regarded the Afrikaans surgeon as an improbable Godlike figure. In Yiddish he called Barnard "the man with the golden hands." Ann Washkansky thought, rather, that Barnard looked like a young Gregory Peck. That would have been great if she had been standing in line for a Saturday-night movie. But this was a man who wanted to remove her husband's heart from his chest. She shuddered at his audacity. Louis, however, was emphatic. "Stop worrying, kid," he always said. "Everything's going to be just fine."

On that quiet Saturday, however, it suddenly seemed to Washkansky that nobody cared. He looked angry and miserable when Barnard approached his bedside. The two doctors on the transplant team who monitored his condition most closely, M. C. Botha and "Bossie" Bosman, had visited Washkansky earlier that morning. They had promised him cheerfully that that they would see him again on Monday.

Washkansky said softly that they had gone fishing—there was no need for him to add the words "while I'm dying . . ."

Barnard tried to reassure him, reminding Washkansky that the entire team was on constant alert. They could be ready for surgery within an hour of a donor being found.

"I'm getting the hell out of here," Washkansky wheezed.

He was too ill to move. Washkansky started coughing and, as usual, brought up blood. His hands were trembling as he pressed a peach-colored tissue to his mouth. He spat and the tissue turned red.

Barnard knew that Washkansky's heart had been reduced to a third of its normal pumping capacity. The second of two massive heart attacks had destroyed most of his left ventricle. After studying the initial angiogram of Washkansky's heart, Barnard had told Schrire that surgery would be pointless. Nothing could save such a heart. And there was serious doubt, now, that the big man would survive long enough for them to even attempt a transplant.

Washkansky, stretched out like a corpse on his bed, asked Barnard if he thought they would soon find a donor.

"Maybe," the doctor murmured. "I hope so . . . yes."

"It was one of those lies you tell," Barnard wrote later, "to keep courage and hope both for yourself and the patient. I had no way of knowing when we might get a heart for him—if ever."

The tension was almost unbearable. By two-thirty that afternoon the man with the golden hands could stand it no longer. He decided to drive home. Another day had disappeared. Barnard could only hope for tomorrow—and pray hard that night for a heart.

Stanford Medical Center, Palo Alto, California, December 2, 1967

That same day, in the early hours of a cold California morning, death closed in on another small white room. Norman Shumway's thirty-five-year-old patient, a potentially ideal candidate for a heart transplant, slid away slowly. He had developed terminal heart disease after a long period of radiation for Hodgkin's disease. Shumway and his young chief resident, the cool and erudite Ed Stinson, were convinced that a transplant could save him. An extensive course of radiation had probably caused his chronic heart failure, but at the same time they believed that his diminished immune system would be too weak to reject a new heart. They just needed a donor.

Shumway stood on the brink—but he would not wish death on anyone. He could not part the blinds, slatted against the gray dawn, in the hope that he might see an ambulance screaming around the bend along Welch Road carrying a potential donor strapped to a stretcher. Shumway was not ghoulish. He was calm rather than frantic. But he was still a man who could not keep a lid on his ambition forever. Shumway needed a heart to save his patient, and to fulfill the destiny he had been inching toward for nine long years. He needed a heart that was still beating and just waiting to be taken. Shumway, having left nothing to chance for so long, needed a slice of random luck to break the heavy spell of waiting.

He might have found a donor more readily if he was still up on the fifth floor of the old Stanford-Lane Hospital in San Francisco, where he and Lower, his close friend, had first transplanted dog hearts in 1958. There were many more downtown trauma victims there than on the sleeker streets of Palo Alto. Shumway knew nothing of Barnard's plans, but as the days grew shorter, he felt a growing urgency.

He tried to amuse his team with shards of black humor. It did not even take the distant howl of an ambulance to prompt another wisecrack. Once, to pass the time, Shumway made a sign with a saying that seemed to encapsulate the curious life of the transplant surgeon. He stuck the wry slogan to the back of his office door. It made him smile while he waited.

WHERE THERE'S DEATH, THERE'S HOPE . . .

Shumway and Lower had moved toward this moment through a radical decade. Beginning eight years before Barnard, they had perfected their innovative surgical technique and also done more than anyone to study ways of countering the menacing threat of rejection. As a result of their copious research, they now understood that the immune system, in an instinctive defense mechanism, would begin to reject and destroy a transplanted heart after seven or eight days. Yet some of their dogs were leaping around, thriving and eating "heartily," as Shumway would quip, deep into their second year with a new heart beating in their chests.

Lower knew that Barnard had copied the technique directly from him while spending three months in 1966 at his lab in Richmond, Virginia. When another South African in Virginia, a lab technician named Carl Goosen, warned that Barnard had told him furtively that he planned to return home to Cape Town to carry out the world's first transplant in a human, Lower had simply shrugged: "How can he?" Barnard had done nothing in transplantation. Even if Lower and Shumway's transplant method could be emulated by a competent surgeon who studied their many detailed research papers on the subject, Barnard would still need years of work before he could equal their practical familiarity with rejection.

Shumway remembered the Afrikaner vividly from their time together in Minnesota. While Barnard had been a relentless worker and a bright operator he'd often appeared, even in the competitive world of American surgery, aggressive and self-absorbed. He was regarded as overbearing by most of his fellow residents. His severe crew cut, those big ears, and a loud and braying Afrikaans accent had not endeared him to the others. Shumway, by contrast, was engagingly laconic. He was the cleverest and funniest of all the outstanding residents at Minnesota. You could tell a joke to Shumway and be assured that he would reply with an even sharper riposte. And Shumway, unlike the more painstaking Barnard, was a brilliant surgeon. Christian Cabrol, a smart and witty resident from Paris, marveled at the way Shumway produced the most beautiful stitching with simple exactitude. Such clarity of purpose and confidence epitomized Shumway both in and out of the operating room. "Norm Shumway," a brooding Barnard once heard Cabrol say, "is serenity."

Shumway and Lower still regarded the race as essentially a friendly private contest. They rarely spoke of Kantrowitz, let alone a complete outsider like Barnard. Their names had been entwined for so long that they kidded each other as to who might win. They knew that when the moment finally arrived they would share, and quietly rejoice, in each other's glory. It would mark a sweet victory and establish cardiac transplantation as a routine medical procedure.

Lower had come close the previous fall, only to be blocked by blood-type incompatibility between his recipient and potential donor. At the start of October 1967, Shumway had stressed his own readiness to operate. He soon found a recipient—the unfortunate man who had swapped Hodgkin's disease for chronic heart failure.

While he searched for a donor, Shumway sensed the need to familiarize ordinary people and the more reactionary members of the medical community with a supposedly bizarre concept. He understood that the world still swooned beneath a ludicrously sentimental notion. The heart, rather than the brain, was regarded as the defining characteristic distinguishing one person from another—the big-hearted hero from the hard-hearted miser, the cold-hearted killer from the young-at-heart pensioner.

Shumway knew that it was just bad writing, and fuzzy thinking, but he lived in the real world. Everyone seemed in thrall to clichés of the heart. No blues singer sang of his broken lung or aching liver; Tony Bennett had not left his kidney in San Francisco. A kidney transplant, while still startling, could at least be approached by most people with some detachment. And so the kidney, and then the more technically challenging liver graft, had inevitably preceded the heart in transplant history.

While he waited, Shumway pressed ahead with his crusade to prepare America for cardiac transplantation. He granted an interview to the *Journal of the American Medical Association* (*JAMA*). Their exclusive was printed on November 20, 1967: " 'We think the way is clear for trial of human heart transplantation,' says surgeon Norman E. Shumway, MD. 'We have achieved a degree of experience with heart transplantation in the laboratory with which we feel confident we can take appropriate care of the patient with a cardiac transplant. Although animal work should and will continue, we are none the less at the threshold of clinical application.' "

Twelve days had since passed and the recipient was close to death, but Shumway held his faith while he continued the long vigil. He had always been a patient doctor.

Maimonides Medical Center, Brooklyn, New York, December 2, 1967

Adrian Kantrowitz, a redoubtable man at six feet, two inches tall and weighing 260 pounds, cut a less serene figure as, again on that very same day, he stared down at the baby with the miraculous hair. They all thought Jamie Scudero was beautiful. His face was perfectly round and chubby while his huge eyes were dark and alert. Whenever the passing nurses paused to look in at Anna Scudero watching over Jamie they would say of her new baby, "Oh, what wonderful hair!" or "Boy, that's what I call a head of hair!"

The surgeon, however, was almost completely bald. He had turned forty-nine in early October. Kantrowitz was at his surgical peak. It did not matter that Shumway was also on the verge of success. Kantrowitz had read the previous week's issue of *JAMA,* but he felt technically and mentally equipped to do what no other doctor had yet dared try.

The operation itself would be relatively uncomplicated, a replica of his hundreds of dog-heart transplants. Kantrowitz knew that the primary battleground would be the fight against rejection. How the human body would react to a transplanted heart remained uncertain. Yet he was convinced that he had been cannier than Shumway and Lower in choosing an infant transplant. His research on puppies echoed earlier scientific findings that an undeveloped immune system was more likely to accept a transplanted organ. Even without any immunosuppressive drugs, one of his frisky dogs was still alive 119 days after receiving a new heart.

Looking down at Jamie Scudero, Kantrowitz forgot about Shumway and Lower. He confronted forces more powerful than any of them. A combination of deadly cardiac flaws—pulmonary atresia with patent ductus arteriosus as well as atrial and ventricular septal defects—lurked deep inside the baby.

Kantrowitz had been at this exact point eighteen months earlier, when he had tried to save the small Gypsy boy by using the heart of an anencephalic baby born to Richard and Rhoda Senz. The raw drama of that night still haunted him, but he was determined to try again. A few weeks before he had attempted that transplant, in June 1966, Kantrowitz had made the front page of *The New York Times* with the news that, during a groundbreaking six-hour operation, he had implanted the world's first permanent left ventricular assist device, described wrongly by some journalists as "an artificial heart," into the chest of a terminally ill sixty-three-year-old woman named Louise Ceraso.

Her breathing and circulation improved markedly after her operation and yet, thirteen days later, with Kantrowitz at her bedside, she died on May 31, 1966. The success of the actual implantation, and his familiarity with death, did not lessen his distress. "When you lose a patient," Kantrowitz said, "you can only feel a sense of failure."

His fierce desire to save hearts remained. Brushing aside the likelihood of yet more international publicity for a modest community hospital in Brooklyn, he pressed ahead with his plan to transplant a human heart. The administrators recoiled in alarm. Cardiac transplantation still seemed a step too far—even for Kantrowitz.

Yet he was driven on by the knowledge that, in 1966, he had been the nearest of all four to grabbing the grail. He had deliberately not revealed any details of his previous human transplant attempt at the surgical conferences where he often met Shumway and Lower. Kantrowitz respected his rivals but he believed that daring, as much as methodical preparation, would be just as vital when the first human heart was finally transplanted. He was convinced that the discrepancy in their characters was one of the reasons why Shumway seemed to have taken a subtle dislike to him. Shumway was more measured while Kantrowitz was decidedly brash. Shumway engaged in discourse with Nobel Prize winners in the California sunshine while Kantrowitz walked among the braided and black-clad Hasidic Jews in a New York ghetto. Shumway was cardiac transplantation's solid pioneer, Kantrowitz the risk-taking experimentalist who planned to salvage the heart on two different fronts—through mechanical assist devices and transplantation.

The race, for Kantrowitz, had been condensed into its own tight little triangle. Shumway at Stanford, Lower in Richmond, Kantrowitz in Brooklyn. While there existed a polite wariness between Kantrowitz and Shumway, Lower was warm and open. Still, Kantrowitz regarded it as natural that even he and Lower did not swap anecdotes about their respective plans. Some details of the race demanded discretion.

At least they agreed that they were all hampered by timid medical committees and ignorant legislators who refused to sanction brain death as a permissible concept in the United States. Kantrowitz would have liked to take a living heart from a brain-dead patient—but the law suggested that he might be charged with murder.

A succinct letter had been sent on November 24 to the same 500 hospitals across America that had been contacted previously by Maimonides in their search for an anencephalic donor: "We are again urgently seeking an anencephalic donor for life-saving purposes. If you have such an infant (or a patient at term with such a live fetus) within the next week, wire or call collect immediately. We are prepared to transport baby and nurse (or doctor) and mother. Be assured that all moral considerations with regard to the baby will be observed. Please accept our thanks for your cooperation last year in a similar situation."

And still they waited. Jamie Scudero's gorgeous head of black hair grew while his heart withered. It was unusually thick and glossy for such a sick infant. On that second day of December, a peaceful Saturday in Brooklyn, Jamie was exactly two weeks old. It felt to Anna Scudero as if she had hardly slept for those fourteen days and nights. Everyone at Maimonides showed her kindness and encouragement—but only Kantrowitz had the courage and power to save Jamie.

He saw Anna again that afternoon on his last round. He was about to return home for the weekend to his own family, to Jean and their three teenage children, whom he had lately neglected. Kantrowitz told Jamie's mother that the call might come at any moment. He urged her not to despair. They would find a donor. The transplant would happen soon—perhaps even that very weekend. "It could be tomorrow," he said hopefully.

Anna nodded as the surgeon stretched out his hand to her. "Tomorrow," she said softly.

"We just need a little luck," Kantrowitz said.

She nodded. Anna had yet to hold her baby, but she could not stop smiling as she looked down at a sign the nurses at Maimonides had placed at the bottom of Jamie's crib: *"If you can't do nothing with my heart, please do something with my hair."*

"Yeah," Kantrowitz murmured. "We're gonna fix his hair. And then we'll give him a new heart."

OUT OF THE COLD

The race began nine years earlier, during the hot and endless summer of 1958, when two young men in masks stood over a tail-wagging dog. In the dingy fifth-floor laboratory of the battered old Stanford-Lane Hospital in downtown San Francisco, Norman Shumway and Richard Lower chose their frisky mongrel carefully. Using extreme cold to bend and slow time in a building that creaked and groaned in the heat, they hoped to make a small slice of history. Shumway and Lower had not known each other for many months but they were already fearless explorers of the heart.

They planned, in another of their quiet experiments, to stop the dog's heart for sixty minutes. But they did not intend to watch aimlessly over a corpse. A heart-lung machine, circulating oxygenated blood through the dog's brain and body, would keep their furry patient alive. Yet while the machine took its place as a life-giving pump, the heart itself would remain utterly still in an icy solution of saline. Denied both blood and oxygen for the entire hour it would become a "dry" field, its relatively bloodless state providing ideal conditions for surgery. Lower had raised an eyebrow when Shumway first suggested that they should try to arrest and then safely restart a heart after sixty minutes. No one had ever achieved such a feat.

Lower whispered a few words to the mutt, tickled it behind the ear, then stroked it gently. He hoped fervently that they would not lose the dog. Shumway, the master of cold, monitored his two liters of isotonic saline. Chilled to between 0 and 5 degrees centigrade (32 to 41 degrees Fahrenheit), the saline would irrigate and protect the dog's heart. Shumway had already primed the humming heart-lung machine with the required three liters of canine blood that, flowing fast and red through the lines of tubing, would circulate oxygen through the rest of the dog, from the tips of its ears to the pads of its paws. This fresh but cool blood, drained from individual donor dogs, had been lowered slightly below normal body temperature to 32 degrees centigrade (89.6° F). Only the heart would turn dead cold in saline. Only the heart, the most voracious consumer of oxygen in the body, even more so than the brain, would have to survive without the basic source of life—oxygen-rich blood.

They knew that this revolutionary technique, which Shumway called "topical hypothermia," could transform the pioneering art of cardiac surgery. If it could be proven to work, there would be no need for the damaging injections of concentrated potassium used to cause cardiac arrest before surgery, and no need to jam the operating site with catheters to infuse the heart with cold blood during surgery. Topical hypothermia would allow the surgeon to cut open and work on the heart in such a way that he would be spared the cluttered tubes and bloody leaks that usually obscured his vision and hampered his work.

Even more significant, Shumway and Lower would have shown it was possible to completely protect the heart for that same length of time. An hour's operating time would open the previously sealed door to far more intricate surgery, allowing for the correction of the most complicated of heart defects. They did not know it then, but their experiment would soon make transplantation a practical reality. That revelation remained, for the moment, hidden even from them.

Lower looked up at the big clock on the wall. Shumway nodded. It was time. He reached for the anesthetic, a solution of pentobarbital sodium. While Lower patted the dog one last time, Shumway silently slid the needle home.

Shumway had become a champion of the cold in Minneapolis, at the Minnesota University Hospital, where he spent much of the 1950s. Apart from witnessing the rise of the world's first open-heart program, Shumway learned to appreciate the power of hypothermia amid the invasive weather. In the freezing and isolated Midwest they spoke proudly of "Minnesota cold." It was the kind of cold that, if you allowed it the opportunity, would turn your skin blue.

In the streets of Minneapolis and St. Paul they delighted in the much re-peated fact that once, in 1885, a reporter from New York had described their twin cities, in print, as "another Siberia, unfit for human habitation." The St. Paul Chamber of Commerce had responded defiantly the following year by launching a Winter Carnival to prove that the region was not only "habitable but that its citizens were very much alive during the most dominant season." That defensive response soon gave way to a haughtier cool. Every year an ice castle, made from the frozen waters of Minnesota's "10,000 Lakes," rose up in shimmering grandeur at their carnival of cold.

The young Shumway came from a slightly milder world. Born in Kalama-zoo, lost halfway between Chicago and Detroit, he had been raised in Jackson, a small Michigan town. While there was often ice and snow in the long, dark months that bridged the years, the winters of Jackson were nothing like those that engulfed him in Minnesota. He arrived as a medical intern in the fall of 1949 and was soon exposed to the raw elements. Shumway didn't care much. He was more intrigued by the idea of working under the inspirational John Lewis and, later, Walt Lillehei.

The two great pioneers of open-heart surgery were compelling men. Lillehei sported sharp suits, alligator shoes, grinning good looks, and a flashy Buick convertible while Lewis, his old medical-school buddy, emerged as the ulti-mate Renaissance man. In addition to being an accomplished surgeon, Lewis wrote and drew beautifully. He climbed mountains, dabbled in early electronic computing, and read Kafka and Joyce in between drinking martinis with Lillehei at Mitch's or the Parker House, where a band played Dixieland jazz all night long.

Unlike Lillehei, who surrounded himself with a large group of junior res-idents, Lewis was an individualist. Shumway described him as a lone eagle, with his refusal to build a team his only real flaw as a surgeon. Yet to the rare intern or resident he regarded as exceptional, Lewis showed great generosity. He loved Shumway's humorous disdain for academic authority. Shumway, in turn, admired the precision of Lewis's thinking and the quality of his jokes. They became a star pairing during their hospital rounds.

Beneath the banter they were fiercely serious; and Lewis burned most whenever he entered the cold, still world of hypothermia. Down in the basement of the University's Millard Hall he encouraged Shumway in the early 1950s to study the physiological impact of lowering the body temperature of an anesthetized dog to around 28 degrees centigrade. With the heartbeat slowed to almost half its normal rate, it became possible to use tourniquets to close off the superior and inferior venae cavae while clamping the pulmonary artery, which sends blood to the lungs, and slice into the right side of a dog's heart. They would then sew shut the incision and release the clamp and tourniquets to allow the heart to resume pumping blood around the body.

They closed the chest in less than six minutes—the time allowed for a quick procedure inside the heart before lack of oxygen caused brain damage. Lewis and Shumway then monitored the dog's return to full consciousness. There were many early fatalities, but gradually they turned a surreal process into a routine procedure.

The most banal cliché of medical aid insisted that, after a person had been injured or stricken with illness, the immediate medical response was to keep the body warm by wrapping the patient in a blanket and serving up a mug of hot sweet tea. Cold was considered the enemy, a killer of tissue. Shumway had seen enough cases of frostbite during the Minnesota winters to appreciate the sentiment. Yet extreme cold did not destroy everything it enveloped. Shumway knew it could also save lives.

Wilfred Bigelow, a Canadian surgeon, had developed the concept of hypothermia in the late 1940s. He had always been fascinated by groundhogs and the way, through hibernation, they survived the bitter Canadian winters. He was intrigued by the natural reduction in heartbeat and the animal's ability to survive underground without food. It was as if the cold ate into time. Weeks and months slid harmlessly past as the slumbering groundhogs remained buried beneath the packed ice and snow.

Bigelow became obsessed with hibernation and the idea that it could help him, as a surgeon, achieve the impossible and work inside a human heart. If the entire body was cooled to a point of near hibernation, would the heart be finally ready for surgery? Bigelow began to experiment, operating on the open hearts of almost a hundred dogs. He lost many, especially those whose body heat was reduced to below 20 degrees centigrade (68° F). Bigelow learned that this was the point from which no dog could be brought back to consciousness. But most of the others, cooled to between 25 and 30 degrees centigrade (77 to 86° F), would wake in water warm enough to steadily raise their temperature back to normal; and they showed no lasting mental or physical deterioration after surgery.

At the same time, hypothermia competed with the heart-lung machine as the best way to allow a cardiac surgeon to shut down the circulation of blood so that he might work on the heart. John Gibbon had toiled for decades in his Philadelphia laboratory as he attempted to build the world's first successful heart-lung machine. In May 1950, *Life* magazine declared prematurely of Gibbon's creation that "this robot, a gleaming stainless steel cabinet as big as a piano, will soon be tested on humans."

It was in Minnesota, however, eighteen months after Shumway's arrival, that Clarence Dennis became the first man to attempt open-heart surgery. On April 6, 1951, at the University Hospital, Dennis operated on a five-year-old while using his own hulking heart-lung machine. The operation went disastrously wrong, making hypothermia seem the more viable option.

On September 2, 1952, Lewis relied solely on total-body hypothermia to open the heart and work inside its chambers. Using an ice-packed tank and cooling blankets, Lewis and Lillehei lowered the body heat of five-year-old Jacqueline Johnson to 28 degrees centigrade (82.4° F). With her heart rate halved, Lewis split open the little girl's chest. After isolating the right side of the heart with clamp and tourniquets, he opened it by cutting through the wall of the right atrium. Three minutes into the operation, Lewis located the hole in her heart. It was a simple ASD (atrial septal defect). Lillehei watched the clock and counted the seconds. Lewis had exactly two minutes to sew it shut and get out of the heart so that oxygen would be able to return to the brain before the six-minute barrier was reached. He stitched this way and that, his hands moving swiftly but calmly.

Two minutes later, making it five minutes since her brain had been oxygenated, Lewis deftly closed the atrial wall. He had a minute left. Lewis checked his work one last time. With thirty seconds remaining he unclamped the tourniquets.

The tiny heart began to beat again, a touch reluctantly until Lewis gently massaged it back into a healthier rhythm. After stitching up the chest, they lowered her into a second tub, one containing warm water. Lewis had done it. He had become the first surgeon to work successfully inside an open heart. The girl breathed. She lived. Lewis and Lillehei clutched hands across her warming body.

Eleven days later, cured and recovered, Jacqueline Johnson went home. The momentous start of open-heart surgery was confirmed the moment Lewis announced the operation at a medical convention later that month. In the wider world, the Minneapolis *Tribune* was the first to break the news. The newspaper praised Lewis's work, which, apart from saving a young life, "seems to give surgeons a method, long sought, of putting the knife into the live human heart in plain sight." By September 30, 1952, even *The New York Times* had joined the chase with a catchy headline: "'Deep Freeze' Girl Making Rapid Recovery." The world's love affair with heart surgeons had begun.

Eight months on, against a backdrop of even wilder public excitement, Gibbon finally became the first surgeon to save a human patient while using a heart-lung machine. On May 6, 1953, in Philadelphia, Gibbon's invention kept Cecelia Bavolek, an eighteen-year-old girl, alive for the twenty-six minutes it took him to repair an ASD and restart her circulatory system. She recovered fully, but Gibbon's next two attempts ended in the death on the operating table of a pair of five-year-old girls. He declared a moratorium on the use of his machine and never operated on the heart again.

Lillehei, almost as brilliant a showman as he was a surgical innovator, was ready to lift the drama to an even higher level. Without a heart-lung machine, and driven by the need to transcend the clock-watching constraints total-body hypothermia forced on the surgeon, Lillehei pursued alternate methods of opening the heart. He opted for a revolutionary and dangerous technique called cross-circulation that he hoped would give him enough time to repair more complex cardiac defects.

On March 26, 1954, Shumway was the young resident chosen by Lillehei to scrub in on a landmark case. They peered down at the table on which thirteen-month-old Gregory Glidden lay. At 10:00 a.m. the baby's chest was opened.

He and his father, Lyman Glidden, both lay anesthetized on two tables set a few feet apart. Lillehei had linked them together with a small oscillating finger pump borrowed from the dairy industry, a beer hose, and a series of cannulae which passed blood from the groin of the man to his son, guiding it up toward an artery and then into the aorta, which transmitted the reoxygenated blood through the little boy before it was routed back into the father's larger body. One heart and a pair of lungs, belonging to the father, kept both bodies alive while Lillehei prepared to open the boy's heart.

For twelve and a half minutes, the father's blood circulated through his son. In that time, high up on the ventricular septum, the wall that divides the ventricular chambers of the heart, Lillehei uncovered a hole he identified as a VSD (ventricular septal defect), a more taxing surgical test than Lewis's and Gibbon's ASDs. Lillehei worked coolly as his small headlamp moved in curious jerks and twitches. The strange tilt of his head, a result of surgery on his cancerous neck four summers before, was permanent. And it made him fear death less than most men.

Twelve silk stitches sealed the VSD. Lillehei closed the outer wall of the heart. They opened the clamps that had shut off the vessels and, in that instant, the little boy's heart began to beat. Nineteen minutes after connecting man and boy they could unhook Lyman and stitch up the hole in his groin. The radical cross-circulation technique had worked seamlessly.

But after a rapid improvement, Gregory Glidden fell ill again. His breathing difficulties were caused by pneumonia rather than a defective heart. Eleven days after surgery he died.

Lillehei was undaunted. On April 23, 1954, Ronald Schmidt's circulatory system kept alive his four-year-old daughter, Pamela, while Lillehei repaired a VSD in thirteen and a half minutes. A week later, on April 30, Lillehei hosted his first press conference. With his immaculate timing and sense of occasion, Lillehei gave an almost imperceptible nod of the head. A side door opened, and a little girl in a yellow dress walked toward her doctor. Her cheeks reddened as she smiled at him. "This is Pamela," Lillehei said.

The small girl was a study in brown-eyed beauty. "Pamela's going to be just fine," he assured the amazed reporters. "Her whole life is ahead of her now. . . ." The man in the alligator shoes grinned at the girl in the yellow dress.

There would be no stopping him and his Minnesota boys now. They were in the heart forever.

By the time Shumway arrived in California, three years later, he had long since abandoned his original ambition of becoming a neurosurgeon. Minnesota had exposed him to the heart. Following Lewis and Lillehei into the most unexplored and mythic organ of the human body was irresistible. The brain, which had seemed so fascinating in the 1940s, could no longer compete with the exhilarating world of heart surgery.

Lillehei, by 1957, had discarded cross-circulation because, obviously, it threatened the lives of two people in the OR. It carried, as Shumway always cracked, the risk of a "two hundred percent mortality rate." Lillehei had since carried out hundreds of open-heart operations while using a bubble oxygenator devised by Dick DeWall—his laboratory assistant and a former general practitioner. With outrageous simplicity DeWall had worked out how a fifteen-dollar pump, a beer hose, a plastic tube, some needles, and two filters could divert blood away from the heart while oxygenating it through his little machine, so that Lillehei could repair not only a VSD but the more complex tetralogy of Fallot.

The machine was ingenious, if not flawless, but Shumway was convinced that in conjunction with his own advances in hypothermia he would at last find a method of making cardiac surgery both safe and relatively "bloodless"— while protecting the heart in a way not even Lillehei imagined possible. By modifying Lewis's method of hypothermia to his own "topical" variation, and concentrating all the cooling around the heart rather than spreading it throughout the body, Shumway would enable cardiac surgery to take its first giant step toward transplantation. He just had to find a setting to match the innovative hothouse of Minnesota—and a place where he would be given the opportunity to finally mold his own team.

The offer of a partnership with a surgeon in Santa Barbara had promised a new start. It proved, however, an excruciating experience. The old buzzard was the worst doctor Shumway had ever met. He was only in it for the money. After six weeks Shumway walked out and went searching for another job— this time at the University of California in San Francisco.

Shumway needed the job, and so, despite being a naturally shy man, he sold himself hard when he met with Leon Goldman, the university's head of surgery. He discussed the extraordinary work he'd witnessed in Minnesota and stressed to Goldman that with such research allied to his clinical experience as a heart surgeon alongside Lillehei, he had a significant contribution to make. Shumway was on a roll when he looked up and suddenly saw that, far from being captivated, Goldman had fallen asleep in the middle of their interview.

At least they stayed awake at Stanford University a few weeks later. Yet it was made painfully clear to Shumway that he had little hope of becoming a heart surgeon in San Francisco. The hospital's cardiac wing was dominated by the seriously conservative Frank Gerbode and the arrogantly skillful Victor Richards. There would be no chance for him to compete for cases with such a distinguished pair. He was offered, instead, the task of running the kidney machine—on the graveyard shift. Shumway would administer kidney dialysis to patients, whether it was at midnight or four in the morning. He was told to forget about heart surgery. It was the machine at night, for him, or nothing.

Needing to support his wife, Mary-Lou, and their three young children, Shumway took the kidney gig, for which he was paid $3,000 a year. He was told there was no possibility of a raise. As a means of earning a little more cash he also did some freelance private work, which was confined to breast biopsies and the mundane removal of gallbladders. It all seemed a very long way from the dynamism of Minnesota, where, as Shumway quipped, you practically had to invent an operation to get a place on a schedule crackling with flair and vitality.

Lower came to Stanford later that year, in the fall of 1957, from a more humble path. He had not been offered a place as a resident after his internship at the University of Washington in Seattle. Lower was not sure he would have accepted it anyway because he was still disturbed by the day he had seen a couple of senior surgeons kill a young woman when they tried to use a dog lung to oxygenate her blood. It was work pioneered in Minnesota, but the Seattle team had neither the skill nor the dedication of Walt Lillehei's crew. After losing their patient, the head surgeon lit up a cigarette and shrugged as if it were no big deal. Jesus, Lower thought, how do these guys live with themselves?

Aiming to eventually become a GP, after acquiring a little surgical experience Lower accepted a residency at Stanford. On night call, one of his duties was to track down the kidney-machine guy, Norm Shumway, whenever one of his patients needed dialysis. His arrival marked a change of luck for Shumway, whose nights, until Dick Lower found him, had been miserable and tedious. Lower, a tall, athletic man who wore glasses, was stunned by the vast size of the kidney machine. It was big enough to fill a large patio. Shumway, in contrast, was an unassuming sight in his baggy clothes, old white coat, and comfortable shoes. Lower was immediately struck by his low-key friendliness. Although six years older than the twenty-nine-year-old Lower, the equally tall and lean Shumway acted more like his friend and contemporary on first meeting.

After a few nights together on the kidney machine, Shumway had suggested casually that they should do some daytime work together in the lab. Lower was thrilled. He was even more impressed by the fact that Shumway was stripped of bullshit. There was none of the conceit or envy that defined so many surgeons. Shumway just wanted to work, but found himself blocked by the men above him.

Although he was regarded as the premier cardiac surgeon on the West Coast, Frank Gerbode's success on the open-heart table was limited. Like most of his peers, Gerbode followed the lead of Dennis Melrose, a South African surgeon based in London, in assuming that the best way to arrest a heart, and work on it in a bloodless field, was to inject it at the base of the clamped aorta with potassium. He lost around half of his patients. Shumway knew it was due to the high concentration of potassium—which, as even Melrose had begun to concede, damaged the heart.

Stanford-Lane Hospital, San Francisco, July 22, 1958

On the fifth-floor lab, with their hour-long experiment about to begin, Shumway withdrew the needle from the dog—a honey-colored mongrel. The anesthetic worked quickly. Shumway checked the heart-lung machine and his icy saline solution while Lower worked skillfully with the knife. He sliced through skin and then cut into the fourth intercostal, the muscles that reside between the ribs, on the right side of the chest. Shumway briefly inserted a cannula, or thin tube, into the right atrium, one of the heart's four chambers, so that he could administer a powerful drug called heparin to prevent clotting.

Lower then peeled back the casing to reveal two lungs and a heart. The lungs were clearly visible, expanding and deflating with the dog's breathing, while the heart remained enclosed in the pericardium. Shumway's knife carved open that protective membrane-lined sac and uncovered the heart. Looking deeper into the cavity of the chest, the wonder of the circulatory system appeared again as a replica of that which appears in man.

The lungs and heart worked together to keep the fire of life burning. While the lungs resembled a pair of bellows, the heart was an inexhaustible pump. The bellows pulled oxygen from the surrounding atmosphere through the mouth and nose, down the trachea, into the lungs, where, mixing with blood, it returned along the pulmonary veins into the two chambers on the stronger, left, side of the heart. From the upper-left atrium the oxygen entered the powerful left ventricle of the heart, which, as the main pumping mechanism, sent freshly oxygenated blood racing along the main arteries and into the dense vessel beds found even in the outermost reaches of the body— keeping alive the tiniest cells.

Once the life-giving oxygen was burned it changed into carbon dioxide, turning the blood a wine-dark red before it was sent back up the circulatory system to pass through two great veins, the superior vena cava and the inferior vena cava, into the right side of the heart. From the right atrium the deoxygenated blood passed into the right ventricle, which, again working like a pump, sent it surging back into the lungs through the pulmonary artery. Blood then filtered through a meshwork of tiny vessels surrounding the numerous small air sacs of the lung, allowing the exchange of oxygen and carbon dioxide. As the carbon dioxide was breathed back into the outside world through the trachea, the constantly flowing blood was replenished and turned crimson again by new molecules of oxygen as yet another journey through the body began.

Shumway had hooked up the dog to a heart-lung machine that he and

Ray Stofer, the lab veterinarian, had stripped down to the bare essentials. Their spinning-disc oxygenator had been transformed into a simple but precise mechanism with few gauges and monitors that could go wrong when the machine assumed the task of pumping and circulating blood. Everything Shumway did smacked of that same stark purity.

Lower sutured the pericardial sac to the edges of the wound around the sternum. This stitching formed a cradle into which catheters were sutured so that the saline could circulate through the heart in a continuous loop. Shumway cross-clamped the aorta, the main artery transporting blood from the heart's left ventricle, and abruptly shut down the heart. The softly whirring machine took over and circulated blood throughout the rest of the body. And then they waited, their eyes flicking back and forth from the ticking clock to the motionless heart.

As in the dog, man's heart was an incredible piece of raw machinery. Shumway described it as "a syncytium of muscle," for it was a shell rather than a solid organ like the liver or a kidney. It was also the world's most reliable pump. In that large and primitive laboratory, empty but for two men and a dog, the contrasting stillness and silence of a frozen heart seemed even more intense.

During the preceding two months, Shumway and Lower had used a series of thirteen dogs, weighing between 14 and 26 kilograms (31 to 57 pounds), to systematically determine the number of minutes a heart could be stopped and stored in saline. Their first five dogs had sailed past fifteen and twenty minutes, until, after half an hour, Shumway and Lower could perfuse the heart again with warm blood, shock it into restarting and gradually wean the animal off the machine and restore it to full consciousness. Shumway eased the barrier up to forty-five minutes with their next three dogs, and the result was another trio of barking mutts to pat and stroke once the dogs came around from the anesthetic.

Their experiments had become mesmerizing in their repetitive success. Yet sixty minutes was a far darker test. Perhaps they were due a failure after such a string of recoveries. Life in California, as Shumway had learned, was not always sunlit.

Lower stared at the small heart, so blue and inert in the saline, and shook his head. The heart looked totally dead. Anyone but Norm would have said there had to be a limit as to how far they could stretch time and deprive a heart of blood and oxygen. An hour extended deep into an obscure place, where, in the end, there could only be death.

It was still too early to test their theory. A mere twenty minutes had passed since the heart stopped beating. Usually so breezy and confident in everything he did, Shumway deliberately averted his gaze from the clock. He had known this one truth since he was a small boy. Time dragged when you were waiting and hoping so hard.

And so they talked instead, about sports and women, books and movies, finding a relaxed and ordinary way of passing the time in the midst of an extraordinary scientific experiment. Norm and Dick, as the two amiable men called each other, seemed curiously modest names for such a pair of medical adventurers. But such plainness suited their characters and surroundings. Their drab workplace, on the corner of Clay and Webster, was never meant to be a place for such grand dreams of the heart.

On rainy nights, in a cramped office deep in the narrow maze of corridors surrounding the laboratory, Shumway was forced to place a battered black bucket on his desk to catch the steady drip. Sometimes he and Lower opened a small umbrella and turned it upside down beneath the largest crack in the ceiling. In the lab itself the big sinks were covered in bare concrete. The plumbing was exposed, while surgical instruments had to be boiled in an old white pot over the gas burner in a far corner of the room. Apart from a new surgical table, it looked as if the Stanford research center had been untouched for the forty years of its existence.

In contrast to the sputniks and rockets blasting into space, Shumway and Lower's quest was stealthy. They had nothing to hide, but it seemed that no one out there could possibly care about their experiments with cooling and stilling the heart. America instead appeared gripped by the novelty of hurtling through that cold blackness the world still called outer space.

It was a difficult quest. The U.S. space program had launched its first satellite almost six months before—on January 31, 1958. But only two more successful orbits were interspersed among five failures before the end of June. The Soviet Union was clearly ahead, having safely launched Sputnik 1, the world's first artificial satellite, the previous October and followed it the next month by sending a passenger-carrying rocket into orbit. The first traveler in space was a dog called Laika.

Shumway and Lower were not yet in the habit of naming their dogs—but they cared for the eventual return to full health of the patient on their table as much as any Soviet space scientist might have yearned for Laika to return to earth in one piece. Laika was lucky. The fate of their own dog seemed less certain. The Stanford mongrel, who weighed an average-sized nineteen kilograms, looked small and terribly vulnerable.

Dick Lower glanced up at the clock. Like Lewis and Lillehei had done almost six years before in Minnesota, during the world's first open-heart surgery, he counted off the minutes. Yet they were no longer racing against Lewis's six-minute time bomb. The heart had been soaking in saline for forty-five minutes. They were moving into new territory.

Shumway and Lower fell strangely quiet in the last fifteen minutes. It was vital to them, and their radical new ambition, that the body stretched out before them should survive the hour and return to life. They would not allow themselves to be stopped by the death of a dog, but, at the same time, it would put a brake on their progress if it was proved that sixty minutes was a step too far.

As the clock's black hands inched ahead they repeated their monitoring—rechecking the myocardial temperature with a tiny thermostat placed on the tip of a 22-gauge hypodermic needle. The dog's body temperature, meanwhile, was maintained by a heat exchanger in the artificial circuit. Arterial pressure remained constant. Only five minutes were left.

They had already decided that they would allow the oxygenator to run for at least another half-hour, as circulatory support, if and when they managed to restart the heart. They had required as little as thirteen minutes of mechanical backup after chilling the heart for three-quarters of an hour. But this would be different.

Shumway and Lower worked quickly when they reached their target. After exactly one hour the aorta was unclamped, blood flow was restored, and the temperature rose steadily while the oxygenator worked alongside in humming tandem. There was little need for words when the heart soon began to fibrillate. It looked good, though they dared not celebrate yet.

Shumway, concentrated and ready, helped the dog with a small electric shock. The heart began to beat instantly. It still meant little as long as the oxygenator kept spinning, providing support to the dog's circulatory system. They did not ask the question out loud, but it echoed through them. Could the heart work alone again?

There was only one way to find out. After waiting and watching for another agonizing thirty minutes Shumway finally said the words: *"Pump off."*

They stared anxiously at the beating heart, waiting for it to stutter and collapse. Lower looked down into the pulsing cavity. He took a breath and smiled. Shumway grinned back at him through his mask as the heart, strong and sure, absorbed the burden of circulation and maintained an even pulse. They had done it. They had taken a frozen heart past the sixty-minute mark and then brought it back to life.

After they had closed up the chest, they waited for the dog to come around. It did not take long. The pooch opened his eyes and, a minute later, alert and breathing easily, flicked out a long pink tongue to lick Lower on the hand.

"Christ," Shumway said, his eyes glinting above his mask as he stared across the steel table at his friend, "we could do anything. . . ."

Three

COLORED HEARTS

Five nights later, on the other side of the world, at the bottom of Africa, Chris Barnard prepared to mark his own cardiac milestone. Early the following morning, on July 28, 1958, at the Groote Schuur Hospital in Cape Town, Barnard would attempt the continent's first successful open-heart operation. Six weeks before, he had returned from his two-and-a-half-year stint at the University of Minnesota, where, apart from being inspired by Walt Lillehei, he had bristled in the company of more sophisticated medical residents like Norm Shumway. Barnard, revealing the ferocious desire that would drive him in the transplant race, was already straining impatiently in his ambition to forge ahead at home.

Only one other surgeon in Africa, Barnard's local rival, Walter Phillips, had dared open a living heart. Nine months earlier, having obtained an oxygenator designed by Denton Cooley, the dazzling Houston surgeon, Phillips had hooked up the machine to a young patient suffering from a tetralogy of Fallot. It was a deadly mistake. Without the necessary laboratory research, Phillips was lost as soon as he cut into the heart. Blood seeped across the floor and the oxygenator spluttered helplessly. After the patient's death, Phillips and his colleagues were ordered not to try any further such operations by

Jannie Louw, Groote Schuur's head of surgery. He instructed them to wait for Barnard's return from America.

The battle for surgical supremacy between Phillips and Barnard had swung heavily in favor of the younger man. His exposure to the miracles of Minnesota brought him a status and breadth of pioneering knowledge against which Phillips could not compete. Phillips was primarily a thoracic (chest) surgeon; Barnard pitched himself as a new king of the heart. The fact that Minnesota's eminent chief, Owen Wangensteen, had arranged for the shipment of a heart-lung machine to Barnard in Cape Town, as well as three years of financial support from the National Institutes of Health in Washington, strengthened his position. Although Barnard and Louw were notorious for their temperamental clashes, the two Afrikaners sealed an uneasy alliance. As Barnard could bring prestige to his department Louw agreed to tacitly support the returning protégé ahead of the unfortunate Phillips.

The imminent prospect of surgery unleashed convoluted emotions in Barnard. His elation at the thought of being the first on an entire continent to emulate Lewis and Lillehei was clouded by the risks he faced. The machine loomed over the operation as both an ingenious mechanical savior and a potential killer. It had arrived by boat two weeks after Barnard flew into Cape Town, giving him and his makeshift team just a month to jell with the machine. Barnard, having worked in the OR under Lillehei as a senior resident, had grown used to working in the company of experts. In Cape Town, however, he felt vulnerable on his own.

Unlike Shumway, who believed so strongly in hypothermia, Barnard had followed Lillehei down the track of perfusion by relying on the primitive heart-lung machine. There was real trauma in relying on an apparatus that could also kill a patient in so many different ways. When it failed to function smoothly, as Barnard wrote, "it was an instrument of death." He listed the grisly dangers one by one: "Bubbles in the helix, a leak in the line, overheating in the warming bath, a slipped catheter, antifoam XC-2-033 in the blood and into the brain—how many hundreds of other leaks, drips, breaks and pressures lurked there, among the separate parts, ready to reduce a human being to a vegetable—or cause his death on the table?"

His foreboding was intensified by Groote Schuur's lack of an autoclave large enough to sterilize the oxygenator's layers of yellow mayon tubing. So Barnard and Carl Goosen, his novice perfusionist, or heart-lung machine operator, had to drive across town to the Red Cross Children's Hospital. Once they had gained access to that hospital's huge autoclave, they had to method-ically wrap their machine in sterile towels for the return journey in the back of Barnard's car. It did not calm his agitation.

Barnard knew that he would have to be awake by four o'clock the next morning so that he and Goosen could start priming the machine by six. His anxiety barely allowed him to consider for long the additional boundary he planned to push aside in operating on a "colored" patient in a white hospital. The "coloreds"—a mixed-race group who had evolved from illicit relation-ships between white colonialists and their indigenous black servants into the third-largest ethnic classification in South Africa—were Afrikaans-speakers. They were still brutally discriminated against, even if their choice of language and relative lightness of skin meant they were regarded as less threatening to the state than the black majority.

Joan Pick, the niece of big Victor Pick, Barnard's laboratory assistant, was only fifteen years old. She was stricken with pulmonary-valve stenosis. It was a potentially fatal ailment, but it could be remedied quickly. Barnard had seen patients cured in Minnesota during surgery under hypothermia. Cooley, the magical Texan surgeon, took so little time that he needed neither hypother-mia nor the machine while clearing the constricted valve.

The choice of Joan Pick as Barnard's historic patient, therefore, had more of a medical than a political dimension. Lillehei's advice had resonated in him throughout the preceding weeks. It was important that he start with something easy, Lillehei insisted, something he knew he could repair. "Nice and simple," Lillehei wrote in a letter from Minnesota. "Nothing too fussy, nothing too flashy. I have every confidence in you. . . ."

Barnard knew that as long as his nerve held and the machine worked he could easily open the girl's narrowed valve and save her life. He just had to stop his arthritic hands from trembling when the moment engulfed him. He felt as if his entire future in heart surgery depended on immediate success. Victor Pick, moreover, relied on him. Attending to the laboratory dogs,

Victor was quietly effective in everything he did. He worked hard, but never said much to the white men jabbering away as they tried to master their new machine.

And so Barnard was struck by the words Victor murmured soon after they had unpacked the heart-lung machine. He spoke simply about the beauty of the cardboard boxes that had sailed across the sea from America. The Afrikaner surgeon looked at the colored technician in bewilderment. Yet Victor imagined the boxes in his own living room—providing furniture for his family in the impoverished colored quarter of Cape Town. Barnard allowed him to take the boxes with a shrug. It seemed hard to believe that anyone could see a new chair, a comfortable sofa, or a pretty table in a bunch of empty boxes.

He guessed that his beloved father would have understood. Adam Barnard, who had died ten days earlier, had given his life to colored people like Victor and Joan Pick. The old pain cut through Chris. He saw his father in the pulpit of his colored church in Beaufort West, a small Afrikaner-run town in the unforgiving Karoo, and he remembered his love and their suffering. He would try, early the next morning, to save Joan Pick—for her sake, for Victor, for his own surgical career, and in memory of his recently buried father.

Adam Barnard came from an illiterate world. Neither of his parents had been able to read or write, and so they'd worked as poor whites in the forests of Knysna, where, among the elephants, they chopped down trees for a living. Adam was twenty-three when he first went to school. He told Chris and Marius that his teacher just shook her head and said, "You're so old. Where do you want to start?"

"I want to start at the bottom," Adam said, "because I know nothing."

He was thirty-four when he finally qualified as a *sendeling*, a junior preacher. Any hopes he might have harbored of eventually becoming a *dominie* (an authorized minister of the Afrikaner Church) were ruined by his commitment to work with colored believers. Chris and Marius were derided as "*die Hotnot predikant's kinders*" (the Hottentot preacher's children). They squirmed when white people avoided shaking their father's hand because it had touched colored flesh.

Adam's work had also intensified Chris's initiation into high school. All the new boys were subjected to the ritual of running down a gauntlet, where they were beaten with belts before having their heads dunked in a pail of cow dung. There was an extra measure of spite in the gibes of "Here's the Barnard kid!" and "Give it to him good!"

Following the lead of his friend Fanie Bekker, who braved the whirring belts at a cocky saunter, Chris took his whipping at a fast walk. He was held down even longer in the cow manure. Chris thought he would suffocate, and so he kicked out and caught one of the seniors in the groin. He had crossed some sort of line—and emerged stinking and defiant with the certainty that he could face down anyone who dared cross him again.

The colored township lay just outside Beaufort West, which itself was reserved for "*Slegs Blankes*" (Whites Only). Sunday mornings, however, brought the races together. In an inexplicable architectural oversight, their respective churches had both been built on the main street of the small town. Dominie Rabie's Afrikaans NGK church, with its granite steeple and huge clock, towered over Adam Barnard's plain haven of colored worship. Both Sunday services started at the same time on Donkin Street. There was an uneasy mingling of white and colored Christians in the center of town before eight a.m. and, again, afterward, when the Afrikaners lingered outside Barnard's church so that they might hear the glorious singing of his congregation. Inside, either Chris or Marius would tap their deaf mother on the arm and turn the hymn-sheets so that she could play the organ in time with soaring voices she could barely hear.

Her deafness contributed to the austerity of their life. While Adam appeared a saintly figure to his two youngest sons, Maria was less forgiving. Chris and Marius often felt that she was grieving over the loss of her only daughter, a stillborn twin of their eldest brother, Johannes, who was twelve years older than Chris. Another son, Abraham, had died when he was three. A "blue baby," a victim of a heart Chris guessed had been ruined by the tetralogy of Fallot, Abraham was mourned by Adam, who insisted on keeping his baby shoes and a slice of cake that still carried the imprint of the boy's tiny teeth in its decayed icing.

Chris and Marius pined for a world beyond their own. On Saturday afternoons they went to the movies, where they loved to watch big-band musicals featuring Jimmy Dorsey or Bing Crosby. But when they stepped out of the *bioscope,* or cinema, they were once more the "Hottentot preacher's kids"—which explained why Chris was so determined to beat the eldest son of the apparently superior Dominie Rabie in a specially organized race over a mile.

The four laps around a grassy track demanded the determination and stamina that always characterized Barnard. He lacked only the speed that distinguished the best milers. Yet his resolve had been enough for him to remain unbeaten over the distance in local schoolboy meetings for a couple of years. Daantjie Rabie, the handsome twenty-year-old son of the revered preacher, was the provincial champion. Four years older than Barnard, Rabie agreed to give the promising schoolboy a 150-yard head start to make the race more equal.

Rabie was still too strong and fast and an exhausted Barnard was overtaken on the final straight. "I tried to stop my tears," Barnard wrote years later, "but they came anyway. In the shower I told myself it was nothing. . . . But I had not won the race against Daantjie Rabie, and for a long time I dreamed of the ten yards separating us, crossing it in a thousand ways. . . . I ran the race over and over again."

That bitter memory drove him on in his profession. His mother had hammered into him and Marius the need to be first. They had always been expected to head everything, from each subject in the classroom to every sport on the dusty fields outside. He had wanted to beat Rabie, however, for the sake of his father—the kind old man Chris and Marius called by the English name of "Daddy."

Their parents eventually saved just enough money to supplement the scholarships the brothers earned to attend university in Cape Town. Chris and Marius were given no choice by their mother—after all the family's sacrifices they were compelled to qualify as doctors. Although separated by four years at medical school, they shared a room in a boardinghouse in Cape Town in 1945 and 1946. Drained by work and their continuing lack of money, which meant they had to walk miles to the university every day, they fought angrily, just as they had done so often as boys. Marius resented his elder brother's refusal to help him in any way; yet Chris was too obsessed with his own work to care much for anyone.

Soon after qualifying as a doctor Barnard produced a staggering piece of experimental research full of the stubborn bravado that would, in later years, bolster him in his struggle with Shumway, Lower, and Kantrowitz. Barnard claimed that he would be able to overcome intestinal atresia, a seemingly incurable congenital condition that causes a life-threatening gap to develop in the bowel. In the largely intuitive way in which he would confront transplantation, Barnard followed a medical hunch that the defect resulted from an insufficient supply of blood to the fetus during pregnancy. To test his theory he needed to recreate the abnormality in an unborn puppy by slicing his way into the uterus of a pregnant dog and removing a fetus, which he would then open up. He would tie off (knot) part of the intestine, so that he stopped the flow of blood into the tiny bowel, sew the fetus back together and replace it inside the uterus of the mother who would then be stitched up herself.

The idea of an unborn puppy surviving such complex surgery seemed ludicrous. However Barnard, with his two colored helpers, "Boots" Snyders and a man he knew only as "Appel," began working with pregnant dogs approximately two weeks from the full term of their gestation. After a nine-month slog, and on his forty-third attempt, a black-and-white mongrel gave birth to a puppy with three black silk stitches in its belly. When Barnard sliced it open and examined the bowel, he drew back in breathless wonder. He looked down again to ensure that his expectant gaze had not tricked him. The puppy was a victim of intestinal atresia—a disease he had bestowed with his knife and scissors.

He then set about correcting the defect. Barnard cut away a small chunk of old intestine and, having increased the blood flow, successfully joined the severed sections of infant bowel. He had not only proved that congenital intestinal atresia was caused by insufficient blood flow in pregnancy but revealed why it had previously been impossible for surgeons to anastomose, or sew together, a bowel in an infant even though they could easily replicate that procedure in an adult. The mistake surgeons before him had made was to at-

tempt to suture together strands of bowel that were still not receiving a sufficient supply of blood. To successfully rejoin a segmented infant bowel, it was
necessary to discard 15 to 20 centimeters (about 6 to 8 inches) of damaged
intestine so that a new juncture, receiving fully oxygenated blood, would be
able to thrive.

Jannie Louw used the innovation in a clinical setting, and the positive results were immediate. By the time Barnard's methodical research had helped
save the lives of ten babies in Cape Town, the technique was being adapted by
surgeons in Britain and America. There was, clearly, a quality and resilience
to Barnard's experiments—borne out by his equally thorough work analyz-
ing 259 cases of tubercular meningitis. He seemed to have the aptitude for
the most onerous tasks. While he had yet to discover the heart, his breakthrough in the less romantic domain of the bowel filled him with an unbreakable conviction in his own ability and brought him to the attention of
those who could transform his career.

John Brock, the head of medicine at Groote Schuur, recognized Barnard's
exceptional drive and potential. When Owen Wangensteen, the chief of
surgery at Minnesota, contacted him, Brock saw a chance for Barnard to fulfill that promise. Wangensteen had been so impressed by the work of Alan
Thal, a dynamic South African doctor in Minnesota, that he asked Brock if
any of his other young countrymen were of a similar caliber. There was only
one candidate.

In December 1955, Christiaan Barnard flew to the city of snow in wonder
and fear. He was thirty-three years old but his gleaming short haircut
made him look younger. On the inside he felt just as lost and lonely as he had
when, as a boy of eighteen, he'd caught a train from Beaufort West, in the vast
emptiness of the Karoo, and steamed through the black night toward the
seemingly giant metropolis of Cape Town and medical school.

Minneapolis was even harder. Minneapolis was another world. He had
never stepped outside of South Africa, and the mere mention of "America"
made him shiver. At least he had heard of Wangensteen, for they used a suc-
tion apparatus named after the Minnesota chief at Groote Schuur. He was

less sure of the geographical details. Confusing Minneapolis with Indianapolis, he wondered whether it was the city where they raced fast cars around a dangerous track.

Staring out of the plane, his gaze switched from the dark sky to the huge white banks lining the airport runway. He had never seen snow before. As he walked down the iron gangway he was hit by a breathtaking blast that explained why they had made such progress with hypothermia in Minnesota. The snow swirled, and an icy wind cut through the only overcoat he could find in the South African summer.

It was warmer inside the terminal, and Barnard fiddled through his pockets in search of money to make a call. As he struggled to identify the nickels and dimes, he remembered his earlier brush with the American dollar during that long and blurring day. He had flown first to New York, where he changed planes for a flight to Minneapolis via Detroit and Milwaukee. It was a schedule from hell and, overwhelmed by the strangeness of America, Barnard made the mistake of overtipping the New York porter who helped him with his bags.

"I ran after him," Barnard wrote later, "and when I caught him he turned about slowly to stare at me. He was a big Negro, and he waited for me to speak first. 'Look I've made a terrible mistake. I think I gave you ten dollars, and I can't afford it. I want to give you one dollar.' For a moment he said nothing. He was much darker than our Cape Coloreds, and his eyes were the color of ebony in white pools streaked with yellow. 'Yes, you gave me ten,' he said, and returned it to accept one dollar. He had not said *'Baas'* or 'Sir.' It was simply 'you'—as though we were equals, and perhaps even with a suggestion that he was superior to me. . . . It was going to be interesting to see how these white Americans lived with their Negroes."

After he finally phoned Alan Thal from the airport, his fellow South African drove over to collect him. They switched immediately to Afrikaans as Thal's car crunched along the skiddy streets, gray with slush and grit and lined with trees turned into eerie white shapes by the snow.

Inside Thal's small apartment Barnard listened to stories about Minnesota and its compelling characters—Wangensteen, John Lewis, Norm Shumway, Richard Varco, and the incredible Lillehei. Barnard could feel the excitement surging through him as he and Thal thawed out over steaming cups of tea.

This was what he wanted—the thrill of the new. It already seemed that after less than a day in America, he was racing toward some secret prize. Wangensteen wanted to see him the following morning. There was no thought that he might need a day to recover from his exhausting journey. It was better that way. It distracted him from his terrible disorientation.

Wangensteen, intrigued by Barnard's breakthrough in intestinal atresia, set him to work in the hope that he might uncover a way of joining a severed esophagus just beneath the trachea. Wangensteen considered gastrointestinal research to be intellectually delicious, but Barnard had had his fill of intestines. He had not left his home, his wife, and two small children in pursuit of experiments on dog gullets.

"Can you handle it?" Wangensteen asked after completing his enthusiastic ode to the esophagus.

Barnard nodded blankly. What could he say? He was just an Afrikaner from the Karoo, lost in America. He trudged back to the boardinghouse on East River Road where the university had arranged his accommodation. Passing the mighty Mississippi, its waters black against the snow, as he later wrote, he "felt very much alone, and this feeling did not leave me."

The weight of America seemed unbearable those first few weeks as he worked on the dog gullet. His first dog died, as did the second. He saw himself killing a long line of American dogs without coming any closer to Wangensteen's aim of fusing a severed gullet.

Barnard kept at it, though, because he did not know how to express his despair to Wangensteen. His loneliness made him aggressive and deepened the impression of arrogance. Barnard noticed with envy how much more deftly Shumway handled Wangensteen. Shumway reacted wryly to the fact that he did not appear high on the list of Wangensteen's Chosen. In the OR he did little more than hold a retractor, and Shumway swore that, one day, if he ever made it to a similar position, he would do the exact opposite and involve his youngest interns and residents in every facet of operating. While Barnard brooded, Shumway covered his disappointment with wisecracks and "a little diddling" in the nurses' room.

Shumway regarded the chief as the archetypal short man who compensated for his lack of height with a swaggering ego. Despite his diminutive size,

Wangensteen tried to look down his nose at men who were far taller than he. Shumway, at six feet, laughed quietly at the sight as Wangensteen tilted himself backward and, using his bifocals, tried to give the illusion that he was peering down at his spiky resident.

Privately, Shumway mocked Wangensteen's violent technique in the operating room. The old boy arrived with a large bag full of so many archaic surgical instruments, it looked as if he was preparing to work on a battered car rather than a human being. Shumway and his buddies spoke of Wangensteen entering the OR "to commit surgery" and laughed when someone quipped that "the chief hates cancer because it kills more people than he does." Lillehei himself had been afraid he would be a victim of Wangensteen's brutal surgery, and he instructed Lewis to protect him when he went under the chief's knife for the removal of a lethal lymphosarcoma on his neck in 1950. Shumway had been part of the gang even then, Barnard noted bitterly, for a pint of his blood helped keep Lillehei alive during the massive transfusions needed in surgery.

Once he had recovered, Lillehei featured prominently in Shumway's most infamous gag. While accompanying Lillehei on his rounds, Shumway decided to alleviate the tedium. As they hovered over the beds of various patients, Shumway took to calling Lillehei by the name of his chief. "That's a good point, Dr. Wangensteen," he'd observe, and nod sagely at a grinning Lillehei.

A few days later the real Wangensteen greeted one of Lillehei's patients. "Good morning," he said, "I'm Dr. Wangensteen."

"Oh no," the knowledgeable invalid insisted as he pointed at Lillehei, "*that's* Dr. Wangensteen."

Shumway sneaked out an advisory arm around his boss. "You know, Professor," he said, "you really should stop impersonating Dr. Wangensteen. You'll start giving our patients the wrong idea about this place."

While some of the young Minnesota residents favored flashy bow ties and smart shoes, Barnard wore the same sports jacket, a thin black tie, a nylon wash-and-wear shirt, old navy-blue trousers, and oversized snow boots. He typically looked troubled and weary, for he rarely left the lab before midnight and, when he got back to the boardinghouse after a two-mile walk through the snow, he would often step straight into the shower, still wearing his shirt, underwear, and socks. He washed his clothes while he showered and then draped them over a chair near a small radiator so they would be ready for use the day after next. His two white shirts soon turned gray.

Barnard's intensity made him believe he could cram Minnesota's academic surgery course into a third of the time usually needed to fulfill its gruelling demands. Wangensteen stressed that all residents were expected to complete a doctoral thesis, while studying physiology or pathology and gaining a working knowledge of two foreign languages. They were also required to spend two years in clinical service and another two in the laboratory. Wangensteen reminded him that the course took six years, though perhaps he could do it in five.

The Afrikaner insisted he would complete the course in two years. In response to Wangensteen's snort of "Impossible," he explained that over a hundred postmortems on tubercular meningitis cases had given him a solid pathology background, and that his thesis would be based on his groundbreaking findings in intestinal atresia. Barnard argued that Afrikaans gave him a strong grasp of Dutch. He would just need to learn German, brush up on his pathology, and write his thesis while working all day in the hospital and many nights in the research lab.

Wangensteen shrugged. Barnard was welcome to take a crack at the impossible.

Whenever he needed a break from the gullet, Barnard wandered across the hall. Vince Gott, who ran Lillehei's lab, answered Barnard's questions patiently while he checked the oxygenator before the next operation. Gott had also begun to develop a technique for pumping blood backward through the veins of a heart so that Lillehei could operate more easily on the aortic valve. It was the kind of inspired thinking that entranced Barnard.

In March 1956, Gott finally asked Barnard to help him run the big machine. The young Afrikaans surgeon's future seemed to unfold before him in Operating Room J. Sitting next to Gott at the table supporting the heart-lung machine, he could not see much of the patient, whom he later described, with a romantic flourish, as a "dark, hollow-eyed youth with a graceful body." Lillehei walked into the room and in that moment made Barnard wish he might become a heart surgeon himself. He dominated the OR with an irresistible authority and power.

Lillehei's headlamp shone directly on the faces of Gott and Barnard. "Ready?" Lillehei asked.

"Ready," Gott said softly.

"Okay," Lillehei murmured as Barnard caught his breath. "Pump on . . ."

Gott flicked the switch and the machine whirred into life. Barnard watched one pump draw out the dark venous blood before it reached the heart, while the other sent freshly oxygenated blood surging back into the body through a tube connected to the left subclavian artery.

"The dark red liquid went through yellow plastic tubes," Barnard wrote, "rolled onward by steel fingers, from machine to patient and back again— blood that would soon fill the empty heart, stir the wakened brain. . . . The immensity of it was staggering, and the longer it ran, the more exciting it became. This was more than a machine. It was the gateway to surgery beyond anything yet known. While it stood in for heart and lungs, vast repairs could be made inside the body. New valves could be put into the heart, maybe even a whole heart itself. We had already begun to transplant kidneys—why not a heart? Or even both heart and lungs. . . . There was no viable end to where it would take us."

Barnard was determined to switch from the esophagus to the heart. Impressed by his relentless curiosity, Wangensteen agreed to transfer him to Lillehei's service. The South African relaxed a little and became friendly with Gil Campbell, a radical researcher who had proved that a dog lung could oxygenate human blood during open-heart surgery. Lillehei had used the technique on a thirteen-year-old black American, Calvin Richmond, who suffered from a VSD (ventricular septal defect), in March 1955. Calvin's mother, who came from Arkansas, had refused to participate in Lillehei's daunting cross-circulation procedure. Lillehei had then tried to find a prisoner in the local jail who might help the dying boy, but all the white convicts refused to allow their blood to mingle with that of a "nigger."

So for twenty minutes the lung of a dog kept Calvin Richmond alive, giving Lillehei and Campbell enough time to repair the VSD. The boy recovered fully. If the racial backdrop was familiar, Barnard was invigorated by the fact that Lillehei's new surgery of the heart was life-affirming. It was not the destructive surgery entailed in ripping out a stomach or a cancerous growth.

Barnard and Campbell met regularly at 6:00 a.m. for pancakes and thick maple syrup, washed down by strong black coffee, at a diner where they played jazz on the jukebox. Those sweet dark mornings helped Barnard. At 6:45 a.m. he and Campbell would head up to the pathology department, where they'd spend the morning studying the latest slides of their research. They were lost in work they loved. Barnard was invigorated by his new routine, and his social confidence returned.

Campbell knew that Barnard was never going to be one of the beer-guzzling boys, just as he would remain removed from the elite gang knocking back the martinis at night as they talked about diseased hearts and new surgical procedures in some plush cocktail bar with Lillehei. Barnard was consumed instead by his own work, and his suddenly determined pursuit of beautiful young women. His first affair in Minneapolis was with a Swedish scrub nurse, Trudy Nordstrom. Barnard charmed her with the same zeal he brought to his surgical experiments. He told her nothing about his wife and children, and Trudy fell heavily for him.

With a Texan resident, Jim Storey, and his wife, Chris and Trudy would drive out to the River Road Inn. It was then that he first heard Dean Martin's "Memories Are Made of This," a song that came to symbolize his years in Minnesota. Their moments together seemed all the more evocative because Barnard knew they could not last.

Trudy was predictably furious when she discovered that Barnard was married and that his family was about to join him in Minnesota. She refused to see him again. It didn't matter much, for he was already secretly involved with Sharon Jorgensen. In between her sociology studies, the twenty-year-old worked in the surgery department's photo lab at University Hospital, where Barnard and Campbell had their research slides developed. She was utterly floored by Barnard.

Louwtjie Barnard, even in ignorance of her husband's latest spate of affairs, was less impressed by Chris's easy charm with women. They drove each other mad most of the time, but she still believed they were inextricably bound by the rural Afrikanerdom of their past. She had met him when she was a young nurse at Groote Schuur and he was still a med student. Louwtjie liked Chris's "big ears and beautiful hands," but she certainly had not fallen quickly for him. She eventually found a love that, because it had not been engendered by a rush of infatuation, was deep and serious. Her earnest affection did not captivate Chris for long.

For Louwtjie, who cursed his callous disregard of her feelings, there was something almost schizophrenic about the way he could turn into the selfless doctor who spent night after night at a dying patient's bedside. She also could not help but admire his ambition, for despite his background he was determined to compete with the world's best surgeons. And so she had supported his American quest. Louwtjie did not know what Chris was chasing, but she understood that something inside him needed to be released or tamed. America, she hoped, might help both her and her husband.

He had at least tried to make a home for Louwtjie and the children, Deirdre and Andre, when they arrived in Minnesota six months after his departure from Cape Town. To supplement his $125 monthly wage so that he could afford a small family apartment near the airport, he had worked on Saturday afternoons and Sunday mornings for his neighbors. He was not too proud to shovel snow from their pavements, or wash their cars.

He failed, however, to make the time to meet his exhausted family when they arrived in Boston. They had to make their own way to Minneapolis. Louwtjie demanded answers to her stinging questions. Why did Americans drive on the wrong side of the road? How could they stand the cold? Why did they put up with the constant noise? Were they living on the actual landing strip? While Louwtjie fumed, Chris complained that his months of menial labor had gone unappreciated.

On Saturday June 9, 1956, in the very week of their arrival in Minnesota, a U.S. Navy jet smashed into three houses less than a mile from their new home. The plane killed six people and maimed fourteen. "That's America for you," Louwtjie cried. "Airplanes crash on houses."

Louwtjie spent most days alone in the duplex. Some of her neighbors dropped in with cookies or newspaper articles about trouble in South Africa. Louwtjie did not like being called "honey," and she was incandescent with fury when it was assumed she spoke Zulu rather than Afrikaans. She was similarly incensed by any reference to apartheid when Negroes were not allowed to live in her Minneapolis suburb.

Barnard, meanwhile, did not rush home at night. He instead visited Sharon Jorgensen, who was typing his Ph.D. thesis. While an oblivious Louwtjie waited for him, he enjoyed leisurely dinners with his girlfriend, lamenting to her the fact that his wife made his life hell. Fascinated by the exotic surgeon, who was fourteen years her senior, Sharon found her sympathies deepened by his repeated wish that he could live with her one day.

The end of Louwtjie's miserable time in America was sealed when Wangensteen's secretary, Leontine Hans, advised her that Chris had a great future in America and that it would be an awful mistake for him to return to a backward country like South Africa. Louwtjie spat out her reply with blunt anger. In South Africa, she said, planes did not crash into houses. In South Africa, her children's accents were not mocked at school. In South Africa, the government did not lie about apartheid. "And," she added as she turned sharply away, "we are not rude people."

Ten months after arriving in America, Louwtjie and the children were on their way home to Cape Town. Chris would join them once his American studies were completed. They hoped it might be a matter of months. He secretly doubted he would see them for another year. If Louwtjie was defiantly dry-eyed, he could not bear to see Deirdre's tears. Chris hoped that they would not see that he, too, was crying. He felt isolated and arthritic—for his condition had just been diagnosed.

Yet Barnard soon felt lucky again. He had a girlfriend and he had the heart. Even though his hands hurt and he missed his children, especially Deirdre, in late 1956 he felt that his life was finally on track. While Shumway did most of the surgery, Barnard worked as Lillehei's senior resident. It was a position that Shumway had previously filled and it conformed to the typical medical hierarchy of a working hospital. While the chief surgeon—in this case Lillehei—remained in overall control of his patients, the senior resident was responsible for the day-to-day care and monitoring of each of those cases. He would report directly to his chief, and occasionally take over from him in the operating room. It was a learning position that carried with it serious responsibilities and exacting duties, and it prepared both Shumway and Barnard for a time when they would lead their own surgical units.

Barnard and Lillehei tended to about forty patients a day, with the majority of those being monitored for preoperative checks through a series of blood tests, X-rays, and primitive angiograms. There was so much detail to be absorbed with regard to each patient that Lillehei's residents were expected to copy down vital information gathered during their morning consultations. On his first day at the head of Lillehei's residency, however, Barnard appeared without a notebook. When Barnard repeated the same approach the following evening, relying on his memory of that morning's findings, Lillehei explained the need to document such information, particularly when it came to listing all the medications that needed to be administered the following day.

Lillehei responded curtly when he saw that, on the third night of rounds, Barnard still refused to make any notes. He instructed Barnard to bring a book with him the next day.

Barnard fired back, pointing out that he had always implemented Lillehei's previous orders to the letter. He had yet to make a mistake or suffer a lapse in memory.

Lillehei merely grunted, and at the next bed Barnard's detailed response was again exemplary. The same pattern continued whenever they shared ward rounds. Barnard stubbornly refused to use a notebook, while Lillehei could not help but marvel at his seemingly flawless memory.

He did not show the same composure during the remorseless pressure of surgery. Barnard's embryonic career almost ended on a day when Lillehei asked him to prepare a seven-year-old boy for a VSD. While Lillehei scrubbed, Barnard opened the chest and circled the inferior vena cava, the large vein that filters blood directly into the right side of the heart. As he became tense, he instructed his young colleague, Derward Lepley, to cut away some tissue from in front of the vein. Blood gushed as Lepley made the incision. Realizing that Lepley had cut a hole in the heart, Barnard panicked.

Screaming with distress, Barnard tried to use a clamp to shut the hole. He tore it still further, and then, in desperation, hooked the bleeding boy up to the heart-lung machine. A red torrent poured from the heart while Barnard cursed and fumbled. When the heart began to fail, he attempted to massage it back into life. Lillehei arrived and drained the cavity of blood and quickly sewed shut both the VSD and the fresh hole in the right atrium. They still could not start the heart.

"Close the chest," Lillehei said quietly.

Barnard expected he would never see a heart again after the last stitch had been pulled tight. He had just begun his wail of guilt, which would culminate in his determination to quit, when Lillehei asked him if he had learned anything during those awful few minutes. Barnard looked at him blankly while Lillehei underlined the obvious lesson. The next time he faced such bleeding he could stop the flood by simply putting his finger in the hole. That would give him time to work out what he might do next. So tomorrow, Lillehei said, you'll go ahead and open the next patient's chest.

The following day, after Barnard had nervously completed the procedure, Lillehei joined him in the OR. His head cocked to the side, the headlamp swinging across the red spread of chest as he studied the looped vena cava, Lillehei tilted his damaged neck so that he could look straight in Barnard's face.

"Good job," he said.

Lillehei ducked his head low, the headlamp shining down into the waiting cavity. Barnard moved closer to the table to watch a master at work. He still had much to learn.

S oon after Barnard's return to South Africa in July 1958, he was called to the small house in Knysna where his dying father waited. As he placed his arthritic hands on his father, he felt the lumps of cancer massing around the liver. He shuddered at the monstrous spread of a disease that obliterated all hope. Old Adam looked into the teeming eyes of his prodigal son. "It's all right," he said softly.

Adam Barnard died a few weeks later. They called Chris just after dawn. He drove all morning and straight on into the simmering afternoon. He was still hours too late. His father lay cold and still in a living room in Knysna, the town where he had been born eighty-three years earlier. Chris's mother told him that just before he stopped breathing, Adam looked at a photograph and said "Ta-ta" to each of his sons.

The funeral was made extraordinary by the sight of colored people in a white church. They were only allowed to sit in the balcony, and, massed together high up in the church, seemingly closer to God, their silent presence was profound in the small coastal town. "They stared at me without smiling," Barnard wrote. "A few of the older men nodded, and some of the women had handkerchiefs in their hands. The preacher would soon talk of my father, but nothing he could say would ever equal this—the mute presence of these Colored people who had come two hundred miles to see the burial of a white minister who had loved them as he had loved his own family."

After the service, "we drove slowly to the graveyard, and many walked. When we reached the gate the Colored people came forward, as though acting on common command—moving in between us and the coffin, and then taking it on their shoulders. There were many of them and, suddenly, the coffin seemed to be floating above all of us. We stood back and watched it go through the gate. The people for whom he had lived were those who now bore my father to his grave.

"There were so many shoulders and so many hands you could not count them. Yet each one carried the weight as though it was a great burden, as though lifting up something more than a little old man. They were carrying a part of themselves to the grave—and with it went all their terrible sorrow."

Groote Schuur Hospital, Cape Town, July 28, 1958

Barnard rose in the dead of night, less than a week later, to prepare for Africa's first open-heart operation. It was just after 4:00 a.m. in the cold and rainy blackness as he hurriedly pulled on his clothes. Unable to sleep, he had shifted restlessly in bed as images of the operation reeled through his head. Barnard had been through each possible outcome over and over again but, rather than calming himself, he felt frazzled and fretful. Louwtjie and the children slept soundlessly as he crept through the dark, not even pausing in the kitchen to make himself any breakfast. Having barely eaten the previous day, Barnard knew that he would not be able to face any food until after the operation. He already felt sick to the stomach.

His bad temper was obvious to Carl Goosen as soon as they met. Goosen, a bright young technician, kept his head down and tried to ignore the histrionics. He could already tell that Barnard would be even more vitriolic beneath the burden of surgery. The two men silently wheeled the Lillehei-DeWall machine into the green-walled operating theater on floor F.

Barnard retreated into the kind of dogged pursuit of success that had epitomized his experimental surgery in intestinal atresia. His work on fifteen-year-old Joan Pick would be much simpler than working on the tiny fetus of a puppy. Once he had connected her to the machine he would just need to expose her heart, open the pulmonary artery, and then make three small cuts to widen the narrowed valve. Once that was done he simply needed to close the artery and remove her from the machine. He would have cured Joan of pulmonary valve stenosis—so long as the oxygenator did not make a fatal slip.

His work in calibrating the machine was fanatically thorough. Time passed swiftly. The machine was ready when he and Goosen were joined in the operating theater by Joseph Ozinsky, the laconic young Jewish anesthetist they all called Ozzie. While Barnard disappeared into the scrub room, Ozzie set about preparing Joan. He spoke to her softly as she was rolled into the room. It was important that she be eased into the ordeal. Ozzie explained again that he was about to send her to sleep. She had no need to worry. Everything would be all right. He spoke in Afrikaans, the language of the "coloreds," and she nodded, and almost smiled.

Her eyes were closed when Barnard and Phillips faced each other across the table. Their old enmity was put to one side as they bent their masked faces and began the cutting. With an "oxbow" incision, slicing from right to left, below the breasts, they parted the sternum and found her heart. Barnard made two holes in the right atrium so that the catheters could drain the used venous blood. Fresh blood from the machine was fed by a thin tube running through a small opening in her right groin and up into her femoral artery.

Barnard nodded curtly to Goosen and the pump whirred to life. With Barnard constantly checking the machine, Phillips moved into the pulmonary artery. The work seemed to be proceeding smoothly until Goosen's voice rose in agitation at a sudden fall in blood supply. When he could not explain the reason for the alarming drop, Goosen was asked by a furious Barnard how much time they had left.

In less then a minute, Goosen confirmed, as calmly as he could, they would either maim Joan's brain or kill her. They had not used any form of hypothermia to help protect the heart. Swearing and sweating, Barnard and Phillips, the bitter rivals, sewed together. Barnard sealed the artery with his final stitch. His voice was wild and high as he gave the command: *"Cut pump!"*

Joan's heart was beating by the time he looked down and discovered the reason for their panic. He had used only one clamp at the bottom of the incision into the femoral artery. The clamp had slipped soon after they had started the operation and blood had seeped out on the floor. It lay in giant red pools around his feet. He knew he would have to use two clamps the next time he operated.

Ozzie eventually lifted the white drapes from the girl's soft brown face. "Joan," he called to her in Afrikaans, "can you hear me?"

Joan opened her eyes to look at him. Ozinsky winked at Barnard. "Okay, Joan," Ozzie said, "the operation's over. Close your eyes."

Joan Pick closed her eyes again. Her brain was undamaged, either by the machine or by any lack of oxygen.

Barnard ripped off his gloves and cap and followed Joan as she was wheeled back to the ward. He could not bear the thought of anyone else making another mistake that might take her from him.

"Go home," Ozzie eventually said. "She's going to be fine."

Barnard refused. Although dizzy with hunger and nervous fatigue, he spent the next four hours at his patient's bedside. He angrily pushed away all offers of rest, food, or even a drink as he repeatedly checked her pulse, urine, body temperature, and the level of blood she had lost. Barnard knew that a dip in any of these criteria would indicate that they had hit trouble. He had come too far to lose her now.

Joan Pick, it would turn out, was destined to make a full recovery. She would live another forty-two years. Indeed, she would live to become a mother, marry twice, and witness the end of apartheid. Although he did not know it then, Barnard had completely healed her heart. When she finally died in 2002, of stomach cancer, a Cape Town doctor would declare that her heart was still "as strong as an ox."

Barnard had brought a raging concentration to his otherwise ordinary surgical skills and a fierce compassion to the aftercare of his patient. He would use those attributes throughout the years of transplantation to compensate for his nerves and technical limitations in the operating arena. He would also feed on the success of that historic open-heart operation.

The surgeon was thrilled when he and Joan Pick made the front pages of every major newspaper the following morning—July 29, 1958. Meanwhile the government, desperate for positive publicity amid increasing international condemnation of apartheid, seized on, as the *Cape Times* described it, "The Miracle Operation."

"The world can say what it likes," suggested Prime Minister Hendrik Verwoerd, the man who called himself the architect of apartheid, "but we have doctors capable of feats that few can match anywhere in the world. To our enemies I would like to point out one key fact. Do they see the color of this girl? She is not white. She is colored. We are separate people but this brown girl was saved by an Afrikaans doctor. Let the world consider that before they attack us again."

Even a young girl's heart was colored by South Africa's devastating racial fixation.

Four

SPARKY'S GANG

Shumway and Lower, deep in a corner of their gloomy fifth-floor laboratory in San Francisco, continued to stretch time. Their fantastic experiments with topical hypothermia became almost boring in their repetitive success. They methodically chilled and stilled a heart in their cradle of saline, then watched as the black hands completed a circle around the unblinking face of the clock. It was easy for them to pass some of the time by talking casually as they pushed the barrier back to eighty or even ninety minutes before they would restart the unharmed heart. But, as Shumway said one slow afternoon in early 1959, while he stared at a motionless heart in the open cavity of a dog's chest, there had to be a more appropriate medical way to "beguile the tedium."

And so, to also divert Lower from his chronic back pain, they entered the realms of fantasy. Shumway began to speculate on the prospect of "bench surgery." Perhaps they could consider the stalled heart in the same way that a mechanic regarded a carburetor that he had removed from under the hood of a car and repaired on a workbench. What was to stop them excising the heart from the chest so that it could be operated on under ideal conditions? As long as it was protected by the icy saline, they could replace faulty valves and sew up gaping holes without being hampered by the flow of blood or the clutter of catheters.

"Next time," Shumway said, "why don't we cut it out and see what happens?"

Lower laughed at such daring. But Shumway was right. The heart was waiting for them. It invited them in. Could they not take it out and put it back? It suddenly seemed so simple. As a test they might remove a heart and then transplant it back into the same dog.

What else could they do with the heart while the minutes crawled past? Who was going to check on them in their obscure lab, which they only had to share on Tuesday afternoons with fourth-year medical students studying anatomy? Alone for the rest of the week, away from the nightly banality of running the kidney machine, they were free to let rip with their surgical creativity. The protection offered to the heart by topical hypothermia meant that they were no longer constricted by any fear that they would damage the organ or be unable to restart it after even an hour and a half of near-frozen inactivity. The only limits were those set by their imaginations. Hypothermia had unshackled them.

Yet, as with all their experiments, there had to be another more immediate purpose. It would not be enough to just remove and then replace a heart in the same dog in the vague hope that it would begin to resemble a portable mechanical part in a living body. Shumway decided that they should attempt to see if their risky feat might eventually cure a ravaging congenital heart defect known as "transposition of the great vessels."

The abnormality arises when the two major vessels that carry blood away from the heart, the aorta and the pulmonary artery, have developed in reverse position. As the most common cardiac flaw identified in the first week of infant life, transposition of the great vessels results in poorly oxygenated blood being pumped to the body. In essence there is a complete breakdown in the traditional function of the two vessels. Freshly oxygenated blood from the lungs, which is sent to the left side of the heart so that it can be pumped as nourishment for the rest of the body, is instead rerouted back into the lungs. Oxygen-depleted blood from the body, meanwhile, returns to the right side of the heart and is immediately sent back from where it came. The baby becomes painfully cyanotic (or "blue," as a result of reduced hemoglobin in the blood), and breathing can be desperately difficult. An associated defect mixes the usually separate streams of blood—which at least helps keep the baby alive. Death, otherwise, comes quickly.

Shumway devised a surgical remedy in which the heart would be excised and then rotated 180 degrees—so that the great vessels would be repositioned correctly. The pair's dramatic plans to transplant these "turnabout hearts" were encouraged by their success in the operating room throughout the winter of 1958.

When the call had first come from Ann Purdy, a cardiologist at the Children's Hospital in San Francisco, Shumway remained calm. Sure, he said, he and his team could handle some open-heart surgery in the OR. They might be blocked by Frank Gerbode and the surgical gang at Stanford-Lane, but they were ready to work on human patients. Shumway and Lower would keep their jobs at Stanford but could scoot over to the Children's Hospital whenever Purdy needed them.

They had solved their initial problem of transporting their heart-lung machine across town by hiring a van from Sparky's Delivery Service. They got a real charge when they roared up in a Sparky van. It was the kind of stunt you would expect from two guys called Dick and Norm. They gently lifted the machine and settled it in the van. With the lab veterinarian and their perfusionist Ray Stofer driving, Shumway and Lower sat in the back and held the oxygenator to stop it from crashing into the sides. Racing up and down the hills of San Francisco, the machine heaved and tilted as the doctors hung on.

Purdy had promised them at least ten patients, at a rate of one a week. Rather than seeking a still unproven transposition, their first case was a basic ASD, which they repaired deftly in a young girl. They struck disaster in their next operation. A tiny piece of heart muscle was sucked back into the machine. It entered the brain of a young boy, killing him. Lower and Shumway were devastated. Even though they had often seen death, they were hit hard. Their luck already seemed to have turned against them.

But Purdy's faith held and she encouraged them to continue. Their next series of cases were successful, with Lower often staying at a patient's bedside for two or three consecutive nights to ensure their recovery. They were on their way, and Shumway grew more assured and relaxed.

"Isn't this just great," he would say as they hunched over an open heart in the OR, "having this much fun and getting paid for it?"

The jokes invariably drove him on. Whenever Lower tried to tie a knot, Shumway would remind him that if he farted again it meant that he was straining too much. He should tie it tight while allowing the work to flow "nice and easy." Lower would grin at the gag before realizing that Shumway had taught him another little surgical trick. Even when they hit unexpected trouble, Shumway would joke his way into calmer territory. When a black-out engulfed the hospital during a difficult procedure, Shumway did not curse or rant. "Hey," he cried out, quick as a flash in the sudden dark as he thought of their stodgy superior, "somebody tell Gerbode to put the lights back on . . ."

Yet their attention inevitably drifted back to the lab. Every stride forward on the fifth floor would make their work in the OR more productive and triumphant. They cranked up the pace of their experiments. Lower began to understand the remarkable complexity of Shumway's character. He had never met anyone as compulsive as Shumway, or as intent on finding laughter in the midst of obsessive work. It was an astonishing combination that, in tandem with Lower's own flexible personality and dexterity in the animal lab, began to produce landmark experiments. Shumway and Lower were about to change the course of cardiac history.

In the midst of their attempts to turn a heart around so that they could overcome a transposition, a new challenge rose up before them. Lower could hardly give voice to the words that echoed through his head: *A heart transplant . . .*

While they were still bent on transposing the great vessels, why did they need to focus solely on one congenital defect? If they could master an actual transplant they would transform surgery. All those irreversibly fatal cardiac diseases and flaws in an adult could be overcome by replacing a dying heart with the still healthy organ transplanted from a human donor who had just been killed by an accidental head injury. While it was still too early to tell, it seemed likely that, using their cold saline solution, they would be able to safely store a heart cut from a fresh corpse for at least an hour. It was impossible to tell how many lives they might save if they could prove that, using topical hypothermia and surgical innovations in the laboratory, transplantation was feasible.

During their first transplant experiment, Lower cut across the base of the dog's atria and divided the aorta and the pulmonary artery. He then removed the entire heart and stored it in a container filled with icy saline at a temperature of 4 degrees centigrade (39.2° F). The little heart felt cold and firm in his gloved hands when, an hour later, he picked it up once more and tried to suture it back into place. Lower forgot about his bad back, and the monotony of waiting, for the challenge of "autotransplantation"—replacing a heart in the same dog from which it had been detached—was immense. The atrial tissues were terribly fragile. There were other problems. A dog's aorta was notably shorter than in a human heart and Lower had little spare tissue to work with as he tried to re-implant the heart. He was also hampered by a knotted mass of veins that crisscrossed each other. It was a bloody mess, with tissue and veins disintegrating in the midst of his frustrated suturing. Even when he and Shumway managed the awkward transplant, their first twenty dogs still died after the rapid formation of blood clots.

They were consoled by the fact that a human heart would be much easier to transplant than its less supple canine equivalent. As a further break, Shumway decided that they should experiment with valve transplants. Why not, he speculated, replace the diseased mitral or aortic valve with the animal's own pulmonary valve? It had long been known, after all, that the pulmonary valve usually remained unaffected by diseases like endocarditis and rheumatic fever.

If Shumway was the more accomplished technician in the OR, he was nevertheless determined that Lower would be given as many openings as possible. The Shumway method, of favoring those younger than himself, was already in practice. And so Lower excised the pulmonary valve and then transplanted it into the descending thoracic aorta. A small segment of an ascending aorta was grafted from a donor dog to ensure that the right ventricle functioned normally. Trial and error, their familiar accomplices, eventually ensured the long-term survival of a long line of dogs following valve transplants. Shumway and Lower were rejuvenated. They were ready for the next step.

While Shumway's breakthrough in topical hypothermia had provided enough time for increased experimentation, Lower produced the inspirational shift in strategy. Instead of attempting the impractical autotransplant, he suggested to Shumway that they should excise the heart without removing the entire arterial system. Lower recognized that if he left a rim of the left atrium, containing the four veins that return oxygenated blood from the lungs, it would be simpler for him to complete the suture. The same principle encouraged him to leave the rim in the right atrium for the benefit of the two venae cavae. With that segment of the original heart in place, it would be easier to attach a donor heart from a different dog. Instead of suturing the veins leading into the heart, they would only need to join the tissue and arteries.

Shumway was impressed by the clarity of the idea. A surgeon would not have to be a technical wizard to attempt such stitching. He brushed aside a reminder that they would still face an immunological hurdle. Alexis Carrel, in the first attempts at transplantation more than fifty years before, had discovered that the immune system instinctively attacks alien tissue. Rejection would eventually set in, the heart would wither, and the dog would die.

Shumway grinned. He told Lower that they would just have to find a dog smart enough not to reject its new heart.

Lower picked out his first series of recipient and donor dogs. There was an instant sense of gratification. It was much easier to sew a heart into a different dog instead of replacing it inside the original animal. He lost his first five transplants, but there were still moments of sustained hope. All of the dogs came around once their transplanted hearts had begun to beat again. Some of the mutts even walked about and wagged their tails. None of them, however, lasted long. They all were dead within a few hours.

Lower worked as though he was on fire with inspiration. And, always, he was guided by Shumway's measured thinking. Yet there were moments when Shumway's own fevered excitement overflowed. This guy, he thought as he watched Lower work, is probably the greatest experimental surgeon since Carrel. They were getting damn close. They were on the verge of what the world would call a miracle.

They felt the first stirrings of elation at the thought that one of their dogs might eventually live for days or even weeks with a transplanted heart. Shumway and Lower were on the cusp of surgical immortality. They knew it.

In the summer of 1959, Adrian Kantrowitz headed east, venturing behind the invisible Iron Curtain to meet an even earlier pioneer of transplantation. Thirteen years before, in 1946, Vladimir Demikhov, the Soviet experimental surgeon, had attempted to switch a heart between two dogs in Moscow. He also carried out the first animal lung transplant a year later. And then, on Christmas Day 1951, without hypothermia or the support of a pump-oxygenator, Demikhov had again transplanted a heart from one dog to another. The animal lived for only a few hours. Demikhov repeated the procedure on twenty-one further occasions over the next four years—with one transplant-dog surviving for fifteen hours. Further details of those cases, shrouded by Cold War secrecy, were confined to the Soviet Union.

Despite his failures it was still extraordinary that Demikhov had advanced so boldly. He worked in isolation from surgical innovators like Lillehei and Lewis in Minnesota, and Kantrowitz's friends and allies on the East Coast, Dwight Harken and Charles Bailey. Kantrowitz identified with the radicalism of Demikhov. Even in his modest base in Brooklyn, at Maimonides Hospital, which he'd joined as the chief of cardiac surgery in 1955, Kantrowitz's originality had blossomed. The National Institutes of Health had recommended him to the U.S. State Department, which organized a group of leading American scientists to represent the country at a trade and cultural fair at Sokolniki Park in July 1959.

A summer trip to Moscow, for Kantrowitz and his wife, Jean, sounded too good to miss. How would he otherwise get a chance to honor the intriguing Demikhov and his mysterious fellow Russians? A delegation, led by Vice President Richard Nixon, with Adrian and Jean as part of the entourage, arrived at Sokolniki Park on July 24, 1959. Nixon staged an impromptu debate on the relative merits of capitalism and communism with the Soviet premier Nikita Khrushchev in front of a model American kitchen at the U.S. exhibition hall. The passionate exchange was beamed across American television.

Kantrowitz's own stimulating encounter with Demikhov would prove a more clinical affair.

At a time when Kantrowitz had yet to explore transplantation, Demikhov invited the American surgeon to scrub in on a mitral commissurotomy—a surgical attempt to split open a blocked mitral valve in the heart. Kantrowitz was startled to hear that such a dangerous operation would be carried out under a local anesthetic. No matter how much anesthetic they pumped into the poor open-eyed guy on the table, they would still be stretching his ribs apart and digging around in his chest. It was terrible to witness, especially when Demikhov tried to widen the mitral valve with a knife. Blood spurted and the patient moaned.

Demikhov called over a nurse and spoke to her rapidly in Russian. She bent her head low and whispered to the groaning man. He was suddenly silent. Demikhov went back inside his heart. They were eventually able to complete the commissurotomy and close the chest of their glassy-eyed patient.

After he had thanked Demikhov, Kantrowitz headed back to the waiting U.S. State Department car. "What the hell did he say in the OR?" he asked his translator, who had been in the operating theater as a spectator.

"Well," the embassy man laughed dryly, "Demikhov said, 'Tell that son of a bitch if he doesn't stop screaming I'm walking out. We've got a big-shot American watching us and I don't want to make a bad impression. Tell the son of a bitch I'll kill him if he makes another sound.'"

Kantrowitz shook his head in wonder. They called *him* a tough guy in Brooklyn, but he was a wimp compared to Demikhov and his stoic patient. If it had been him with his chest splayed open, under only a local jab, he would probably still be screaming. He would remember his Russian afternoon whenever another timid American doctor told him he was crazy.

Jean Kantrowitz knew that meeting with such a reckless giant of world surgery would only embolden her husband. Like Demikhov, he feared nothing. She had sensed that eleven years earlier, in the summer of 1948, on a warm evening in Manhattan, when her life had changed forever. After bumping into him on a crowded sidewalk, Jean looked up and thought that she was standing in front of an Olympic swimmer—except that he was far too interesting to be just a sportsman. She knew the difference. She had gone with a ballplayer for a while. But this guy, Adrian, whom she dimly remembered meeting two years before, called himself a surgeon. He had suggested, after chatting awhile, that he could give her a lift home. She laughed when she saw his car—a light green DeSoto convertible. Its soft cream top, in a little gesture of romance, was already rolled down. Jean wondered what some of her old friends in Trenton, New Jersey, would think if they could see her.

She had never heard anything as outrageous or ambitious as the plan outlined to her that night. Jean smiled in awe as the big man next to her told her that, one day, he would operate on the human heart. It was a breathtaking change from her last beau's promising a couple of tickets for a Dodgers or Yankees game. He dazzled her with his conviction that an extraordinary surgeon would create an artificial heart that could sustain life once a patient's own damaged organ had been removed from the chest. Adrian Kantrowitz, then a few months from his thirtieth birthday, seemed like he could do anything.

His parents, like hers, were Jewish immigrants. Adrian's father came from Russia, his mother from Latvia. Unlike Jean's family, they had made a very comfortable life for themselves in New York. His mother had been a costume designer for the Ziegfeld Follies on Broadway, and his father was a doctor, a successful general practitioner. Back in 1921, when Adrian was just three years old, his mother had decided that he and his brother, Arthur, five years older, would also become doctors. She was elated when Arthur eventually announced his plans to enter Columbia University and become a physicist. "That's to do with enemas, isn't it, Artie?" she beamed. When she learned the disappointing truth, Mrs. K. pinned her medical hopes on her younger son. Adrian, as affable as he was ingenuous, did not let her down.

In December 1943, having squeezed a six-year course into four years, he graduated from the Long Island College of Medicine, a modest institution that, alongside some grander university names, had been ordered by the U.S. Army to churn out as many young doctors as possible. After a nine-month internship at the Brooklyn Jewish Hospital, he had been assigned to the 97th Infantry Division, a unit of youthful soldiers about to face military combat for the first time. Despite his own youth and inexperience, Kantrowitz was made a battalion surgeon in Europe.

The 97th Division crossed the Western Front early in 1945. Most days Kantrowitz's main task was to stanch bleeding. He resorted to the simple brutality of clamps, shutting down the spurt or seep of red from the whimpering soldiers. He could then deal with the causes of those distressing sounds. Kantrowitz always tried to comfort the men as quickly as possible. None of the fancy new painkillers he had read about in New York were available to him. And so he pumped them full of morphine. He would then hook up primitive intravenous fluid-feeders so that plasma or saline entered the most wounded bodies.

During the war another American surgeon, Dwight Harken from Boston, had performed the previously unthinkable—a form of surgery on the heart. On June 6, 1944, Harken found a shard of metal lodged deep inside the right ventricle of a dying soldier in Cirencester, in the English countryside. Using a Kocker clamp, he tugged the shrapnel toward the opening. It moved forward slowly before, suddenly, it stuck. Harken, afraid of killing his patient, hesitated.

"For a moment," he wrote later to his wife, Anne, "I stood with my clamp on the fragment that was inside the heart, and the heart was not bleeding. Then, suddenly, with a pop as if a champagne cork had been drawn, the fragment jumped out of the ventricle, forced by the pressure within the chamber. . . . Blood poured out in a torrent. . . . I told the first and second assistants to cross the sutures and I put my finger over the awful leak. The torrent slowed, stopped, and with my finger *in situ*, I took large needles with silk and began passing them through the heart muscle wall, under my finger, and out the other side. With four of these in, I slowly removed my finger as one after the other was tied. . . . The only moment of panic was when we discovered that one suture had gone through the glove on the finger that had stemmed the flood. I was sutured to the wall of the heart! We cut the glove and I got loose. . . ."

The patient recovered. Harken eventually opened a slit in the wounded hearts of 134 men, clearing the shrapnel from each and sewing shut the incision. He did not lose one solider. World War II had forced through advances in medicine on a massive scale, from the rapid development of antibiotics to the sustained use of anesthesia and large-scale blood transfusions. It had also, thanks to Harken's courage and brilliance, transformed the wild concept of "blind," or closed-heart, surgery into a practical possibility. He had proved that the heart was a far tougher muscle than that frail thing forever breaking in bad poetry and cheap love songs.

After the war Kantrowitz became friends with both the dynamic Harken and the Boston surgeon's fiercest rival, Charles Bailey from Philadelphia. The two older men were chasing a surgical cure for mitral stenosis, a narrowing and scarring of the mitral valve in the left ventricle that often occurred after cases of rheumatic fever. They both believed it would be possible to cut into a beating human heart, locate the mitral valve by feel, and then insert either an index finger or a small surgical instrument called a valvotome into the blocked opening. It would be a technique loaded with menace for the patient—yet Harken and Bailey were racing to be first.

After his first three attempts had all ended in the death of his patients, Bailey realized that his renegade work was about to be banned from hospitals across America. Before any moratorium could be declared he secretly scheduled his last two attempts for the same day—June 10, 1948. Bailey would operate on a thirty-year-old man at the Philadelphia General Hospital at eight in the morning. Regardless of the outcome, he would repeat the same blind procedure on a young woman at two p.m. at Philadelphia's Episcopal Hospital.

Bailey lost his morning patient to heart failure even before he could split the mitral valve. He left his assistant to close the chest and stalked out of the operating room to take a hot shower. Bailey then dressed himself in his smartest suit. He had another case, perhaps one which could cost him his medical license, waiting for him across town.

Using a buttonhook knife and then his finger, Bailey opened the mitral valve belonging to Claire Ward, a twenty-four-year-old mother who had been warned by her own doctor that to be operated on by "that cowboy" meant almost certain death. Knowing that she was going to die soon anyway, Claire took the risk.

Within a week Bailey showed off his radiant patient at a meeting of the American College of Thoracic Surgeons. They could not know it then, but Ward would live for another thirty-eight years, the triumphant first survivor of a closed-heart surgical procedure Bailey dubbed mitral commissurotomy.

Six days later, Harken completed his own first successful mitral-valve opening. Over the next three years, amid many more deaths, each struggled to prove that mitral commissurotomy was completely justified. Harken regarded these early losses as "the pain of the pioneer." Kantrowitz, meanwhile, learned much about their contrasting characters. Harken believed it was his personal responsibility to impart the grim news of a fatality to the patient's family. Bailey insisted such trifling chores should be handled by his juniors. Kantrowitz swore that he would always follow the Harken way, especially after he had witnessed one of Bailey's supposedly routine commissurotomies.

In the midst of his finger-fiddling, Bailey tore the wall of the aorta. Blood poured from the patient's chest. Death was inevitable. Kantrowitz exclaimed in despair, at which point Bailey turned round and said, his stare cool and unblinking above his mask, "Adrian, if you're going to be a heart surgeon you've got to remember one thing. The blood on the floor is not your own."

Louis Leiter, the kindly chief of medicine at Montefiore Hospital in the Bronx, was bemused when Kantrowitz announced his intention in the fall of 1949 to devote himself to the heart.

"You're mad," Leiter said, as if on cue, reminding Kantrowitz that he was a highly promising doctor who might one day have a family to support. But Kantrowitz insisted, and later told Jeannie that, if nothing else, Harken and Bailey had taught him that "If you're going to do something new, it isn't new and it isn't good until they say you're out of your mind. . . ."

With the heart-lung machine still years away from completion, Kantrowitz was in the midst of devising a scheme to expose the left side of the heart, including the mitral valve. Instead of following Harken's and Bailey's model of closed-heart surgery, he intended to operate on the mitral valve with direct vision in a temporary bloodless field. Leiter sighed and smiled. He was a tolerant man, and so he took a gamble and offered a three-hundred-dollar research grant and unlimited use of the animal laboratory during Kantrowitz's six-month hiatus from his surgical residency. The lone proviso was that, before he returned to general surgery as their senior resident, Kantrowitz could work only on cats. The noise of barking dogs would be too disturbing to the rest of the hospital.

Kantrowitz needed a lot of cats; and so he and Jean began to explore ways of finding the cheapest possible supply. They decided to follow two distinct paths. The first led them to various homes for lost or abandoned animals. Adrian and Jean would take turns to step through the doorway with the claim that they wanted to adopt a cat. In their second option, along the garbage-filled streets of the Bronx, they faced some tougher customers. The Bronx cats lived on wasteland or in crumbling apartment blocks. There was not a single puss of the fluffy type that played with ribbons or little balls of wool. These were howling alley cats that ran the streets as if they owned them.

Jeannie did not mind. She accompanied Adrian when he went cat hunting. While he dragged a large burlap bag over his massive shoulder, she carried food and milk in an attempt to entice the mewing and hissing strays. They eventually took to arriving in the dark with a two-dollar trap in each hand. The traps were sold by a company called Havaheart—a detail that made them laugh as they skulked down the alleys. Each device was two feet in length with a door at either side of the wire cage. Once the cat slipped through the opening in search of food, the doors closed behind it. Sometimes they got lucky and could take a cat away with them to the lab. More often, having laid their traps, they would race off into the night. In the morning, Adrian would rely on various janitors to call and tell him whether a cat had been caught in their traps. He paid them a quarter a cat.

The work was slow and studded with failure. Cat after cat died on the table. Kantrowitz might have been discouraged had he not been so driven to operate on the mitral valve with direct vision. Each time he lost a cat, he was able to identify the reason. The first fifty-three cases ended during or soon after surgery, with only seventeen cats surviving the procedure for periods ranging from two to twenty hours. Yet Kantrowitz became increasingly familiar with the workings of a heart, recognizing its feel and texture and learning how he might stop and start it again. His next six recipient cats all recovered from surgery and survived for a minimum of thirty-six hours. Cat number 56 was still eating well and functioning normally after ten days, while number 59 was sacrificed immediately after the procedure. An autopsy revealed that its heart was clear of any abnormality or surgical damage. Kantrowitz could at last believe he had been right all along—but he needed one last burst of definitive success to provide his clinching evidence.

He had no new cats, no money, and only a few days left before he was due to begin his general surgical residency, on January 1, 1950. Once that reality descended upon him, he would, perhaps for years, have few opportunities for research. Two days after Christmas he went back one final time to his favorite adoption home and looked carefully at the cats presented to him in their cages. Kantrowitz saw a beautiful inky-black cat that was slightly larger than usual. It stared straight into his face.

When Kantrowitz pointed out the animal to the young attendant, he was told he had selected the home's most famous occupant. The big black cat had belonged to Marge and Gower Champion, the husband-and-wife dance team whose starry exploits on Broadway had just resulted in a lucrative Hollywood contract. Their first major movie together for MGM would be *Show Boat*. The cat appeared to be the only casualty of the dancing duo's triumph. Just before Christmas, as they prepared to move from New York to Los Angeles, the Champions had decided they would be unable to care for him while they wowed Hollywood.

"I'll take him," Kantrowitz said as he stroked case number 60, his "champion cat," knowing this would be his last chance to achieve a coup in cardiac research before he returned to the less exhilarating world of the gallbladder and the intestine.

On December 29, 1949, they filmed the operation, producing the first visual record of a mitral valve. Kantrowitz felt good as he sewed the chest shut, already talking softly to the cat, saying the name they would always use for him—Sixty.

"We better take this cat home with us," Adrian said to his new wife.

Sixty was no ordinary cat. He was one remarkable feline. And he soon proved that his extraordinary brain had come through surgery wholly unscathed by any lack of oxygen.

"Jeannie," Adrian hollered a few days later, "look at this damn cat!"

Sixty had perched himself on top of their open toilet seat, a look of concentrated bliss on his face as he emptied his bladder. Marge and Gower Champion had trained one hell of a cat.

Kantrowitz had his proof. His experiment had been vindicated, and from that moment on, he felt as if he could do anything with the heart.

Stanford Hospital Center, Palo Alto, California, December 23, 1959

That Wednesday afternoon, in their bright new laboratory in Palo Alto, forty miles from San Francisco, Lower and Shumway selected a two-and-a-half-year-old mongrel. He had a lively look about him that seemed to say that he was ready for the historic challenge of cardiac transplantation. It had taken a while for Shumway to feel similarly frisky. He had been made to swallow an insult dished out by Garrett Allen, the newly appointed head of surgery at Stanford, who had recently organized the division of the university hospital into two separate units—the existing branch in San Francisco, and a medical-school offshoot in Palo Alto, a neat and small California town with a Spanish name that meant "tall tree."

Allen had offered Shumway the opportunity to temporarily head the cardiac division in Palo Alto until a "big name" could be appointed in his place. Shumway fumed silently but decided that, while Allen hunted for his hot shot, he and Lower might as well get out of the decaying downtown lab on the corner of Clay and Webster and try something new in the plush world of Palo Alto. They might even show Garrett Allen what they could do if given a chance.

Their latest experiment unfolded before them with dizzying possibilities. If Shumway and Lower could keep a dog alive with its transplanted heart, they would have taken the next giant step toward replicating the feat in man. Their breakthrough in hypothermia remained the bedrock on which that extraordinary aspiration was built, but they needed to prove to themselves that it was surgically possible to cut out a beating heart from one body and transplant it into another. If they could shock the heart back to life so that it pumped blood through a new host system with its original vigor—for days rather than just hours—they would have removed the final technical doubts about such surgery. Shumway was well aware that rejection would set in after a week—but that mighty battle could wait. They first had to conquer a surgical mountain.

Shumway chose another mongrel as their donor dog. While they were roughly the same size, each weighing about 19 kilograms (42 pounds), the two dogs were very different cross-breeds. They still both looked small and delicate as they were prepared for anesthesia. Once again it seemed strange to Lower that even an ordinary mongrel would offer him a heart that presented a greater challenge to his surgical skills than its human counterpart. If he could perfect the stunt in a dog, he knew how much easier it would be to adapt the technique to the more pliable human heart. He pulled down his mask and stretched his fingers into the thin latex gloves. It was almost time.

Lower looked over at his friend. Shumway winked at him over his own mask as the two dogs slipped away into unconsciousness. The donor dog would disappear painlessly into death. The more important mongrel, the recipient dog, had already been attached to Shumway and Stofer's heart-lung machine. The animal's temperature was gradually lowered to 28 degrees centigrade (82.4° F) as Lower emptied his mind of everything but the exacting task ahead of him. He reached for his knife and began the cutting.

Shumway attached a respirator to the endotracheal tube to provide ventilation and assist the recipient dog in its breathing. The heart and great vessels were then exposed by an incision that ran in a long straight line down the length of the pericardium. The edges of that sac, which encloses the heart, were sutured temporarily to the cavity in the dog's chest to form an operating well. With the oxygenator carrying out the work of the heart and lungs, Lower was ready to excise the recipient dog's heart.

He clamped the aorta and the pulmonary artery. His hands were as steady as his unflinching gaze.

Lower made another incision in the pulmonary artery so that, while blood was drained, the dog's lungs would be decompressed and removed from the operating field. He separated the heart by slicing into the posterior atrial wall. It was as if he were cutting into the now silenced heartbeat of the recipient dog—for it is normally the echo of the atrioventricular valves closing shut to prevent the backflow of blood into the atria that produces the familiar beating sound of the heart. The right atrium was severed at the base of the superior vena cava and the inferior vena cava—the two great veins that drain deoxygenated blood from the upper and lower parts of the body. Lower cut the left atrial wall along the entrance of the pulmonary veins before, finally, separating the heart from its body by dividing the aorta and pulmonary artery above the valves. The heart, like a boat released from its moorings, was loose.

With Shumway watching over him, he lifted the heart from its cavity. All that remained were the posterior atrial wall receiving the inflow of the venae cavae and the pulmonary veins—with a ridge of atrial septum, the thin muscular wall in the heart, separating them. Lower had removed the first heart in less than two minutes.

The crater in the recipient chest was empty, and the dog, now without a heart in its body, was kept alive by the machine. Norman Shumway and Richard Lower had been in this position often enough before for the element of wonder to have long since disappeared from the stark sight. It would be different, they knew, the first time they looked down into the chasm of a human chest. But for now, they were stimulated instead by the need to fill the gaping hole in their dog with a donor heart.

The second anesthetized dog lay motionless on the adjoining table. Shumway repeated the same technique of excision and, working more cautiously with the heart they would transplant, completed the task in little more than three minutes. The heart was immersed in a saline solution chilled to 4 degrees centigrade (39.2° F). Cold seeped through the heart, and within a further three minutes the myocardial temperature had dropped from 28 to 12 degrees centigrade (82.4 to 53.6° F).

Lower picked up the heart. It did not seem as if he was holding a miraculous source of life. The dog heart felt cold and slippery in his hands. He held it firmly but gently as he looked down. Blue and inert, it was otherwise unmarked by any obvious defect. Lower's gloves were tinged with blood as he lowered it into the waiting chest of the first dog. It made a neat fit.

Shumway joined the atrial walls and the atrial septum of the donor heart to the posterior atrial wall of the recipient dog in one long and continuous loop of a suture. A catheter was inserted and bronchial blood filled the left side of the heart. They then sewed together the ascending aorta and pulmonary artery. Shumway knew that the fragility of the dog's aortic tissue made this the most taxing segment of the procedure—but Lower's work was precise. The transplanted heart was lodged firmly in place. They had completed the most difficult part of the procedure.

The aortic clamps were removed to restore blood flow to the coronary arteries. Almost instantly the myocardium, the heart's muscular wall, began to pink up with the influx of warming blood. Shumway was about to return the heart to life. Using electric paddles, he shocked the transplanted heart. The fibrillation stopped and, simultaneously, the heart began to beat rhythmically in its new body. Their elation was curbed by the memory of past disappointments. The oxygenator kept spinning, supporting the change of heart for five minutes. Shumway gave Stofer the nod. The dog was unhooked from the machine. Even unaided, the pumping of the transplanted heart was obviously strong.

Lower and Shumway grinned at each other behind their masks. If the dog survived for at least a day they would be able to claim the world's first successful heart transplant. They began to stitch shut the chest. Shumway looked at the clock. They had been at work less than an hour.

R oy Cohn, the acting chief of surgery in Palo Alto, was exhilarated by the success of Lower and Shumway's transplant experiment. Their dog had done fantastically well with his new heart. "Reborn" on December 23, his tail-wagging energy and playful barks made him look like a mutt who truly believed Christmas was coming. Appearing at a local television station, KTVU, Cohn had highlighted the colossal achievement on the program *Doctors' News Conference.*

While Alexis Carrel and Charles Guthrie had first transplanted a puppy's heart into another dog's neck, fifty-four years before, in 1905, it was very different from the Stanford case. The Carrel–Guthrie dog, which had not survived more than two hours, kept its original heart intact. A few other surgeons, most notably Vladimir Demikhov, had tried variations on that technique, but Cohn proudly outlined the essence of his colleagues' innovation. For the first time in the long legacy of scientific experimentation, an animal had been returned to normal activity with its circulation supported solely, day after day, by a transplanted heart.

San Francisco's television and radio stations, as well as the city's newspapers, were entranced. "A young Stanford surgeon has successfully transplanted a living heart from one dog to another," George Dusheck of San Francisco's *News-Call Bulletin* reported on December 30, 1959. "The dog is still alive one week later. The daring experiment was carried out by Dr. Richard Lower, working with Dr. Norman Shumway, at Stanford's new Palo Alto medical center. Other surgeons have attempted similar transplants; the animals have all died within hours. . . . Dr. Lower's accomplishment is, as Dr. Cohn put it, 'a technical stunt.' Nobody expects the dog to survive permanently."

Yet in the final paragraph of the report, headlined "Stanford Surgeon Switches Heart in Dog—It Lives," the *Bulletin* hinted excitedly at the broader possibilities for humanity: "Dr. Lower's feat, therefore, is a demonstration that when the problem of host immunity reaction is solved, the surgeons will be ready to install healthy hearts (presumably from victims of other diseases) in place of diseased hearts."

The sudden interest in the two young surgeons irked Garrett Allen, who was still searching for his big name to replace Shumway. Arguing that the surgery was too controversial, for Lower had received abusive letters from dog lovers and fringe groups campaigning against animal experimentation, Allen ordered that the still healthy history-maker should be put down.

Shumway and Lower were too fond of their tough mongrel to obey Allen's instruction. They also knew it was vital that the dog should be allowed to live until the inevitable signs of rejection emerged. Only then would they be willing to end the dog's life in order to conduct an autopsy that might explain why this experiment had worked so spectacularly when the five previous attempts at the same procedure had all failed.

Shumway could have done without the hysteria surrounding their otherwise cool and diligent work. Yet he was happy to welcome the interest of another young doctor. On a cold but glittering winter's day, Eugene Dong arrived at Shumway's office in Palo Alto. There were no leaks in the ceiling, but it was still an austere and cramped office, ten feet by five, with just enough space for two metal desks and two chairs. A small window in the far left corner over-looked the surgical wing of the new medical school.

Dong, a Chinese-American nearing the end of his internship at Bellevue Hospital in New York, had traveled across the country to Stanford in the hope of being offered a surgical residency. Shumway believed in interviews about as much as he did in media coverage and so he dispensed with the formal question-and-answer routine. He talked instead in his laid-back style to an aspiring resident who had fallen under the spell of the heart. Dong made it clear he would take any job they might be able to offer him.

Knowing how much he and Lower could use another ardent heart man, Shumway suggested that, with his support, Dong should apply for a fellow-ship to work with them. He was pretty sure the American Heart Association would grant Dong's application. Shumway wrapped up the formalities with an intriguing invitation to visit a special patient.

His office was just a few doors down from the square and comparatively airy laboratory, which measured thirty feet by thirty feet. Lower and their fa-vorite mongrel were in the lab together. The dog bounded over to greet Shumway and Dong. After introducing Dong to Lower, Shumway recounted the full extent of the animal's transplant history. He was approaching the end of his seventh day with a new heart.

Dong wore heavy-rimmed glasses. As he watched the dog jump and skip around the lab, Dong's eyes seemed to be standing on stalks of surprise be-hind his thick lenses.

"That's amazing," Dong said softly.

"Yeah," Shumway nodded. "We could have some real fun here. . . ."

On the last morning of the year, and of the decade, the story made *The New York Times*. Under the headline "Dog Stays Alive with a New Heart," the report stated that "two young surgeons have successfully trans-planted a living heart from one dog to another. The mongrel male dog was alive today, a week after the operation. The experiment was carried out at Stanford University's new medical center by Dr. Norman Shumway, 36 years old, and Dr. Richard Lower, 30."

Shumway and Lower might have made the big time, but they were reflective rather than ecstatic. Eight days after the transplant, early signs of infection had hardened into rejection. The dog's immune system had begun to attack its new heart. They guessed that the dog could live for a few more days, maybe even another week, but they needed to open it up and check the heart before the condition of the tissue was totally ruined.

And so that Thursday afternoon, at exactly 2:25 p.m., on December 31, 1959, with the dramatic decade of the sixties waiting to burst open, the two friends put their little furry pal to sleep for the last time. They sliced down the center of his chest and removed the transplanted heart so that they could begin a new year by studying it under a microscope. If there was a streak of sadness in them, at the loss of a patient they had cared about so much, there was also an undercurrent of jubilation at the extent of their success.

A few minutes before the dog finally closed its eyes, Shumway had taken an EKG of the heart. It looked normal. It looked good. They were suddenly sure that if they had a way to prevent rejection, the transplanted heart would have beat on for years. The possibilities, as Shumway had always promised, were endless.

Before they reeled out into a darkening December afternoon, in search of a drink and an early start to New Year's Eve, they completed their last task of the day. They reviewed the office memorandum that had been prepared by Stanford University. "On Wednesday December 23, 1959," the internal hospital memo began, "Shumway and Lower performed an unusual heart transplant operation. They took a heart from a dog and put it into the body of another dog, using a new surgical technique for this procedure. . . ."

They filled out the date and time of death, and Shumway, relieved at the brevity of the description and the absence of any grand rhetoric about the future, added one last sentence, a personal quote from him as team leader. It was typically understated: "I expect this experiment to be the beginning of a very fruitful study."

Five

HEADS AND HEARTS

 Two days later, on January 2, 1960, John F. Kennedy announced the beginning of his campaign for the presidency. "The most crucial decisions of this century must be made in the next four years," he warned. "How to end or alter the burdensome arms race, where Soviet gains already threaten our very existence; how to maintain freedom and order in the newly emerging nations; how to rebuild the stature of American science and education . . ." Kennedy's voice also rang out in anticipation of "the decade that lies ahead—the challenging, revolutionary Sixties." He had been "reminded of the exhortation from *King Lear*: 'I will do such things, what they are I know not . . . but they shall be the wonders of the Earth.'"

After a ten-year struggle through the paranoid 1950s, transplant surgery was about to be accepted as a medical "wonder." Richard Lawler, a Chicago surgeon, had carried out the first successful kidney transplant back in May 1950. Some called it a "miracle," but many had vilified Lawler for "playing God" when he grafted a kidney from a recently deceased woman into forty-four-year-old Ruth Tucker. While his patient inexplicably escaped acute rejection of her transplanted organ and lived for another six years, Lawler was, in his own words, "ostracized by much of my profession. . . . Some of my good friends wouldn't even talk to me for fear I would contaminate them." A devastated Lawler withdrew from transplantation forever.

Other surgeons could not be deterred. On December 24, 1954, in Boston, Joseph Murray crossed the ethical line stipulating that a doctor should "do no harm" to a patient. Murray removed a kidney from Ronald Herrick in order to save his identical twin, Richard, who had been dying of Bright's disease. Five years down the track, on Christmas Eve 1959, the healthy twenty-seven-year-old brothers celebrated the anniversary of their transplant and the fact that public controversy had been replaced by the glow of a festive story— Richard Herrick had even married the nurse who'd looked after him in the hospital. Transplant surgeons were bolstered in their quest to achieve the ideal of routinely switching kidneys and livers between ordinary people—not just identical twins, whose shared DNA meant they avoided the otherwise predictable threat of rejection.

Lower believed that Shumway's work in hypothermia, even more than transplantation, would epitomize Kennedy's decade of brilliant promise. He was convinced it would eventually earn his friend the Nobel Prize. Lower saw how easily Shumway related to established Nobel Prize winners at Stanford. Joshua Lederberg, the great geneticist who had been awarded the Nobel in 1957, and Arthur Kornberg, the pioneering biochemist who'd just equaled that achievement in December 1959, had both been enticed to the new campus in Palo Alto. Shumway would occasionally sit with them in the university lunchroom. He may have been a sharper joke-teller but he was still their intellectual equal. Lower began to tease him about his comfort in such heavyweight company. "Gee, Norm," Lower would say, "you look so good next to Lederberg and Kornberg, I'm gonna give you a new name . . ."

And he did. Lower would shout out in the Stanford cafeteria whenever he saw his pal shyly picking his way toward their table. "Hey, Shumberg," he yelled, "over here!"

Chris Barnard was hungry. He was ravenous. There were no Nobel Prize winners for him to share a sandwich with in the stark Groote Schuur canteen in Cape Town. Table Mountain soared gloriously above the hospital, an obvious reminder of the Cape's natural beauty. Yet to Barnard, sur-rounded by highly competent but no truly inspirational doctors at the bot-tom of Africa, the medical terrain looked notably flatter and more barren.

He was sure that the task of scaling medicine's unconquered mountains could be achieved more easily on the flip side of the globe—in Europe or, es-pecially, in America. While he knew that his best South African contempo-raries were a technical match for most surgeons around the world, there was no medical genius in residence to press him on toward greatness, no one close at hand to rouse him with towering ambition or colossal achievement. He still looked toward Minnesota.

Barnard and Walt Lillehei exchanged dozens of letters. Since the triumph of his first open-heart procedure eighteen months earlier, when Lillehei had guided him from afar, Barnard had grown as a surgeon. He lost few patients, compensating for his lack of surgical flair with a voracious determination and compassion for their aftercare. Barnard related details of his medical progress to Lillehei amid increasing complaints of isolation in his own country.

"It can seem like a desert cut off from the rest of the world," Barnard wrote to Lillehei in January 1960. "Even the medical journals, which I read cover to cover, arrive months after they come out in America. I sometimes worry what I am missing because I feel like I am falling behind old colleagues who seem to be doing such great things. Without your contact I live in a dif-ferent world. Minnesota seems very far from here."

In the grip of the Cold War, and haunted by the threat of nuclear cata-strophe, America was on the verge of cultural transformation. Anything and everything seemed possible. From the dream of man walking on the moon to transplanting human organs, from sexual liberation to racial struggle, from the beat generation to rock and roll, America crackled with electrifying change. Barnard, meanwhile, came from a blinkered country where there was not even a single TV set. Television, considered a subversive force in South Africa, was banned by the state.

Nelson Mandela, on trial for treason in Johannesburg in 1960, wrote co-gently of Prime Minister Verwoerd's "grim programme of mass evictions, po-litical persecutions and police terror." In an attempt to rally his dispirited people, Mandela suggested, with undue optimism, that Verwoerd's elevation to power was "the last desperate gamble of a doomed and hated fascist autocracy—which, fortunately, is soon to make its exit from the stage of history."

Verwoerd accused Mandela and his party, the African National Congress, of plotting a "communist-backed revolution." Mandela was demeaned as "a puppet of Moscow." If most white South Africans smugly swallowed that lie, Barnard was restless and edgy. His frustration, however, was strictly professional, rather than even vaguely political. He yearned not for an end to apartheid but for the medical impetus that might transform his career.

And so he was stunned one morning at the start of a new decade when, smoking a cigarette over his newspaper in the hospital canteen, his eyes locked on an eerie photograph from Moscow. Vladimir Demikhov sat next to a healthy-looking Alsatian that had the upper part of a puppy's body grafted onto its neck. The puppy's head was clearly still being controlled by a working brain. A surreal and monstrous image captivated Barnard. He had been intrigued by Demikhov ever since, back in Minnesota, he'd heard that the Russian surgeon had attempted to transplant a heart from one dog to another in Moscow in 1946. The heart had begun to beat, but Demikhov's dog had soon died. The dark mysteries of a heart transplant remained beyond Barnard's scope—for he was unaware then of the breakthrough made a few weeks earlier at Stanford. Barnard was certain, however, that he, too, could replicate an upper-body graft from one dog to another. He raced from the canteen to the animal lab, where he persuaded a talented young medical resident, John Terblanche, to assist him. Within five hours of starting surgery, Barnard and Terblanche had duplicated Demikhov's sensationalist stunt. The smaller head of a puppy, also grafted onto the neck of a larger dog, turned to both the left and right. Barnard's colored lab technician, Victor Pick, did not know whether to laugh or run from the lab in fright. The surgeon himself was mightily impressed by his own bizarre first attempt at transplantation. He called in his more dubious chief, Jannie Louw, to witness the sight of a two-headed dog lapping water from two separate bowls.

A few weeks later, photographs Barnard had taken of his creation hit the front pages of the South African newspapers. Having contacted the press himself, he had become a minor surgical celebrity. Louw, digging deep into their shared religious Afrikaner past, pasted a personal warning on the wall of the Animal House: "Do Not Toy with the Delilah of the Press!" Barnard tore it down.

He was already determined to widen his scope of surgical reference by visiting Demikhov in Moscow. The American and European explosion of interest in kidney transplantation had concentrated his mind; and Demikhov was said to have done more animal experiments in organ grafting than any surgeon in the world. Barnard did not care what the South African government thought. He would fly to the Soviet Union. Barnard would do anything in the pursuit of transplant knowledge. He needed to escape the feeling that he was drowning in darkness.

A deeper despair soon spread across South Africa. On March 21, 1960, madness descended when white policemen opened fire on a crowd in the township of Sharpeville, an hour south of Johannesburg, killing sixty-seven black people. International condemnation of the massacre was unprecedented. Even the U.S. State Department, usually reluctant to voice any criticism of apartheid, expressed a hope that black South Africans would "obtain redress for legitimate grievances by peaceful means." The United Nations was more forceful in its criticism, with only Britain and France abstaining from a resolution that blamed apartheid for the killings. South Africa, almost overnight, had become a pariah state.

The stock exchange in Johannesburg collapsed, and white South Africans, already unnerved by the warning made by the British prime minister, Harold Macmillan, that "the winds of change" were sweeping across Africa, began to arm themselves. Barnard's own tribe, the ruling Afrikaners, retreated into the "*laager*" mentality they had called upon when their ox-wagons formed a circle of defense in past sieges against the Zulu and British armies. While he understood the local mentality, and resented any foreign criticism of South Africa, Barnard could not risk losing touch with the outside world.

As soon as his application for an Oppenheimer grant for international medical research was awarded later that month, Barnard began planning both his return to Minnesota and his first trip to Moscow. He needed to visit the country that had opened the heart to him. He also yearned to find something new to pursue in surgery with a maverick like Demikhov.

Barnard wrote to the director of the Soviet Ministry of Health in late March:

"I plan to visit the U.S.S.R. from May 18–29 and would be very grateful if you would arrange for me to visit your research centers in Moscow, where they are working in the fields of cardiac surgery and the transplantation of tissues. If there are research centers elsewhere in the Soviet Union which you feel I should visit, I would be happy to do so, as I would like to meet as many of your best surgeons and research workers as possible."

With reference to his own experience in Cape Town, Barnard stressed his open-heart unit's "very good results. . . . In addition I am engaged in surgical research work and we are particularly interested in the field of cardiac surgery and the transplantation of organs."

While he awaited the Soviet response, Barnard also pined for his young girlfriend in Minneapolis. He still wrote a couple of times a week to Sharon Jorgensen, whom he described to close friends as "very blonde and very beautiful." As the last few weeks of summer in Cape Town slid away, Barnard began to dream even more ardently of Minnesota. The Cape winters were often gray and miserable, while springtime in Minneapolis, as Barnard wrote, meant that "along the Mississippi the trees were a splashy bright green—brighter than anything we knew in South Africa. In the fields there were wild flowers."

If only he could see Sharon, and then meet Demikhov in Moscow, Barnard was sure that he would find his way again.

He returned in time for the Minnesota spring he missed so badly. Barnard had been away for two years, and in that time he'd transformed cardiac surgery in South Africa. His achievements enabled him to return with a little swagger in his step. The approval of Wangensteen and Lillehei bolstered him still further. Lillehei encouraged him specifically, arguing that the opportunity to run his own show, and to face monumental surgical battles, was worth far more than being a support member of a cardiac team in a far grander hospital in America. South Africa was not the end of the world, no matter how remote it seemed to Barnard. He was not even thirty-eight yet. There was still time for him to make it—as long as his hands held up.

His rheumatoid arthritis had been diagnosed four years earlier. He had felt it first in his feet when he'd taken his children, Deirdre and Andre, ice skating in Minneapolis in the raw winter of 1956. While they had swept around him in smooth little arcs, shrieking with joy at the hiss and scrape of their skates, he had clung instead to a cold black rail. "Why don't you let go and skate?" a little American girl had asked him mockingly. "Are you chicken?"

Barnard had not been able to answer. It had felt as if his feet were in a roaring grate of fire. He'd tried to blame his ill-fitting skates, but when his hands began to throb a few days later he saw a specialist at the university hospital. It was then that he heard the terrible news of his ailment. His feet were soon so fat and inflamed that he struggled to pull on his shoes. The joints in his fingers hurt almost as much. Louwtjie, his long-suffering wife, had helped him on those frozen Minnesota mornings. She had buttoned his shirts, fixed his tie, and slid a sports jacket over his aching shoulders. Barnard had realized then that there were certain things only a wife, rather than a young mistress, could do for him.

Those moments together had been among their most tender in a prickly marriage. Chris and Louwtjie tried out a variety of remedies, ranging from guava leaves to brake fluid which she swore had cured the ailments of many neighboring farmers when she'd been a girl in South-West Africa (now Namibia). Whether or not it was thanks to the brake fluid, his agony lessened after a few weeks in Minnesota. The specialist suggested that Barnard had a peculiarly high tolerance for the more debilitating effects of the illness. He was not usually bothered by pain during surgery, and so he expected he had some time left before becoming hopelessly stiff and twisted. Rheumatoid arthritis, however, had made him, unlike some surgeons, aware of his own fallibility.

His downbeat memories had been sparked by the fact that his reunion with Sharon Jorgensen had made him feel surprisingly old and confused. Barnard was shocked that she was no longer smitten with him. Sharon did not blame him for choosing to live with his family in Cape Town rather than with her in Minneapolis. The fact that she regarded it as the correct decision wounded him. She did not rage or accuse him of breaking her heart. Sharon, rather, was full of rational good wishes for his happiness and success. At twenty-two she was already moving on with her own life. Barnard, a sucker for melodrama, felt as if she had coolly plunged a knife into him.

He buried himself in work, trusting that his trip to Moscow would dredge up more sustained hope for his career. The Soviet Union, keen to spread its global influence to Africa, had become vociferous in its condemnation of apartheid—and so, while granting Barnard entry, his visit was more closely monitored than it might have been before the Sharpeville massacre. He still enjoyed ritual early morning vodkas with Demikhov and listening to him speak, through an interpreter, of his early kidney and heart transplants. The laboratories and operating theaters were frighteningly primitive, but the extraordinary Demikhov encouraged Barnard to dream.

Why should an American, Demikhov asked, be the first to walk on the moon? Why could it not be a Russian, or, as Demikhov said, slapping Barnard on the back, a South African? Demikhov roared when Barnard explained earnestly that South Africa did not have a space program. Okay, okay, Demikhov laughed, a Russian would have to walk across the moon first. But why, then, did the world's greatest surgeon have to be an American?

Barnard grinned as he knocked back his vodka. Demikhov could be a model for him to follow away from America. He looked around the bare room in which they sat. The facilities he used in Cape Town were far superior. If Demikhov had come this far in Moscow, despite communism, why could he not go even further?

"Nothing is impossible," the Russian said through his interpreter. *"Nothing . . ."*

Clearwater Hotel, San Francisco, October 10, 1960

Early that Monday morning, with a cold and dense fog curling round the bay, Sparky's boys slipped back into town. Norm Shumway and Dick Lower carried three stapled pieces of paper and a box of slides. Their lecture— "Studies on Orthotopic Homotransplantation of the Canine Heart"— would be delivered at a forum of the American College of Surgeons in San Francisco.

The Surgical Forum had been instigated in 1945 by Owen Wangensteen as a way of allowing young surgeons interested in experimental research to present and publish their work. In the intervening fifteen years, especially with the cardiac breakthroughs achieved in Minnesota, the status of the forum had risen markedly. Yet the 8:30 a.m. Monday lecture, reserved for the arcane and the unknown, was not a prestige slot. They didn't care. Lower felt nervous enough at the prospect of reading out his first paper in front of the thirty or so surgeons who usually turned up at the early lectures, and Shumway hated any kind of fuss.

But Shumway was already tussling suspiciously with a small degree of fame. In a two-page investigation into "Progress in Transplants" on June 27, 1960, *Time* magazine had acclaimed his work at Stanford. "The first serious attempts to transplant organs by modern surgical techniques began in the early 1900s, when pioneering Dr. Charles Claude Guthrie, working at St. Louis's Washington University, created two-headed dogs by grafting. Today most of the surgical techniques have been perfected. Such surgeons as Stanford's Norman E. Shumway, Jr., have developed grafting to the point where a dog with an unrelated dog's transplanted heart is up and hopping around within twenty-four hours, but it dies within three weeks."

Shumway dismissed the report, mainly for its failure to mention Lower. He also thought it ironic that no reference should be made of Lower's most obvious predecessor, Alexis Carrel, who had attempted the first cardiac transplants in conjunction with Guthrie. At least the omission in *Time* was novel; for in medical circles it had become almost de rigueur to exalt Carrel, while glossing over Guthrie's contribution. Their brief partnership had fractured, the strain between the two surgeons exacerbated by Carrel's receiving the Nobel Prize.

If he and Lower clearly led the modern cardiac transplant race, Shumway knew they were not completely alone. Watts Webb, who worked with James Hardy, a relentlessly ambitious academic surgeon in Mississippi, had reported a dozen heart-lung transplants in dogs in 1958. The longest survivor had lasted for seven and a half hours. And, besides Hardy and Webb, there were sure to be others who would chase what the American surgeon Marcus had called, in 1951, an impractical but "fantastic dream"—replacing a terminally diseased heart with a transplanted organ taken from another body.

The race had begun to gather a slow but steady momentum. Even the unnamed journalist at *Time* closed his article with a guarded prediction: "In the field of transplants, the great target is the heart. Some victims of atherosclerotic coronary disease (the leading killer in the United States today) might be saved if they could receive a transplant of a healthy heart from, say, a traffic accident victim."

The forum's moderator and a projectionist soon joined them in the small ballroom. Moving slowly, the moderator looked as if he could not remember what he had drunk at the previous night's cocktail party. Shumway winced at the obvious sight of a grim hangover. The projectionist, by contrast, appeared as bored as he was sober while he scanned the rows of vacant seats.

"Standing room only," Shumway quipped.

The moderator smiled weakly and sank into a seat. He looked at his watch—8:25 a.m. In the five minutes remaining, the moderator steadied himself while Lower ensured that the slides were loaded correctly by the projectionist. At 8:32 the four men looked around the empty room. The moderator indicated that he could wait a few more minutes in the hope that someone would turn up. And yet no one came. Lower finally rose and headed for the podium.

"A technique has been developed," he said, as he looked up from his notes, "for replacement of the canine heart with a homologous heart. The recipient animal can be expected to survive for several days during which time the denervated, transplanted heart appears to function normally."

Lower nodded to the projectionist, who, with a whirr, brought up the first slide on a screen above the small podium. Staring at the grainy sight of a dog's opened heart, the moderator clutched the sides of his chair. Only the smell of a greasy breakfast would have tested him more than that graphic series of dog heart photographs. Lower explained his surgical technique precisely until, shortly after 8:40, he reached the symbolic heart of his own paper. Everything they had been working toward during their daring experimentation was contained within four simple sentences: "In a series of ten consecutive transplantations, six of the recipient animals lived for six to twenty-one days. The recovery from anesthesia was uneventful. During convalescence the dogs ate and exercised normally. The pulse rate was variable and increased moderately with exercise."

Lower knew that neither the moderator nor the projectionist would enter a debate about transplantation of the canine heart; and so he read his and Shumway's conclusions with brisk authority. With the transplanted heart appearing to be "completely normal," Lower suggested that, if the problems of immunological rejection could be conquered, "it would continue to function adequately for the normal life span of the animal."

Lower paused, indicating to the moderator that their first-ever presentation of a landmark medical discovery had reached its end. And then the surgeon said two polite words: "Thank you." The moderator did not linger with either praise or even a basic expression of interest in their transplant success. He had his hangover to nurse. If they had not been expecting to meet the Nobel Prize committee quite yet, neither had Shumway and Lower anticipated such utter apathy. They shrugged and gathered their materials.

Their work was not totally ignored. Scanning the surgical papers submitted on that opening day of the Surgical Forum, John F. Allen, the science editor of the *San Francisco Examiner*, decided to make a small news-splash the following morning. "Six whole hearts have been transplanted from one dog to another by a group of Stanford surgeons," he reported on October 11, 1960. "Doctors Lower and Shumway, having pretty well perfected the surgical technique involved, now are concerned with the problem of long-term storage of the hearts, looking toward the day when a young human heart from an accident victim can be kept long enough to be transplanted into a man whose own is worn and failing."

The Soviets, engaged in a race into another dark, forbidding place, outer space, edged ahead of the Americans when cosmonaut Yuri Gagarin became the first man to travel through space, on April 12, 1961. After a 108-minute orbit of the earth, the Soviet rocket reentered the atmosphere. Seven kilometers above Kazakhstan, Gagarin was ejected and returned to earth by parachute.

Twenty-three days later, on May 5, 1961, Alan B. Shepard was launched on a suborbital flight that lasted fifteen minutes. The first American in space traveled in a Mercury-Redstone capsule named *Freedom 7*. Yet the Soviet flight had circled the mysterious blackness of space for ninety-three minutes more than the Americans. Such statistics counted in the Cold War, and so, twenty days after Shepard had been launched into orbit, John F. Kennedy, in the first year of his presidency, stated his determination to win the race that mattered most: "I believe that this nation should commit itself to achieving the goal, before this decade is out, of landing a man on the moon and returning him safely to earth."

That same month, Victor Cohn, the Minnesota science writer who had reported on many of Walt Lillehei's medical innovations, had written a speculative story syndicated across America that predicted another evocative race. It was the third article of a series—*1970: Your Fantastic Future*—in which the country's leading science writers described "the world you will live in by 1970." Cohn began his story with a forecast: "*'May 1, 1970—A surgeon today successfully transplanted a human heart from an auto-crash victim to a patient whose heart had been failing.'* A news story like this is possible sometime in the next ten years. Work on transplanting human organs is being pushed in a hundred centers in the US, Britain, France and Russia. 'It may be that we're on the threshold of success,' predicts an outstanding surgeon. . . . Drs. Norman Shumway and Richard Lower of Stanford University recently made heart transplants into six dogs, and the dogs ate, romped and barked for as long as twenty-one days. . . . The great heart race has begun."

Adrian Kantrowitz, having read Shumway and Lower's inaugural paper, was about to join the chase. The talk at Maimonides Hospital, where he was now chief of cardiac surgery, swirled around all that he and his cosmopolitan team of researchers planned to do—with pacemakers, artificial hearts, electronic stimulators, U-shaped ventricular assist devices, and finally, even transplanted hearts.

For a small community hospital in a Jewish quarter of Brooklyn, it seemed a little too much to absorb. Yet Kantrowitz ignored the limitations surrounding him. He had already done battle with the ruling hierarchy at Maimonides over a single case, which proved his readiness to brush aside any opposition to his dynamic thinking and dramatic surgical innovations.

The big man had known he was heading for trouble from the moment he saw the slight and pretty girl in the football helmet. She cut a strangely com-

pelling figure as she drifted down the hospital corridors in baggy white paja-
mas with her head encased in the bright yellow protector. Rose Cohen was
not a refugee from the psychiatric wards afflicted by some deranged delusion
that she was a quarterback who might be tackled at any moment by a gang of
heavily muscled men with violent defense on their minds. She suffered from
a more physical, but no less disturbing, disorder.

"Stokes-Adams," Kantrowitz said, naming the anomaly of inconsistent
electrical conductivity in the heart that results in a temporary loss of pulse and
struck down Rose three or four times a day. Her loss of consciousness would
be so sudden and profound that each time it looked as if she had simply
dropped down dead. Although she would regain her senses after thirty or forty
seconds, Kantrowitz knew that the heart block would eventually kill her.

The Maimonides specialists, among them the distinguished cardiologist
William Dressler, were at a loss as to how they might treat her. And so
Dressler, determined that Rose should not be taken first by a fall that cracked
open her skull, reached for the helmet. She was instructed that the only time
she did not have to wear it was when she lay in bed.

Unlike the elderly Dressler, Kantrowitz was convinced that an obvious
surgical solution could be found. He was intrigued by the delicate and natural "electrical engineering" that drives the heart's relentless yet complex machinery. Beyond the fact that an ordinary heart needs to beat about 100,000
times every day, an exquisite array of electric pulses means that each chamber acquires its own distinct rate under varying conditions. As heart block
occurs when there is a break in the electrical connection between the upper
and lower chambers, Kantrowitz was convinced he should insert a pacemaker
into the chest of Rose.

Kantrowitz had produced one of the world's earliest implantable pacemakers with his own brawny hands in 1958. His version was based on the model of
an electronic metronome he had seen in *Popular Mechanics.* He'd gone down
to Canal Street, in lower Manhattan, where a cluster of little electronics shops
sold the parts needed to build a transistor radio—or, in Kantrowitz's case, a
prototype of the internal pacemaker.

Using a transistor and a few capacitors, Kantrowitz's crude metronome
had worked inside his dogs in the research lab. He was sure it would duplicate

the same function in Rose Cohen—who, unfortunately, was still Dressler's patient. Pointing out that she was a young woman in her twenties, Kantrowitz suggested politely to the old cardiologist that life inside a football helmet was not much of a life at all. Dressler nodded dismissively, as if he expected Kantrowitz to know that the alternative, a fractured skull, was even less appealing. Hoping to win their polite argument, Kantrowitz outlined the success of his internal pacemaker experiments. He listed his small triumphs in pacing the canine heart and claimed that the same technique could be applied to a human patient suffering from heart block.

Dressler was outraged at the thought of placing "a battery" in his patient. "Over my dead body," he sneered at Kantrowitz.

The surgeon, for once, remained silent. A day later, his assistants approached Dressler's residents and reiterated the validity of the idea. The young cardiologists at Maimonides were quickly convinced and agreed that Rose's family should consult with Kantrowitz. Dressler marched down to the administrative office, where he lodged a formal complaint against "that crazy man." He did not even need to say Kantrowitz's name. The administrators were already fearful of the uncharted territories in which Kantrowitz worked. They were far more comfortable with the conventional judgment of Dressler.

The surgical residents who witnessed the scene went back to Kantrowitz and told him about Dressler's protest. "Yeah?" Kantrowitz said in his heaviest Brooklyn drawl. "So? What are you waiting for?"

Certain that they could save Rose Cohen's life, they poached her away from Dressler. She sat in bed, her helmet resting on the small table next to her, and listened while Kantrowitz explained his plan to her and the whole Cohen family with friendly clarity. "Do you think it might work?" Rose asked quietly.

"Yes," Kantrowitz replied.

"All right," Rose said. "What have I got to lose?"

Kantrowitz implanted his device and the results were immediate. The pacemaker worked beautifully, and the Stokes-Adams attacks disappeared. Rose was ecstatic. Dressler was predictably despondent.

When Rose collapsed again in hospital, Kantrowitz remained calm. He placed her under the X-ray machine and found the reason for her falling to the ground. One of the wires had broken. With her heart beating regularly, they were approaching almost a million cycles after a week's worth of work in the chest—no ordinary wire could survive that tempo. A more resilient replacement lasted a little longer before it broke and Rose lapsed into unconsciousness. When it happened again—after they had carried out yet another repair and implantation of the pacemaker—Dressler began to mutter darkly about the wisdom of the helmet.

Kantrowitz had a better idea. He called up General Electric in Syracuse and told them about his work. Intrigued by his daring, as well as by the commercial potential, the corporation sent over a couple of their best engineers. They stared in disbelief at Kantrowitz's pacemaker. It was the worst engineering they had ever seen. There were any number of things wrong with it.

Kantrowitz laughed in delight at their candor. "Okay—but can you fix it?"

"Sure," the first man, Jerry Suran, said. "It's a great idea. It just needs to be built by a proper engineer."

A few weeks later, General Electric produced the first Kantrowitz pacemakers, each one weighing four ounces and consisting of five batteries, two transistors, three resistors, and a capacitator. Kantrowitz took Rose Cohen back to the operating table. She woke up and felt fantastic. Days and weeks passed until Rose was well enough to go home. Her condition was completely resolved—and she would live for more than another twenty years with that same device ticking in her chest. Even Dressler was impressed. Kantrowitz suggested that, one day, they ought to write a paper together, about Rose Cohen and other future cases. They would call it "Observations in Patients with an Implanted Cardiac Pacemaker—Clinical Experiences."

Kantrowitz had won the battle of the pacemaker but it was too early to tell who might win the war at Maimonides—especially now that he had announced his readiness to move into the uncertain realm of cardiac transplantation.

Although typically open in acknowledging the influence of Shumway and Lower's San Francisco paper, Kantrowitz decided to target a different patient population—infants born with a fatal cardiac defect.

For research, he would concentrate exclusively on the transplantation of hearts between puppies rather than fully grown dogs, in the hope that their undeveloped immune systems would not be as affected by rejection. Even more striking, Kantrowitz chose not to fight rejection with immunosuppression drugs. He believed that the uncertainties surrounding rejection meant that any cocktail of antirejection medication would be based primarily on guesswork. The battle against rejection would ultimately be won by the likes of Shumway and Lower, but Kantrowitz appreciated that it would take years of research. He was more consumed by the dream of salvaging a new life while carrying out the first human heart transplant—and choosing a baby as a recipient patient seemed to offer a better bet for long-term survival.

Kantrowitz also favored using total-body, rather than topical, hypothermia, as it would enable him to operate for up to an hour without a pump-oxygenator. Knowing how often the still recent invention of the heart-lung machine could go awry, Kantrowitz felt more comfortable in reducing a supposedly unnecessary risk during a procedure that Shumway and Lower carried out relatively quickly. A different danger lurked. While profound hypothermia could extend the time he had to operate, brain damage was a constant hazard. And an intractable hemorrhage or an air embolism caused by a faulty application of profound hypothermia spelled certain death. Kantrowitz still preferred to rely on himself and his new surgical partner, Yoshio Kondo, rather than on a machine. Kondo, a technically solid and extraordinarily diligent Japanese surgeon, was the ideal partner in Kantrowitz's great transplant quest. While the ideas were formulated by Kantrowitz it was plain that, at least in the earliest trials, they would be executed principally by Kondo.

In an experiment crammed with jeopardy, their first nine attempts at transplantation failed. For their tenth try a random pair of puppies, obviously similar only in weight, were both anesthetized and prepared for surgery one night in Brooklyn in early 1962. The recipient puppy was put in a tank of ice water, which lowered its temperature to 26 degrees centigrade (78.8° F). At that point, the cooling of the donor puppy began. The two temperatures were stabilized when the recipient fell to 19 degrees (66.2° F), while the donor puppy reached a more moderate 30 degrees (86.0° F).

Kondo performed his surgical excision on the donor dog and placed the heart in the same cold saline as used by Shumway. The heart was chilled at 4 degrees centigrade (39.2° F) for twenty minutes before transplantation, while the recipient puppy remained in its own ice tub. The young dog was covered with a sterile vinyl sheet that left enough space for the chest cavity to be opened by Kantrowitz, who avoided using the Lower technique of forming the pericardial sac into a well. With clear vision in a bloodless field, he quickly removed the heart—and then Kondo replaced it with the donor organ. They used silk sutures to fix the new heart, and then, to purge any lingering air bubbles, flushed the left atrium and ventricle with saline before the final stitch was made.

After almost forty-five minutes of circulatory arrest, the clamp and tourniquet were removed and the puppy was immersed in another tank of water, warmed to 42 degrees centigrade (107.6° F). Kondo massaged the tiny heart as the puppy's body heat gradually rose to 28 degrees (82.4° F) after a further twenty minutes. The heartbeat was then restarted with a shock of 110 volts and the body temperature climbed to 36 degrees (96.8° F). Kondo closed the chest cavity and 50 millileters of fresh blood was transfused back into the puppy.

Kantrowitz was hopeful all through the first postoperative day, though their previous nine dogs had been lost within forty hours after transplantation. It was still too early for him to start celebrating. The small puppy, however, was almost defiantly optimistic as it padded around the laboratory and accepted a liquid diet. After they had sailed past another twelve hours the tiny survivor was offered solid food as a reward for its resilience. It dug into its first decent meal with relish.

The days passed, and with the puppy eating and ambling around its quarters in seeming contentment as its new heart pumped steadily, Kantrowitz suddenly knew the exultant truth. They had done it. They were on their way. They were already racing toward the ultimate prize—a human heart transplant.

"Yoshio," Kantrowitz said softly to Kondo, "let's do another. Today. Let's go."

Six

CHANGING TACK

The big bold headline in the *Palo Alto Times* on March 26, 1963, was typically corny: "'Heartless' Mother." A grainy photograph of the mother, surrounded by her sleeping brood, startled the residents of that quiet California town on an otherwise ordinary Tuesday morning. The heartless bitch in question, known as Maisie, was a dog whose heart, the previous year, had been "completely removed from her body and stitched back into place seventy-seven minutes later." Maisie, Shumway and Lower's latest heroine, had just given birth to seven healthy puppies.

Another story beaming with local pride and national significance ran in the *Times* the very next day. "A team of surgeons at Palo Alto–Stanford Hospital has achieved the nation's lowest mortality rate for open heart surgery," their reporter Jack Viets revealed. "In the past three years the surgical team, headed by Dr. Norman Shumway, has performed 258 open heart operations. They have lost just eleven patients. . . . The team believes that open heart surgery today is about as safe as surgery for stomach ulcers."

Shumway was never one to court "newspaper fame," but his 95.7-percent success rate in the OR was cause enough for him to grant a brief interview to Viets. His real research interest, in transplanting hearts, was evident. "We have the surgical technique now. We will be ready when the problem of rejection is solved. But I am hopeful that we will be transplanting human hearts within the next decade."

The Stanford men were way out in front. Beyond perfecting the surgical art of transplantation, and preparing for the battle against rejection, they had already proved it was possible to store a heart in cold saline for at least seven hours without damaging the organ. They were moving steadily toward one of the emerging dreams of the twentieth century. Alongside the glorious fantasy of space travel, the heady notion of transplanting a human heart had begun to take hold of America. The surgeons who achieved that miracle—and it appeared certain to be Shumway and Lower—were destined for medical immortality.

Gene Dong and Ed Hurley had became key members of their tight and imaginative team. Dong, with his thick glasses and quick wit, determined the physiological function of the transplanted heart and studied ways of detecting the early onset of rejection. Hurley, favoring sensible spectacles and a crew cut, played the straight man alongside three jokers as he carried out the bulk of animal transplants and supplied Dong with his research material.

With Shumway and Lower increasingly involved in clinical surgery in the operating room, the onus of leading and monitoring Stanford's transplant experiments was assumed by Doug. He dictated the direction of their research and wrote the many indispensable grant requests for federal money. If Shumway's name remained at the top of each application for program funding, the principal investigator in the lab had clearly become Dong.

Despite immersing himself in work, Dong could not forget the racism his Chinese-American family had withstood for two generations. Dong had seen the shadows when he and his wife had moved to Stanford from New York in 1960. He had dressed himself in his best suit and gone in search of accommodation in the neighboring suburb of Menlo Park. Dong approached the door of every house where a sign—"Room to Rent" or "Room Available"— was either stuck on a board in the front yard or plastered against a window. He knocked with renewed hope each time, only to find that another room had been mysteriously filled ten minutes earlier.

Three years later, there was nothing sweeter for Dong than Shumway's expectant grin that he would make a massive contribution with the seriousness of his work and the quality of his joke-telling. Dong eventually proved, by measuring everything from cardiac function to renal side effects, that a heart removed and then replaced in the chest of that same animal remained unaffected. But his most significant test awaited: to predict failure of the heart by rejection.

After a kidney transplant it was easy to assess the organ's function by simply checking the output of urine. And as soon as trouble appeared there would be time to turn to dialysis. The heart was different. Failure, when it came, was quick and complete. Dong needed a noninvasive method to gauge rejection. He soon introduced an episodic form of treatment—for his experiments suggested that, through careful monitoring of specific medication periods, he could slowly reduce the volume of cortisone injections until the first signs of rejection were detected.

Dong was obsessed with the idea of transferring all their data to a computer— even in 1963, he had seen the future. He eventually raised the $70,000 they needed to buy their first hulking machine for the lab. Even though it offered a mere 8,000 bytes of memory, and required a paper-tape input without a floppy disc, he thought he had glimpsed heaven. Dr. Dong became one of California's first computer wizards. Shumway and Lower thought it mildly screwy, but recognizing their friend's zany brilliance, they allowed him to surf his waves of computerized thought. It did not take him long to process all their laboratory research and prove unequivocally that cardiac transplantation was devoid of physiological problems.

Hurley was engaged in a bloodier battle—with autotransplantation. In order to supply the organs that Dong studied, it was Hurley's task to excise the heart from an animal and eventually stitch it back into place. Like Lower four years previously, Hurley began by using the dog as his initial model. While he had enough success to keep Dong busy, there was invariably so much bleeding that he lost many dogs. Hurley considered switching to sheep or baboons, but he was not convinced that even their tougher aortic tissues could withstand the cutting and stitching.

It would take a burst of lateral thinking from Shumway to change the pattern. Driving home one evening along the Peninsula, he saw some calves standing meekly around their mother in the fading sunlight. Shumway knew that placental cross-circulation in calf twins might mean they were equally compliant in immunological terms. They could provide Hurley and Dong with an alternative transplant model. Shumway suggested that the runt of the pair, known as the freemartin, should receive the heart of its stronger sibling.

An intriguing idea that, Dong complained later, had been born in hell. Dong and Ray Stofer, their resourceful vet and perfusionist, were charged with finding enough bovine blood to prime the heart-lung machine before Hurley started the actual calf transplants. At first they sat back and grinned when the manager of a San Jose slaughterhouse cheerfully confirmed that they could take as much blood as they needed. It was then, however, that the simplicity of their brief ended.

Stofer and Dong, supported by a few lab technicians, drove up to San Jose whenever Hurley was due to begin another transplant. They would march into the bloody yard with large-bore tubes and bottles clinking in their hands. Pulling on rubber boots and plastic aprons, they looked like a group of scholarly butchers as they headed toward the line of freshly culled animals. The sounds and smells of the slaughterhouse reminded them of the severity of their work.

An even more disturbing sight twirled above their heads. Most of the cattle corpses towering over them weighed in excess of 2,000 pounds. Their hind legs were trussed and connected to a dangling hook. Stofer and Dong would climb small ladders to get up to eye level with a bulging jugular vein. They would make an incision and then tape the tubes to the side of the animal's huge neck to direct the blood down into the waiting bottles. Sometimes, if they had not been sufficiently careful, the tubes would slip free and Dong and Stofer would be drenched in blood spraying from the spinning corpse.

The grisly work was not confined to the slaughterhouse. Inside the laboratory Hurley had to keep his calves upright, in harnesses, to control the release of gas formations in their stomachs. A neck brace also lifted their heads and helped them breathe naturally. There was still too much blood and death, and ultimately the freemartin experiments were abandoned because the weaker twin could rarely withstand perfusion. Dong and Stofer, however, remained chained to the slaughterhouse, for it was decided that Hurley should explore autotransplants in calves.

Working with stronger and more pliable aortic tissue, Hurley seemed to be closing in on his first survivors. He had just taken one calf off the aortic cross-clamp when Shumway's head popped around the door. "Hey, Ed," Shumway said amiably, "how's it going?"

Before Hurley could provide an upbeat answer he was mortified to see that he had stitched the pulmonary artery to the distal aorta. It was a common mistake because, unlike in human and canine hearts, the vessel walls in calves are of similar thickness. Shumway skimmed over the error, but Hurley was devastated to lose another calf.

He persevered and soon had his first forty-eight-hour survivor. It helped that he had stayed awake for most of the previous two nights to nurse the calf through some rough patches. When the animal looked comfortable, Hurley went down to the cafeteria for breakfast and reflected wearily on his triumph. Half an hour later, on his return to the lab, Shumway was waiting for him.

"You'd better go see your calf," Shumway said softly. "It's dead."

Hurley's calf was utterly still. Alone in the lab, and apparently in panic, it had strangled itself in the harness.

There were no further trips to the San Jose slaughterhouse for, after Shumway stepped in, the calf transplants were discarded. With Shumway's greater experience and surgical precision backing him up, Hurley soon conquered the autotransplant in the notoriously difficult canine model. Most dogs survived the procedure and returned to complete health, enabling Hurley, Dong, Stofer, and Shumway to write another seminal Stanford paper—"Isotopic Replacement of the Totally Excised Canine Heart." It seemed as if they could do anything if they just tried long and hard enough.

In the adjoining room, Lower worked mostly with Ed Stinson, who had joined the lab as a second-year medical student in 1961. In between his lectures and exams, Stinson exhibited a capacity for research and an intellectual curiosity that convinced Shumway that he had found the man who would eventually lead the Stanford cardiac program in the future human transplant era. They had met after one of Shumway's rare lectures to a small group of students. Stinson was different from everyone else. He was immediately captivated by transplantation and sought out Shumway to inquire about a part-time lab job. Beneath the layers of shyness and seriousness, Shumway sensed something exceptional in Stinson and set him to work alongside the man he already knew to be the world's finest experimental surgeon.

Lower taught Stinson calmly and methodically—so much so that the serene atmosphere entranced most surgeons who visited Stanford in the hope of learning more about their unique transplant program. Watts Webb, who had already tried heart-lung transplants in dogs, worked with James Hardy, the acclaimed Mississippi surgeon. Webb was stunned to see Lower and Stinson sewing and stitching with such ease in a tranquil lab. Things were different in Mississippi. Hardy, one of Shumway's rivals in the race to a human transplant, was habitually surrounded by a horde of twenty surgeons and technicians in a jostling and frenetic atmosphere.

"I can't believe it," Webb said after he had watched Lower and Stinson talking quietly as they transplanted another heart. "But this is much better."

"Sure," Lower said. "It's the way we like it around here."

Kantrowitz was on fire. He was ablaze with ideas and theories, and at last he had the money to explore them. Throughout the late 1950s and early sixties, Kantrowitz had produced innovative work that was rewarded with regular grants for small projects from the National Institutes of Health. Robert Ringler, deputy director of the National Heart and Lung Institute, had long admired the originality of his thought. When he heard that the fiscal year-end was approaching, with millions of dollars still available for medical grants from Washington, Ringler had made a discreet call to Maimonides. Kantrowitz was advised that if he were to submit a competent proposal, his surgical unit would be one of the fortunate few to land substantial NIH backing for the next five years. It would allow him to follow his imagination, unfettered by financial constraints. His wife, Jeannie, stayed up night and day and, working in conjunction with a grant expert she had hired, produced a document deemed worthy of a few of the millions the NIH had earmarked for surgical research.

The money was poured straight into Maimonides' financial trust, which meant that Kantrowitz could appoint skilled surgical research assistants to help him in his quest. And they came from around the world—from Japan and Norway, Switzerland and Haiti, Cuba and South Africa. Chris Barnard, in this way, would lose one of his best assistants to Kantrowitz.

Raoul de Villiers, who had worked for years alongside Barnard in the research lab, had resisted his invitation to set up a private practice together in Cape Town. De Villiers knew Barnard's background better than most, for he, too, came from a poor Afrikaans family. His father, just like Adam Barnard, had had only a meager education and also endorsed the Calvinist doctrine of hard work and abstinence. Barnard and de Villiers had little else in common; they did share a similar taste in beautiful young women. This caused trouble between the two Afrikaners when the young woman in question, Suegnet, was already engaged to de Villiers. Barnard persisted in pursuing her, conceding defeat only after Suegnet repeatedly rebuffed him. She and Raoul pitied Louwtjie Barnard when her husband resorted to chasing a more amenable nurse. Barnard seemed addicted to risk.

Raoul and Suegnet soon married, and he was desperate for a change. He had been made two overseas offers. The first came from Oxford; the second was from a doctor in New York. He might not have heard of the American, or his small hospital, but an extraordinary vitality filled the letters he received from the Maimonides Hospital in Brooklyn. He stared down at the name scrawled at the end of each letter and wondered what kind of man he might find when he finally met Adrian Kantrowitz.

The de Villiers family arrived in New York on a broiling summer night, their ship docking just as darkness spread across the city. Several doctors from Kantrowitz's lab were waiting for them as they disembarked. The overwhelmed Afrikaners were swept through the humid and crowded streets, noise and color engulfing them as the car inched toward their hotel in Brooklyn. It was hard to take in the fast words of welcome, and the promise that Adrian and Jean Kantrowitz would treat them like family alongside all the other international researchers who had joined them. The big man, they were promised, would be unlike anyone they had ever met before.

When they met, de Villiers was struck most by the size of Kantrowitz—and how different he was from Barnard. The New Yorker resembled the surrounding city. Kantrowitz was big and brash and constantly on the move.

De Villiers loved the way he would bellow, *"C'mon, let's go!"* as if they were a crack army unit about to storm enemy-held territory.

Kantrowitz was as inquisitive as he was irrepressible. De Villiers was staggered by the ceaseless invention and unbreakable will driving each experiment. Regarding Kantrowitz as a perpetual investigator and a constant optimist, de Villiers slipped smoothly into the Brooklyn rhythm. It helped that his and Suegnet's apartment building, just around the corner from the Kantrowitz home in Flatbush, housed a talented pair of Japanese doctors.

Yoshio Kondo and his wife had also found the transition from Tokyo to be comparatively easy; yet their countryman, Yuki Nosé, young and single, felt overwhelmed. Arriving with only a smattering of English, he had expected that he would rapidly pick up the language while devouring fat American steaks and driving around in a fast car. Yuki was stunned. His arrival coincided with Yom Kippur, the Jewish day of abstinence. He was even more bewildered by the mass of black and bearded Hasidic Jews surrounding Maimonides. At least the sound of Yiddish seemed closer to Japanese than did the indecipherable English of other Brooklyn locals.

Distraught after two days in America, he went to see Jean Kantrowitz. In barely comprehensible English, interspersed with a couple of newly acquired Yiddish words, Yuki managed to suggest that his accommodation violated his contract. He announced that he would take the next flight back to Japan.

"Yuki," said Jean, who had welcomed him to Brooklyn with a bottle of scotch, "calm down."

Yuki Nosé did as he was instructed. He got hopelessly drunk and discovered that his Yiddish actually improved with every enlightening glass of Teacher's.

He eventually took great delight in telling de Villiers how he managed to cope without sex. When he got "hot," Yuki said, he took the subway down to Coney Island and ran straight into the cold water. It kept him under control. He was also helped by the fact that his research in the Maimonides lab, working with Kantrowitz on some of the world's earliest ventricular-assist devices, was fascinating enough to take his mind off sex much of the time.

If he was drawn instinctively to the mechanical pump as a way of saving the most hearts, Kantrowitz's immersion in transplantation was swift and persuasive. He identified his rivals as David Blumenstock's team in Coopers-town, Jim Hardy's unit in Mississippi, the Hanlon and Willman partnership in St. Louis, and, out in front of everyone, Shumway and Lower. Kantrowitz was convinced that his team alone could catch the Stanford program. Shumway and Lower were technically ready to proceed with the first human case—and yet they were held back by a variety of concerns, ranging from the definition of death in the donor patient to unresolved immunological problems in the recipient.

Kondo and Kantrowitz, meanwhile, proceeded with the transplantation of puppy hearts. Without any immunosuppression treatment, their two longest survivors were still alive and healthy after 57 and 112 days. That second puppy, a German shepherd that received the heart of a female terrier, would eventually live for over 200 days.

They met at seven each morning, when Kantrowitz, Kondo, Nosé, de Villiers, and the others began their working breakfast, and slogged straight through until six every evening. Kantrowitz would grind on while the others returned to Flatbush. And once a week, late on a Friday afternoon, in what Adrian and Jean called their "Carbohydrate Rounds," they would all party together and drink and talk and joke, in a variety of accents and languages, about their work—and Yuki Nosé's continued attempts to master Yiddish and find himself a girl.

The parties often spilled over into the night and they would end up at the Kantrowitz house, where towering ambitions and declarations of resolve raged. Kantrowitz's posse shared the same grand ambitions as the youthful Kennedy administration. Expressing his certainty that he would transplant a human heart, and his hope to be the first to do so, Kantrowitz echoed JFK's resolve to put an American on the moon in the next decade.

Only once did a shadow fall over the team—for thirteen days in October 1962, when the Cuban Missile Crisis threatened nuclear confrontation between America and the Soviet Union. Even Kantrowitz fell ominously quiet as he watched Kennedy on television. The young doctors from across the world sat silently around him, scanning his face for some sign that the threat would soon pass. And when it did, with the whiskey flowing and their voices rising in excitement, it felt as if nothing would stop them.

And all the while, alongside Adrian, the dominant presence at the center of each party, Jean held everything together. Suegnet de Villiers, watching Jean closely, could not stem her admiration. Whether she was driving across New York every afternoon picking up her kids from swimming or the library, or trying to teach Yuki to roll his *rs* and say "Raoul" rather than "Laoul," or "intravenously" rather than "intlepenisly," Jean brought order to the Kantrowitz camp.

Adrian had the vast and soaring mind, but Jean supported him. They seemed extraordinary together, and sometimes thinking of Cape Town and home, Suegnet could not help comparing all they had with the broken relationship of another heart surgeon and his wife. Chris Barnard, whether he was chasing a nurse or Suegnet herself, appeared ferociously needy. Kantrowitz, in contrast, seemed destined for greatness. Even wearing one of his most colorful Caribbean beach shirts at home in Brooklyn, Kantrowitz exuded an indestructible ambition. As his team gathered around him he would fill everyone's glass and say quietly: "*C'mon, let's go!*"

Chris Barnard struggled to control an occasional shake in his hands during surgery. The nervous tremor eased whenever, through sheer force of will, Barnard calmed himself sufficiently to make another competent suture. Canny enough to realize that his first assistant, Rodney Hewitson, was a far superior technician, Barnard refrained from venting the darkest of his moods on the two men closest, and most important, to him at the operating table— the unflappable Hewitson and his equally composed anesthetist, "Ozzie" Ozinsky. The rest of his team was not so fortunate. Barnard raged at the merest hesitation or the slightest error.

He could not stop his hands from shaking even more helplessly after the emergence of the surgeon as superstar was confirmed on May 3, 1963. In his Cape Town office six weeks later, Barnard held an imported copy of the specific issue of *Time* magazine that featured a glamorously intense cover portrait of a man in a surgical cap and gown, his mask hanging loosely around his neck. The image was accompanied by a stark inscription: *Surgeon Francis D. Moore.*

Barnard knew that, as the chief surgeon at Boston's Peter Bent Brigham Hospital, the site of so many breakthroughs in kidney grafting, Moore certainly belonged in the American medical pantheon. He was also engaged in experimental liver transplants between dogs that led *Time* to trace a legacy of surgical pioneers stretching from Harvey Cushing and Robert E. Gross to Dwight Harken and John Gibbon; and from Walt Lillehei and Joseph Murray to Francis Moore and Norman Shumway.

In Cape Town, so distant from Boston and Stanford, Barnard felt his throat constrict at the mention of so many surgeons with whom he was acquainted. He could obviously accept Lillehei's position among the elect, but the appearance of Shumway in that exalted list ate into him. Shumway was a fine surgeon, but he was the same age as Barnard. They had both been Lillehei's senior resident. And so it seemed acutely painful that Shumway should be celebrated in *Time* while Barnard's own name remained unrecognized outside cardiac circles.

In a thirteen-page celebration *Time* suggested gushingly that "under the bright lights that illuminate the surgical incision with brutal clarity, the achievement of the surgeon and his assistants becomes one of the greater glories of science. Man may strain ever further into space, ever deeper into the heart of the atom, but there in the operating room all the results of the most improbable reaches of research, all the immense accumulation of medical knowledge are drawn upon in a determined drive toward the most awesome goal of all: the preservation of one human life. In hospitals all over the U.S. surgeons now make a routine performance of lifesaving procedures so radical that they were almost unimaginable a few years ago. There is hardly a place in the human body that surgeons have not been, hardly an operation too daring for them to perform."

It was as if death no longer stalked the OR. According to *Time* the modern iconic surgeon appeared almost invulnerable. His only flaw was an understandable arrogance. "The great surgeons's egoism is reflected in a selective amnesia. Practically any one of them, asked to name the three greatest living surgeons, has difficulty in thinking of two others. Individualists down to their physical characteristics, great surgeons show that even their skilled hands need be of no particular design. Like a pianist's they may be long and slender or broad and powerful."

It was transplantation, however, that inspired a national weekly news-magazine to wax poetically over surgery and its practitioners. While stating wrongly that a heart was technically more difficult to transplant than a liver, *Time* hailed the cardiac breakthrough of Shumway. "But would anybody in his right mind dream of cutting out a human heart? Yes, say the Stanford en-thusiasts. In certain cases it may be the best way to give some newborn chil-dren a chance of a normal life."

The Mayo Clinic's John Kirklin, who had always played the role of the cautious moderator to Lillehei's exuberant hustler, tried to temper the adula-tion. "Surgery is always second best," he cautioned. "If you can do something else, it's better. Surgery is limited. It's operating on someone who has no place else to go."

Kirklin was another surgeon Barnard knew well. For a couple of years in the mid-1950s there were only two medical centers in the world where open-heart surgery was practiced, and both were in Minnesota. And so it was one of medicine's curiosities that its most radical branch of surgery should have emerged in the parochial Midwest, for a mere sixty miles separated the Mayo Clinic in Rochester from the University of Minnesota hospital in Minneapo-lis. "It must be due to the severe climate of Minnesota," Shumway had joked in his best meteorologist's voice, annoying Barnard in the process.

In 1962, on another visit to Minnesota, Barnard had spent far more time in Rochester than Minneapolis. He had been dazzled by the pyrotechnics of Lillehei's mind, but he needed to grasp Kirklin's patient efficiency. Barnard, once more, borrowed judiciously from an older American doctor and hitched what he found to his own distinct character.

Time, however, would not be undercut by Kirklin's sober analysis. "Today, patients who have no place else to go are vastly more fortunate than their predecessors. To virtually all of them, surgery offers more hope than it ever did before. And to many of them with heart defects or in need of transplants—those for whom there never was any place else to go—surgery now offers the first and the best hope of all."

The greatest surgeons in America were already racing toward the fluttering white tape of victory. Fame and glory awaited them. Barnard faced only obscurity and disappointment at the bottom of the world. It could have been different. Prompted by Lillehei, the Albert Einstein College of Medicine in New York had approached Barnard in 1962 with a comparatively lucrative contract to join their cardiac division. Torn between his desire to gain a foothold in American surgery and his more emotional desire to remain in South Africa, Barnard would ultimately reject their offer in February 1963. Three months later, as *Time* slid from his fingers to the floor, he wondered if he had not made the most terrible mistake of his life.

Adrian Kantrowitz drove a small segment of the surgeon's popular image as a heroic and gunslinging pioneer by establishing Maimonides Hospital as the second most prolific cardiac transplant unit in the United States. He was even more interested in his own new inventions, such as the U-shaped assist device and the intra-aortic balloon pump, which he devised to save patients suffering from acute heart failure. Maimonides' cardiac campaign actually contained three tiers: mechanical assist devices, transplantation, and artificial heart research, which Kantrowitz left to another academic Japanese surgeon, Tetsuzo Akutsu.

Raoul and Suegnet de Villiers, who returned to Cape Town after their yearlong contract with Kantrowitz, marveled at the scape of his ambition. Thanking them for all they had brought to his team, Kantrowitz reminded them, with a wink and a laugh, to keep an eye on his future progress. "Next time you see me," he said in a parting as serious as it was playful, "you might just be looking at the cover of *Time* magazine."

When he got home, it seemed to de Villiers as if nothing had changed in Cape Town. Barnard still stalked the labs and corridors of Groote Schuur, ranting at his technicians and charming those nurses who remained outside his furious orbit. De Villiers slid back into the old routine, switching between the Animal House and the operating theater, avoiding Barnard as well as he could. He did not reveal the breadth of experimentation being undertaken at Maimonides—for he knew how adept Barnard was at pilfering ideas.

Kantrowitz's theoretical knowledge, and the sheer expanse of his surgical imagination, were unmatched in South Africa. Even Barnard would have been startled by the diversity of research at Maimonides. And yet it was not totally dispiriting to be back in a South African hospital. Having seen Kantrowitz and his team in the OR, de Villiers was convinced that Groote Schuur offered greater clinical proficiency. Kantrowitz would always be more of an intellectual innovator than a surgical stylist. As much as he would refuse to admit the truth to Barnard, if de Villiers's own heart had to be opened, he would prefer his fellow Afrikaner, rather than the exuberant American, to wield the knife.

After a while it became obvious to de Villiers that more significant shifts were unfolding at home—inside the country, in the hospital, and in Barnard himself. Nelson Mandela sat in a Pretoria jail, awaiting another trial the Nationalist government promised could end only in him being hanged or imprisoned for life on Robben Island. A similar fate awaited his fellow ANC activists—Walter Sisulu, Govan Mbeki, Ahmed Kathrada, and Dennis Goldberg—who had been captured in the Johannesburg suburb of Rivonia in July 1963. The arrests had been made as a direct result of the notorious Ninety-Day Law, which enabled the security police to detain anyone without trial for at least three months. Their interrogation and torture had shattered the ANC's secret network so completely that all its leaders were either jailed or exiled. South Africa was in the unremitting grip of apartheid.

They tried to resist the absolute color bar at Groote Schuur. Cardiologists and heart surgeons insisted on treating white, black, colored, and Indian patients, sometimes allowing different racial groups to share the same ward. Marius Barnard, who had just returned from three years as a GP in Rhodesia, was more liberal than his brother, and he was relieved to learn that Chris had not bowed to government pressure to make open-heart surgery an exclusively white privilege. Having decided to become a surgeon himself, Marius was offered an opening in the cardiac department by Chris—the fraternal bond for once overcoming their chronically strained relationship.

Chris Barnard was not quite in the midst of a midlife crisis, but de Villiers could see that surgery no longer consumed him. Even women could no longer compete with his latest passion, which was to cajole and drive his teenage daughter to sporting greatness.

There were times, as she skied over the silvery water, when it seemed as if Deirdre Barnard was a beautiful stone skipping flat and hard across the mirrored surface of the lake. Her father would count the number of leaps and tricks as she bounced across the water in one loop after another. The difference was that he did not watch her from the shore, whooping in amazement at his own throw, but from over his shoulder as he drove the boat that pulled her across the lake on her water skis.

Deirdre turned thirteen in 1963. She had grown taller, stronger, and more confident than the "little *pik* of a thing, a river reed with a blonde tassel on top" he had first watched ski on a family holiday in Knysna, three years earlier. He knew nothing about waterskiing then, but, as he wrote later, "it did seem beautiful. A curious sort of wild freedom was obtained, within a very tight frame. Bounded by the laws of nature and the power of a machine, it existed on top of water, at the end of a tow line."

Barnard and his friend Hentie van Rooyen had built a small speedboat, named *Louwtjie.* He also studied the rules of the sport and taught Deirdre how to perform the three events that made up competitive waterskiing: tricks, slalom, and the jump. Their initial progress was slow because the surgeon was just as much a novice as the schoolgirl. Then Deirdre cut her knee open and her father had to stitch the wound shut—his hands shaking again, this time like an intern's, as he tried not to hurt her. Her eyes filled with tears, but, blinking hard, she did not allow them to fall.

He bought her expensive skis and, because she was so vulnerable, made her wear a crash helmet and a life jacket, as if it could protect her from further harm. She improved dramatically. Deirdre was so thrilled to be spending so much time with her dad that she would have done almost anything to please him. She had never before seen him so interested in her. As she dazzled and he studied, Barnard became increasingly obsessed with the idea that he could turn his daughter into a star.

It was a curious fixation and revealed the looming doubt within Barnard himself. The possibility that he would become a world leader in cardiac surgery seemed remote on those days when he felt adrift in a politically reviled, if obscure, country. He poured his frustrated aspirations into Deirdre.

"I spent every minute away from the hospital [with her]," he remembered. "Sometimes my arthritis pained so much I could barely lift the sandbags needed to set the boat deeper and so create a larger wave for a trick. Deirdre was always willing, always laughing—and always a delight. By this time I was wholly water-borne. When she flew across the water I was with her."

Barnard entered her in the 1963 South African Championships and she easily won the senior title. No one could believe it. Deirdre had trounced experienced skiers twice her age. She became the youngest female in the country's history to receive the mystical green-and-gold Springbok blazer given to those white South Africans chosen to compete in international sports.

He asked for extended leave from Groote Schuur in order to manage South Africa's junior waterski team at the European Championships in Spain. Deirdre was the ace in that squad. If the sports boycott against South Africa had yet to bite, the outside world's disdain for apartheid was such that Deirdre often described herself as an Australian when her accent prompted questions in Europe about her nationality. The shame of apartheid ran deep in a compassionate and intelligent girl.

Deirdre finished second in the European juniors and then agreed to compete for the senior title in France. She came seventh in the slalom and ramp events, and tenth in the tricks competition. Even her father was satisfied with her first senior international appearance. "She was obviously a coming champion," he wrote. "It now seemed only a matter of time before she made it. I told myself that we were all born with a certain amount of ability, and a champion not only had an extra amount, but also stopped at nothing in the drive to become first. If Deirdre lacked anything I was prepared to give it to her. I had enough, I thought, for both of us—with some to spare."

Barnard would wake Deirdre before dawn every morning so that they could be on the lake by six; and he then returned home early from his surgical duties so that he could drag her across the water for at least three hours in the late afternoon. Barnard had stopped writing to Lillehei. He dreamed less of becoming the Demikhov of Africa. He no longer worried about keeping up with his former colleagues from Minnesota. Waterskiing, rather than cardiac surgery, now defined his world.

He was convinced Deirdre "had the making of a world champion. At that point I was hooked onto her career. I did not know how far I would eventually go in heart surgery. We were constantly at work, experimenting with valves and new techniques, but so were many other teams in hospitals around the world. Maybe we would make it, maybe not. There was no doubt, however, about this little girl. She was something incredible. Feeling this way, I bought her a skin-tight white suit, and on the water she looked like a nymph moved by invisible winds."

Deirdre had become a certified aqua-star, the finest waterskier in South Africa, who was on her way to becoming one of the best in the world. Barnard's new ambition meant that Louwtjie saw him more often than she had in previous years. He might have been a speck on the water, but at least she knew that he was with Deirdre rather than hunting down another woman. Louwtjie considered those years at Zeekoevlei as amongst the happiest her family had known. Only the isolation and turmoil of their younger son, Andre, ate into her contentment. Chris was so consumed by Deirdre's waterskiing that he had no time left for Andre. While he showed no jealousy toward his sister, the acutely sensitive Andre yearned for his father's attention. The scars were hidden but, inside Andre, they were growing.

There was also something disturbing about the intensity Barnard showed toward his daughter. He was forty-one and she was fourteen, and even if he had never read *Lolita*, he wrote of her with a certain Nabokovian obsessiveness. "Every day I would leave the hospital to pick her up at school. It was Rustenburg Girls High at Rondebosch, and I waited at the corner in the car with the boat on its trailer. She would come out, wearing her school uniform—black skirt, two inches below the knee, black stockings, and lace-up shoes, dark blue shirt with blue blazer, and a derby hat. Her blonde hair was carefully pinned up so as not to touch the collar. If it did you were fined two pennies. Half-an-hour later the same little girl was in a next-to-nothing swim-suit, her hair tumbling down to her shoulders, racing across the water at 30 m.p.h. and laughing as she always did when we played together—at least in this first period."

His desire for international success allowed him, in a monumental adjustment for a man of his ego, to concede that "people began to speak of me as Deirdre Barnard's father. Somebody in the family, at least, was going to make it."

Deirdre was increasingly overwhelmed by her father's craving in their early-morning training sessions. "You've heard about 'crying buckets,'" she wrote many years later, "but have you ever heard of a lake made up entirely of tears? There were plenty of mornings when I believed what my mother said—that Zeekoevlei was made up completely of tears and all of them had been shed by me."

Seven

MISSISSIPPI GAMBLING

University of Mississippi Medical Center, Jackson, Mississippi, January 23, 1964

 James Hardy, a big man with an even bigger name in surgery, was hooked. He wanted to be the first. He had been the first man to carry out open-heart surgery in Mississippi. He had also been the first surgeon in medical history to transplant a human lung. Hardy now longed to be the first to give a human being a new heart. He loved the way the words ran together on the page, or simply rolled out of his mouth in the slow drawl of his southern accent.

"The world's first lung transplant . . . the world's first heart transplant . . ."

Hardy worked most days to an absurdly detailed schedule of tasks, which he listed in his spidery handwriting:

5:00—Arise, plug in coffee
5:15—Correct children's spelling
5:30—Mentally review a.m. operations
6:00—Awaken children/quick breakfast
6:15—Leave for hospital

6:30—See sickest patients
6:45—Speak to op. patients and relatives
6:50—Begin 10 minute surgical scrub
7:05—Begin first operation (My hair is gray)
11:00—Rounds
12:00—Mortality & Morbidity conference
1:00—Class with students
2:00—See patients in clinic
4:00—Review laboratory data
5:00—Check sickest patients
6:00—Home for supper
7:00—Hospital. Write? Read?
9:00—Evening resident call
10:00—Bed (May have to get up)

Hardy was forty-five, the same age as Kantrowitz, four years older than Shumway and Barnard. His most significant surgical contribution had occurred seven and a half months earlier when, assisted by Watts Webb, he had transplanted the left lung of a patient, who had suffered a massive myocardial infarction, into a fifty-eight-year-old man, John Russell, whose left main bronchus was riddled with cancer.

Russell was on death row, having been found guilty of murder by a Mississippi jury. At the rate the disease was spreading, cancer would get him before the chair. Russell had been offered the option of a lung transplant, and when he accepted, his death sentence was commuted by the governor for his "contribution to the cause of humanity."

On June 11, 1963, Hardy and Webb transplanted the lung. It expanded and worked effectively as a respiratory organ for eighteen days. Yet Russell died on the last day of June from renal failure. Hardy's histological study revealed only minimal evidence of rejection. Their success had been limited, but Hardy could claim his first. He hoped the heart would be next.

Hardy knew it would cause them trouble—especially in the South, which was dominated by religious conservatives. A transplanted heart would uncork all the old suspicions and vehement accusations of doctors who "dared to play God." Mississippi, he noted wryly, was renowned more for its muddy river rather than its open-minded attitudes. It reveled in its own form of apartheid.

"Almost every village and town developed its White Citizens Council," Hardy wrote, "the purpose of which was to maintain segregation, ostensibly under law. Nonetheless, economic boycott and social ostracism were commonly the lot of those who exhibited even the slightest evidence of moderation in racial relations. . . . If the offense was considered extreme, the Ku Klux Klan might surface for more definitive persuasion of the recalcitrant citizen."

Hardy admitted to growing concern as most state newspapers and both local television stations "maintained the same defiance of the federal government and rang with the slogan *Segregation Forever*. Governor George Wallace was doing the same thing over in Alabama. The negative effects of this policy were pervasive in numerous directions. For instance, when the most militant forces tried to close the public schools to prevent integration, many women banded together quietly and sought to prevent this disaster. My wife was among them and I was frankly uneasy about our safety."

Hardy felt the stigma of Mississippi keenly. He had not received one out-of-state application for a surgical residency in years. The Society of University Surgeons also withdrew its plan for a southern rendezvous and explained to Hardy that two of its members were black and would "naturally feel uncomfortable" in Jackson. Hardy was advised by state troopers to hide his Mississippi registration plates whenever he drove north to medical conferences in cities like Chicago and Detroit. In Washington, D.C., he had understood the sentiment when black bellhops had refused to carry his bags up to his hotel room. Like Chris Barnard, at the bottom of Africa, Jim Hardy was defined and often judged by the racial policies of the place he called home.

In 1961, he had found more reason for hope when Robert Marston became the dean of the Medical Center. "One night," Hardy reported, "Dr. Marston brought in a crew and tore down the wall that had separated the white and colored sections of the hospital cafeteria. All the drinking fountains in the building were stripped of the 'white' and 'colored' signs."

Hardy turned to Marston when he needed permission to transplant a heart into a human at the start of 1964. The dean had supported Hardy and

Webb's landmark lung operation and quickly gave his backing to the new aim, on the condition that stringent criteria should be followed. Marston insisted that, as cardiac transplantation was still so experimental, Hardy could only consider a patient who was already close to death and had no other hope of survival. He would also have to refrain from removing the beating heart of a brain-dead patient. As Hardy assumed that too much damage would be done to any heart harvested more than a few minutes after it stopped beating, he agreed that any possible transplant would have to wait until a suitable donor and recipient patient were both close to the point of death. Only then, with family permission, could he proceed with the transplant at the exact moment the donor's heart lost its pulse.

The chances of such a coincidence occurring in a small hospital in Jackson were remote. And so, realizing how far he trailed Lower and Shumway, Hardy resorted to more extreme measures. He had been encouraged by the progress made by Keith Reemtsma, a surgeon at Tulane University School of Medicine, who'd grafted a chimpanzee's kidneys into a forty-three-year-old dock worker in November 1963. And so, determined to be first to the heart, Hardy ordered the purchase of four chimpanzees. If their kidneys could be transplanted into a man, who survived for nine weeks, Hardy saw no logical reason why a chimp heart should not be used in the same way. He pointed out to some of his more dubious staff that chimpanzees and humans share approximately 98 percent of the same chromosomes.

The chimps were kept in the basement of the university lab, where they were fed well and exercised regularly in the hope that they might one day save a human life and help Jim Hardy make a little more history. The day soon came.

On January 21, 1964, a sixty-eight-year-old white man was referred to Hardy by a community hospital. His lower left leg was black with gangrene, his face mottled with blood clots. Both conditions had been caused by his heart's inability to pump enough blood around his system. He had been found two nights earlier in his home at Laurel Trailer Park on the outskirts of Jackson. Neighbors confirmed that his name was Boyd Rush. They described him as a retired upholsterer and "a deaf mute." Rush was in a comatose state with only a faint pulse. Having suffered from hypertensive cardiovascular disease for years, he had been stricken by a heart attack in his trailer. Hardy was the only man in Mississippi who thought he might save Boyd Rush.

On January 22, Hardy amputated the gangrenous portion of Rush's leg and prepared for transplantation. The following afternoon his chief cardiologist concluded that "life expectancy can be measured in this case by hours only." If they could keep him alive with a new heart for days, weeks, or even months, Hardy would be able to claim that his experiment had extended a life. Rush's sister, Mrs. J. H. Thompson, agreed to sign the consent form, which confirmed that: "I agree to the insertion of a suitable heart transplant if such should be available at the time. I further understand that hundreds of heart transplants have been performed in laboratories throughout the world but that any heart transplant would represent the initial transplant in man."

Destiny seemed ready to play its part. A brain-dead trauma victim lingered in the ICU, the shell of his body functioning through the aid of a ventilator. His family gave their permission for his heart to be used in a transplant. With no brain, they reasoned, some other poor soul might as well benefit from his heart. That Thursday afternoon, January 23, his physical state worsened and for an hour Hardy wondered if he had found his transplant match. He still instructed his team to prepare the largest chimp just in case their luck ran out.

Time seemed to accelerate. Just after eleven that evening, Rush went into shock and Hardy swept him into the OR. Rush's blood pressure had plummeted to sixty. After establishing that the heartbeat of the prospective human donor was unlikely to subside for another few hours, Hardy instructed a surgical team in an adjoining room to anesthetize the chimp. Moving quickly, he opened Rush's chest. The heart stopped just before they began the cardiopulmonary bypass. The machine took over and Hardy knew that there was no turning back. Only a transplant could save Rush from death on the table.

Hardy faced the four surgeons assisting him. He looked into the eyes of each man as he spoke of the scorn they would face for transplanting a "monkey heart" into the chest of a Mississippi retiree. Hardy also reminded them that if they aborted the transplant they were literally sealing the death of their patient. Hardy said he would ask each of them to vote in an informal poll. The majority would hold sway.

He asked the question quietly and solemnly: *"Are you prepared to proceed?"*
The surgeon next to him nodded. He had voted with Hardy. The third
doctor wished to abstain. He would not oppose the operation but neither
could he voice his support for inserting a chimp's heart into a man. Two more
votes needed to be cast. If they both said "no" then they would be deadlocked.
There was a slight hesitation before the two nods came. Yes. And yes again.

In the room next door they cut open the chimp and harvested the heart.
Hardy excised most of the human heart, using the Lower-Shumway technique,
and then stepped back to stare for a moment. "It was an awesome sight," he
wrote later, "to contemplate the empty space that the patient's greatly enlarged heart had occupied."

The chimpanzee heart looked still and small in the cold saline of a metal
container. Hardy began the suturing. The minutes passed and one of the surgeons spoke later of the sound of a trolley leaving the adjoining OR. At least
they did not have to see the terrible sight of the chimp, its chest raw and
empty beneath a bloodied white sheet, as it headed toward the hospital in-
cinerator. They turned back to the man they were trying to save.

After three-quarters of an hour, Hardy had completed his stitching. He
looked up at the clock. It was just after two a.m.—the dead of night in Mississippi. He gave the signal. They waited, the seconds feeling long and heavy,
until the animal's heart began to twitch inside the man's chest. The quivering
did not settle into a steady beat, and so Hardy, the sweat rolling down him,
used a defibrillator to shock the chimpanzee heart. It immediately worked
and, in Hardy's words, "a forceful beat was restored and supported a blood
pressure of 90 to 100 mmHg."

They stood around and watched, unsure whether or not they were witnessing a miracle or an aberration. "At least we're in business," Hardy said.

They did not remain in the transplant business too much longer. After
an hour the heart, which was far too small for the man it was meant to support, simply stopped. It had faltered during the previous half-hour and only
spluttered back into life when attached to a pacemaker. Even that was not
enough. Hardy used his hands to try and massage the transplanted organ
back to life. But the heart died, and with it so did Boyd Rush. The transplant

was over. Hardy had a first, of a kind, involving a chimpanzee, but he had still failed.

Two weeks later, on February 8, 1964, Hardy arrived at the Sixth International Transplantation Conference in the plush surrounds of New York City's Waldorf-Astoria Hotel. He could feel the icy disdain. Publicity surrounding his disastrous attempt had made Hardy's work seem chaotic and even duplicitous. The day after the transplant, on January 24, an Associated Press story had been splashed across the nation's newspapers. Hardy had shuddered to read the opening sentences, which claimed that "Surgeons took the heart from a dead man, revived it and transplanted it into the chest of a man dying of a heart failure today. For an hour it worked—perhaps the first successful human heart transplant in the world."

The error had been lifted straight from an ambiguous statement released by the hospital's director of public information—which neglected to mention that the donor was a chimp rather than a human. Hardy was furious that the truth had been so absurdly twisted. The AP report confirmed that "the dimensions of the only available donor heart at the time of the patient's collapse proved too small for the requirements of the considerably larger recipient. 'This disparity must be minimized in future operations,' a spokesman said. . . . The hospital declined to disclose the names of the surgeons, the names and ages of the donor and recipient, and withheld details of the arrangement and circumstances leading to the transplant."

The next day, January 25, *The New York Times* printed a more accurate headline—"Chimpanzee Heart Used in Transplant to Human"—after the humiliated Mississippi Medical Center was forced to reveal the previously omitted details of the case. Hardy had not won the race, as he had hoped; rather, he had become embroiled in a freak show that focused on the use of a chimp and the deceit of the hospital. "The publicity, the outcry and the criticism were enormous," he remembered years later. "Public media reporters seemed to come out of the woodwork. We hunkered down and waited it out."

Hardy worked hard on his lecture in the hope that he might salvage his own dented credibility. He had his defense ready. "Much knowledge was gained by this first transplant in man," he wrote. "First, the heart could be readily transplanted in man and a forceful beat restored. It was clear that the transplantation of a healthy human donor heart, when transplanted into a human being in reasonably stable metabolic balance, might well provide additional years of life. . . ."

Sitting calmly on the conference stage in New York, he waited to be introduced by Wilhelm Kolff, the venerable creator of the kidney machine. As he reached the end of his preamble, Kolff turned to Hardy and quipped, bizarrely, "In Mississippi they keep the chimpanzees in one cage and the Negroes in another cage, don't they, Dr. Hardy?"

The impact of this remark on an already unsympathetic audience, who knew that Kolff had endured the Nazi occupation of Holland, was profound, and Hardy was stunned. Kolff protested afterward that he had merely been joking, in an effort to lighten the atmosphere, but Hardy took it personally, later reflecting that "For one of the few times in my professional career, I was taken aback and did poorly. The audience was palpably hostile. . . . I gave our experience as it happened but there was not a single hand of applause thereafter. It was a dismal day."

Hardy withdrew from the race. "I had noted," he said, "that when one loses his academic post, for whatever reason, he is not likely to get another one of comparable significance. I decided to wait until Shumway and his group transplanted a heart in man."

Shumway's dominance in the field of cardiac transplantation was underscored in New York. In the wake of the hysteria surrounding the Mississippi fiasco, Shumway presented a conference paper that same day, February 8, that he had written with Lower. Their title, "Special Problems in Transplantation of the Heart," was typically straightforward and downbeat. Shumway made a salutary warning about the fever of "the race" and underlined the need for years of vigilant research.

"The purpose of this report," he said pointedly, "is to identify some problems which require solution before the golden moment in tissue transplantation is upon us." Shumway looked up and paused, as if purposely to slow the headlong tempo of those racing behind him. He knew that Kantrowitz was in the audience, as were Hardy, Blumenstock, Hanlon, and Willman.

Shumway identified four areas of particular difficulty: preservation of the heart; post-transplant circulatory support; early detection of rejection; and case selection. He sounded like a wise general urging caution among his more impulsive captains. "Perhaps the cardiac surgeon should pause," Shumway said finally as he looked out into his hushed audience, "while society becomes accustomed to resurrection of the mythological chimera."

The applause, so conspicuously absent after Hardy's awkward performance, swelled loudly, and even Kantrowitz brought his own hands together. Shumway's cogent assessment had been undeniably impressive—particularly in the way he opened up the definition of death. It was an antiquated piece of legislation which regarded a heartbeat, rather than brain activity, as the one true signifier of human life. Shumway and Kantrowitz both lamented that ludicrous "boy-scout definition of death." Until it was overturned, their chances of successfully transplanting a human heart were limited.

As much as he admired Shumway's lucidity, Kantrowitz could not help but think that such moderation had been cast aside by Dwight Harken, the first surgeon to operate on the heart with consistent success when he removed pieces of shrapnel amid the madness of World War II. And Walt Lillehei had been ready to risk everything when he proceeded with the first cross-circulation experiments. You had to take that sort of gamble, Kantrowitz believed, to make history. He suspected that another two years of work in cardiac transplantation were needed. Yet it sounded as if Shumway would have preferred it if they all agreed to delay the first transplant another two decades. Kantrowitz was not prepared to wait that long.

He imagined that Shumway secretly delighted in his patriarchal role— which contrasted neatly with Kantrowitz's Brooklyn persona. Shumway, Kantrowitz imagined, could already visualize his own place in history but was far too bright to spell it out in public. Kantrowitz, too, was smart. He, too, dabbled in secrets. He understood that, even if the express purpose of these gatherings was to share information, there were some secrets you simply never divulged. And, even if Shumway downplayed the idea of a competition, or a race, Kantrowitz saw it differently. They were rivals. They were racing. Jim Hardy had already pulled up lame. Shumway was far in the lead.

But Kantrowitz was flying. He and Shumway, in the end, were not so different after all. They were both bent on being first.

Just after dawn on the wintry morning of June 12, 1964, Nelson Mandela began his first day of life imprisonment on Robben Island. In between breaking rocks in a lime quarry, day after day, Mandela would write furtively of his certainty that, one day, freedom would come. "In my lifetime," he promised, dreaming of the day he would leave the island, in a moment which would signal liberation for the whole of South Africa, "I shall step out into the sunshine, walk with firm feet." Until then, on that miserable hump of rock and soil in the sea, on an island that had once been home only to lepers and madmen, Mandela faced more than ten thousand days in jail.

Robben Island lay a mere seven and a half miles from Cape Town, where Chris Barnard, at the same time, lost himself on the water. He was in a speedboat, towing his teenage daughter in his wake across the Zeekoevlei. Barnard hardly ever thought of Mandela, or of any of the men on that island. Waterskiing mattered more to him. He was typical of his time, and of his people. Apartheid, and the easy luxuries it brought white South Africans, made it simple to forget—no matter the closeness of any dark and terrible suffering.

Yet at Groote Schuur, Barnard stepped out of the bubble. He saved lives day after day—black lives and colored lives and Indian lives and white lives. How many of those liberal English-speaking South Africans who sneered at Afrikaners like him while claiming to deplore apartheid from the comfort of their suburban homes could say the same? He didn't care what they thought. Barnard always had another grand ambition kicking around in his head.

He had read avidly of Hardy's escapade, feeling a strange empathy with a man he knew from past surgical conferences. Hardy came from Mississippi—America's enduring corollary to South Africa—and yet he had transplanted the first lung. Barnard thought that Hardy's idea of using a chimp heart had been "pretty damn good." He could see himself trying the same thing one day—although he would choose the larger baboon as a more suitable candidate. Hardy, like Demikhov in Moscow, gave him hope. Perhaps you did not have to be in New York or Boston or Palo Alto to take a tilt at history. Barnard had the itch again to get into transplantation. He liked his dream of the first kidney graft in Africa. And then, maybe, he might be ready for the heart.

Barnard and John Terblanche, a research fellow who had assisted him on his infamous two-headed dog transplant, began serious renal experimentation in the Animal House. They mostly swapped dog kidneys, in preparation for Barnard's setting up a transplant unit in 1965. Yet their relationship was strained. While Terblanche considered Barnard easily the most obnoxious man he had ever met, he also thought him brilliant.

Barnard seemed to have a remarkably intuitive gift—especially when it came to the heart. In a constant stream of correct diagnoses, he was able to pinpoint the cause of a patient's decline or improvement through gut-feel rather than an analytical assessment of reams of data. When asked by a cardiologist or fellow surgeon to explain his reasoning, Barnard would just say, "The heart doesn't look right." Pressed for an exact meaning, he rarely offered a more precise explanation.

Bob Frater, a South African surgeon he had enticed from the Mayo Clinic in Minnesota back to Groote Schuur, wrote that "the subsequent behavior of the heart bore him out. He was clearly integrating information on the sizes of the heart chambers, the tenseness of the atria and the great arteries, the contractility of the ventricles and the cardiac rhythm. This tendency to inductive rather than deductive reasoning was carried through to the post-operative period. Although obviously there can never be any reasonable proof of anything more than coincidence in these happenings, it was notable that he would often arrive at a patient's bedside, without being called, at precisely the moment when the patient's condition changed for the worse."

Barnard, for all his waterskiing mania, had not lost his touch. He could feel the old urge to shine as a surgeon rising up in him. It was still hard. While he and Terblanche carried out some tentative cardiac transplants in dogs, Barnard had yet to conquer the technique. He had no survivors among his few attempts. He decided, instead, to focus on the kidney. Terblanche led the laboratory program while studying for his surgical board examination—in which he excelled. An envious Barnard accused him of succeeding in his studies at the expense of their research. The two men parted bitterly. Terblanche was excluded from the lab and sent back out on ward rounds, while Barnard now faced working alone. He also intensified his time on the water.

The world-championship fantasy dictated his life so thoroughly that he and Louwtjie had sold their house in Pinelands and relocated to Zeekoevlei, on the fringes of Cape Town. It did not matter that he now faced a much longer commute to the hospital, or even that Deirdre and Andre would need to take a train and then a bus to get to school each morning. They now lived on the water's edge, with their own mooring berth.

Barnard had been appointed chairman of the national waterski committee and helped organize the South African championships at Zeekoevlei in 1965. He gladly accepted the onerous task of laying down the buoys on the lake—with only a single helper. "There was a howling gale the day this had to be done," Deirdre Barnard recalled years later. "It was the most terrible weather. Rain came pouring down, the wind howled and the water was very choppy. I kept thinking they'd give up, but they didn't. . . . He was oblivious to everything and everyone around him, including me. I could see him, I could have called out to him if I had wanted to. Yet he was removed from me and I was suddenly very conscious of the fact that, although he was my father, we inhabited totally different spaces."

The tension deepened and the cracks widened. Barnard himself was not sure how much more Deirdre could take, because between her crying and the days of silence that passed between them, he sometimes felt as if he were torturing her. And then there would be another kind of day, a wonderful day when they flowed on the water and it seemed as if she suddenly believed in the dream again. Deirdre worked then with such concentration that he could almost see himself in her. He could be persuaded, in those moments, that her longing was as profound as his own.

Barnard had set his sights on Canada in 1967. Deirdre would be seventeen and ready to take a shot at the world championships. He had less than eighteen months to shape her destiny. But that year, 1965, had seen considerable progress amid the strife of his relentless training program. She had just returned from Australia, where, in a world-championship trial, she'd finished second in both the slalom and the jump, and fifth in the tricks competition. Her performance gave her a top-ten world ranking. They were right on target.

And so he had been correct, after all, to insist that she should fly to Australia despite a middle-ear infection. The specialist had argued that the only way he could clear and safeguard her hearing would be to open up both eardrums—which would have prevented her traveling to Australia.

"Hell, man," Barnard remembered saying, "she's going anyway."

"I advise against it," the specialist cautioned, "not with both ears opened."

"We're opening nothing," Barnard glowered as he wheeled his daughter out of the office.

He placed his trust in a gloriously unscientific home remedy Louwtjie's family had used for generations. They boiled the feet and leg joints of a sheep in a giant pot on the top of the stove. It was an evil brew, but Louwtjie carefully skimmed off the oil that had risen to the surface. They let it cool and then poured the oil into Deirdre's infected ears. It was not a treatment Lillehei or Shumway might have prescribed in Minnesota or California, but Barnard was not surprised when, the following morning, the humming in his daughter's ears had stopped. The pain had also gone. Barnard was tempted to phone the quack who had tried to stop them from flying to Australia—just to remind him that they lived in Africa, where, sometimes, ancient cures were more effective than conventional Western medicine.

Deirdre returned to Australia early in 1966. After winning the Victoria State Championship she replicated the feat in the Moomba International, where she jumped 115 feet—thirteen feet beyond the world record. Unfortunately the mark was not ratified, because the Moomba lacked championship credentials. Barnard's ecstasy was tempered by his suffocating determination. "Deirdre's picture was in all the papers," he wrote. "I was wreathed in her glory—and my son, Boetie [Andre], began to suffer from a sense of exclusion. I felt it . . . yet the urgency of Deirdre's training inevitably rode over everything else, demanding she receive most of my time. Everything was geared to one goal: she had to be made a world champion."

They were closing in on his fantasy; and Deirdre began to dread the thought that she might disappoint him. And so she tried harder than ever—

even as she secretly thought more and more of boys and dancing and, especially, of a morning when she would be able to turn over in bed at dawn and go back to sleep for a few more hours in the downy warmth, rather than shivering and yawning as she pulled on her wetsuit at the edge of the lake.

The wealthy and grateful son of one of Barnard's patients, a woman in whom he'd successfully implanted a pacemaker, surprised him with a new eighteen-foot, 225-horsepower speedboat. The surgeon, who had always taken a hospital salary rather than money from his patients, did not need convincing that he should accept the gift. He did not have the spare cash to buy himself a new suit, but he had a boat with the power and the speed to drag Deirdre to the next level. His old boat, the *Louwtjie*, was traded in, as his wife and daughter watched quietly. He settled quickly on a name for his sleek new model: *Pacemaker*.

Deirdre, inevitably, was less besotted than her father. She could not hide her feeling that so much else in life mattered more than waterskiing. "It was about then," Barnard said, "that I began to worry about Deirdre ever reaching the top. She was, I feared, too nice a girl. She did not have the killer instinct needed to become a world champion. She would be beaten and laugh about it. When I am beaten I may laugh—but I also cry inside. But not Deirdre. She would cry if she saw an overloaded donkey, or a Colored child alone in the street. If I shouted at her she would cry, too. But if she lost she would laugh it off. . . .

"Deirdre had the natural ability to become a champion. Besides this, it required drive and discipline, and I had thought I could make up for any she lacked. But it was becoming clear you could not transfer that to someone else. Champions were hungry people. They were made that way, and what they had could not be transferred, especially the hunger. You had it or you did not have it."

Chris Barnard knew he had the hunger. He felt as if the craving was eating him alive. He could no longer rely on his daughter to feed it. As he had done so often before, Barnard looked to the country that had an insatiable appetite like his own. He turned to America and decided to immerse himself in kidney transplantation with the most stellar American leaders in that field. He would call David Hume in Virginia. He would call Tom Starzl in Colorado.

He would even call Norman Shumway in California. Barnard was no longer proud. He was desperate.

D avid Hume had been racing for years. And yet his compulsion was undimmed. He stormed through the Medical College of Virginia, the hospital in Richmond where he was chief of surgery, with ruthless bravado. There were not enough hours in a day to contain either Hume or the breadth of his work. Midnight ward rounds were a typical feature at MCV. The lights in his laboratory also burned endlessly, for Hume seemed determined to fulfill the description of him as a "restless genius"—first made by his mentor, Francis Moore, the surgeon *Time* had decided was famous enough to adorn their front cover in 1963. Hume yearned for that same level of recognition. While his work in kidney and liver transplantation, and in the control of rejection, was renowned in international medical circles, only the heart could deliver the kind of public awe Hume felt any transplant program led by him deserved.

His seminal work in kidney transplantation in the early 1950s, at Harvard, had established his reputation. He had been wounded, however, by the loss of his first eight patients and the fact that even his most memorable early success ended in the death of a young man less than six months after he had received his new kidney. Leaving Boston for Richmond in 1956, Hume was determined to recover and build the world's greatest transplant unit.

Hume and Starzl, his closest equivalent in liver grafting, were charismatic and ferociously bright pioneers. They were more gung-ho than either Shumway or Lower. Hume was one of those guys, Lower observed wryly, who thought it a sign of weakness if you admitted to needing more than four hours' sleep a night.

When Hume slumped in his office early one morning, after he had worked through the night, a colleague felt instant sympathy. Hume's eyes were sunken into his usually beaming and handsome face. His skin was gray with fatigue. Yet when the man asked him if he was all right, Hume insisted that he was "feeling great." He had a busy day ahead of him, an exciting day. Hume, though on the point of collapse, looked as if he believed utterly in his rejuvenation.

In 1965, Hume had decided that Lewis Bosher, his chief of cardiac surgery, was not a man who could deliver transplant glory to Richmond. He was not even in the race. At least Kantrowitz, Blumenstock, and the Vallee-Willman team in St. Louis were attempting to catch Shumway and Lower. Bosher was not even in the blocks. After they argued once too often about the need to join the chase, Bosher was demoted and Hume set out to transform MCV's cardiac service.

It did not take him long to decide who he wanted to lead the heart race in Richmond. Hume went for the best man in cardiac transplantation. He called up Norm Shumway and invited him down to Richmond. Shumway was amused and intrigued. Hume was remorselessly intelligent—if a little too much of a playboy for Shumway's taste. He was a charmer but, unlike many suave men, he burned with conviction. Hume was determined to create a medical legacy in Richmond. Shumway was making his own kind of history at Stanford, but for an hour or so, he was tempted.

He could not, in the end, escape the central flaw in Hume's character. Hume was stubborn to the point of being, in Shumway's laconic phrase, "sorta pig-headed." He was a compulsive meddler, a trait epitomized by his determination to get a grip on a heart disease called "the second aneurysm." Despite being a renal specialist, Hume insisted on being called to the OR whenever there was an aneurysm—a dilation in the wall of an artery, usually the aorta, which can result in internal bleeding or a stroke if untreated. Shumway decided that working with Hume would be akin to life under Owen Wangensteen. He had done that once before, without much fun, in Minnesota.

"Okay, Norm," Hume sighed when he accepted that he was never going to wear Shumway down. "Who do I go for next?"

Shumway knew how much he would miss him, for they had done their best work together, but he valued their friendship more highly. "You've got to go for the top guy," he said. "You should ask Dick Lower." Shumway paused and then grinned. "Lower's the guru."

Hume moved fast. Lower knew that Shumway had recommended him, and so, in the fall of 1965, there was little need for debate. At thirty-six, the same age Shumway had been seven years earlier when he became cardiac chief at Stanford, Lower had a chance to run his own show. How could he resist? He would shake his friend's hand and head east to a new life.

They would keep in close contact, Dick and Norm, but the old team had broken up. It was now between them—they were racing each other. Within another two years, they were certain, one of them would gracefully edge ahead of the other and emerge as the first man in history to transplant a human heart.

Eight

THE PRINCE

In the spring of 1966, Adrian Kantrowitz appeared unstoppable. His team had just received a $3 million National Institutes of Health grant—then the second-largest in medical history. Only Michael DeBakey, the most famous cardiac surgeon in America and a master power broker in medical politics, could claim a heftier chunk of NIH and FDA financial backing, almost $4.5 million. Kantrowitz was ready to take on Shumway and Lower in the transplant race while, simultaneously, meeting DeBakey head-to-head in the battle to develop a groundbreaking ventricular assist device. The big man was set to take on the world.

DeBakey was celebrated for his repair of aortic aneurysms and aortic dissections—just as he was feared and loathed for his standing as the most powerful man in American medicine. The dark, tough son of Lebanese immigrants who had settled in Louisiana, he had once been even more of an outsider than Kantrowitz. But his ambition was as ferocious as the scalding temper with which he terrorized the operating room. It was said that De-Bakey was too busy to ever attend a party, unless he was sure that a congressman might be present from whom he might squeeze another million-dollar grant for his work at Baylor Medical Center and at the Methodist Hospital in Houston. He was also happy to open his doors to television cameras and glossy publications like *Life* or *Time*. DeBakey knew how the gleaming wheels of money and celebrity worked, and he played the game with brutal efficiency.

With the transplantation race having been slowed by the reaction to Hardy's chimp experiment, and by Shumway's measured response, DeBakey invited a *Life* reporter and photographer to trail him for a year as he prepared to implant a left ventricular bypass. DeBakey had failed in his first attempt three years earlier, installing a heart assist pump in a doomed operation; but on April 21, 1966, he implanted a temporary auxiliary device. His patient died on the fourth day, but that didn't discourage *Life* from devoting ten pages of color photographs and bold text to DeBakey's mechanical adventure.

Kantrowitz had already emerged as his main rival when, two months before, in February 1966, he had inserted a smaller left ventricular device that he hoped might serve as a permanent implant. His patient had been a poor choice, however, and died on the first postoperative day from pulmonary complications and bleeding caused by his liver disease. The U-shaped device, which Kantrowitz had invented with his brother Arthur, a physicist, had worked perfectly. It was based on Kantrowitz's renowned "counterpulsation principle"—an approach driven by his obsession with increasing coronary blood flow when the heart relaxes in diastole and the aortic valve closes. Kantrowitz had developed the inspired technique of using a pressure pulse in the root of the aorta to augment the flow of blood and send it surging through any narrowed or damaged arteries. He believed that a mechanical device would augment the work of the damaged heart by pumping blood during the heart's natural cycle of relaxation. In some cases, he was sure, the rejuvenated heart would eventually resume a large part of its normal function.

The pump functioned beautifully in May 1966, when Kantrowitz's U-shaped mechanism helped sixty-three-year-old Louise Ceraso's diseased heart to circulate blood through her body. She responded well in the first week, and Kantrowitz imagined sending her home, the world's first recipient of a permanently implanted left ventricular assist device. On the seventh day, Ceraso began to have small strokes, culminating in her death on May 31. When the pathologist opened her up in the autopsy room he discovered large blood clots in both arms of the assist device. Ceraso had survived longer than DeBakey's patient—but the Houston surgeon had been right, after all, in arguing that a temporary implant was more practical than the permanent model.

Kantrowitz was passionate about the L-VAD (left ventricular assist device), which he was certain could save many more lives than transplantation. He knew transplants had the potential to rescue patients from terminal heart disease and, once rejection had been defeated, provide them with another twenty or thirty years of active life. That fact explained why he was in the business. Yet even the single-minded Shumway conceded that the demand for new hearts would always outstrip the supply of donor organs. They agreed it was unlikely they would ever transcend a plateau in medicine where more than 10 percent of patients requiring transplants could be offered a new heart. If Shumway was determined to perfect the procedure, Kantrowitz continued to explore mechanical assist devices as an alternative to transplantation. Once an effective L-VAD had been developed, it could be mass-produced and used to save an unending line of cardiac patients.

Transplantation was different. Having transplanted hundreds of hearts between puppies since 1963, Kantrowitz and his team were technically ready to make a human attempt in June 1966. He turned to his chief supporter, Clarence Dennis. Having been Wangensteen's research partner for years, and an inspiration to Lillehei, Dennis had deep roots in Minnesota. After failing with the world's first two attempts to use a heart-lung machine in 1951, Dennis had moved to New York. He became chairman of the Department of Surgery at Downstate Medical Center, which doubled as Maimonides' academic base.

At Downstate he listened to, and watched over, Kantrowitz's brainstorming sessions with genuine interest. Dennis was used to radical ideas from Minnesota, and so he saw immediately how Kantrowitz's transplantation experiments in the laboratory had prepared him for a human trial. He offered his unequivocal backing.

The Maimonides committee of administrators and doctors, however, were in shock. They had barely recovered from the previous weeks' publicity, led by the front page of *The New York Times*, which had engulfed Kantrowitz's cardioassist device. This latest ambition was far more unsettling. Kantrowitz, naturally, was insistent. He had lives to save. He had history to make.

William Neches was twenty-seven years old and asked everyone to call him Bill. Neches, an unassuming junior resident at Maimonides, had identified the undisputed kings of medicine—the surgeons who carried themselves with an imposing grandeur. Some were icily remote, while others exploded with fury. Neches understood. They were the men whose very hands saved or lost lives.

Bill Neches would walk instead with the princes—the pediatricians, the gentlest doctors, who care for the smallest broken and ailing bodies. As a Jew born in Brooklyn in 1939, he felt at ease serving his residence, as a pediatric cardiologist, in the heart of an Orthodox enclave. Appropriately, the hospital was named after Moses Maimonides, the great medieval Jewish scholar and physician who had established the concept of medicine as a natural science. It served the surrounding community of Hasidic Jews, in a neighborhood stretching from Borough Park to Flatbush.

But Maimonides Hospital also tended to a variety of other ethnic groups. The Hungarian Gypsies of Coney Island, like the Hasidim, maintained a hermetic culture with customs and laws unique to them. Only sickness and the threat of death could force them to open themselves to the world. And now they were frantic. Miller Stevenson, a tiny baby they regarded as a future leader of their traveling clan, was dying. The Gypsies were ready to do whatever was needed to save the boy they hailed as a prince.

Miller Stevenson had been born at the hospital on May 11, 1966. It was a sun-filled Saturday that, for the Gypsies, soon darkened. The diagnosis of congenital heart disorders frightened and angered them. Bill Neches was called in to explain the assessment of the senior cardiologists. Howard Joos, the chief of pediatrics, a kind and serious Harvard-trained pediatrician, could not talk to the Gypsies with the same warmth as Neches.

The young doctor unraveled the complex defects that engulfed the infant.

Neches used simpler words than those in the written diagnosis of the cardiologists who identified five distinct possible cardiac malformations: transposition of the ventricles, pulmonary valve atresia, patent ductus arteriosus, atrial septal defect, and ventricular septal defect. Each was troubling in isolation. Together they comprised a terrifying list. Neches knew that to save such a heart Kantrowitz could only try something so extreme that they did not yet dare say it out loud.

Nine desperate days after the birth, Neches persuaded a small deputation to sit down with him. He would have preferred to face the parents alone but he met, instead, with the baby's mother and two grandfathers. Pauline Stevenson, at twenty-seven, was the same age as Neches. Her father-in-law, Wando Stevenson, and her father, John De Mitro, were equally distraught. Pauline and her husband, Robert, already had three daughters. Their fourth baby, Miller, was their first son, a boy in whom so much hope had been invested by the Gypsies.

While she was pregnant they had traveled around the fringes of Boston. It was only in the last few weeks that they'd opted to settle, amid the faded amusement rides and clattering roller coasters, in Wando's basement apartment in Coney Island. He took them to Maimonides for the birth.

Neches tried to sift through their doubts and suspicions. They had no need to worry about money, he stressed, for they would be covered by a state aid program. The relief of Pauline and the men filtered through the room. Neches could, over the coming days, prepare them for the moment when they would finally be ready to hear a dramatic new word.

Transplantation was one of the reasons why Neches felt exhilarated to be working under Kantrowitz. He had watched the surgeon from afar, dazzled by a giant marching through the hospital with a large entourage of doctors in his wake. Yet Neches discovered that Kantrowitz was a humorous and considerate man. He was also an extraordinarily lucid teacher.

Although Neches had never seen an anencephalic baby, Kantrowitz trusted him to take responsibility for the potential donor hearts. A letter drafted by the surgeon and signed by Howard Joos and by William Pomerance, the director of obstetrics at Maimonides, had been sent out to five hundred hospitals across the country in April 1966:

Dear Doctor,

We are prepared to study the problems of orthotopic cardiac homo-transplantations in human babies, and I hope that you will want to help us locate the case material which we will require. Our surgeons have perfected the technique in puppies during the last several years. . . . A donor infant will also have to be large enough, probably at least five pounds. As recipients we will seek newborn infants with lethal congenital malformations, whose life expectancy is not longer than a few months and whose malformation is not subject to currently available palliative or corrective surgery. Informed parental consent will, of course, be necessary. . . .

Before an actual transplant could be attempted, Neches had monitored some of the anencephalics flown into JFK and La Guardia. He met the specially chartered planes, and then, in an ambulance, Neches and the stricken babies had sped across New York.

His first two patients, rather than monsters, had been Baby Striley and Baby McLaughlin. Anencephalic babies were usually left alone until their hearts stopped beating. Neches was used to a more diligent kind of care. With only two or three pediatric cases a month at Maimonides' cardiac wing, Neches had become accustomed to a special relationship with the sick babies. Pediatric respirators had yet to be invented, and so Neches and his fellow residents would monitor an infant in twelve-hour shifts. They would manually remove the breathing tube when necessary and pump a large and awkward adult ventilator by hand.

He brought the same level of care to his anencephalic babies, in an attempt to see how much longer their hearts might survive beyond the typical forty-eight-hour life span of such infants. The time difference appeared negligible, endorsing Kantrowitz's claim that there was no prospect of salvaging an anencephalic. Ironically, while they could never exist as ordinary human beings, they were often born with healthy hearts.

The first two babies delivered to Maimonides followed the pattern. When their hearts stopped beating, the organs were harvested, cooled, perfused, and eventually resuscitated. The technique, devised by Lower and Shumway, worked. A human heart transplant would be possible. But they knew it would be more likely to succeed if Kantrowitz could take the heart while it was still alive.

On June 28, 1966, they were ready. Coaxed by Neches and Kantrowitz, Robert and Pauline Stevenson had accepted the idea of a transplant for their son. They knew that nothing else would save him. They stared down at the typed Authorization of Heart Transplant form as it was read aloud to them:

> The parents of Miller Stevenson, an infant presently hospitalized at Maimonides Hospital, do hereby authorize and request Dr. Adrian Kantrowitz and whomever he may designate as his assistants to perform a heart transplant upon our child named above. We understand that the hospital will try to obtain a normal heart from whatever source is available and will surgically transplant this heart into our child's chest. We understand that this is a new surgical procedure and that great risks are involved and that there may be a greater risk of infection than in other types of surgery, and that our child's body may reject the transplanted heart. We also understand that the prognosis is poor at this time and that the hospital and doctors have made no representations nor given assurances as to the success or result of this procedure.

They gave their address, for the sake of formality, as 2828 West 24th Street, Brooklyn, and scrawled their names on the lines reserved for their signatures.

Bill Neches, meanwhile, having returned early that morning from JFK, watched over a different baby on the far side of the Aron Building. This baby, with its perfect torso, two arms and two legs, ten fingers and ten toes, had flown 2,500 miles through the night. He was barely a day old.

Richard and Rhoda Senz, like the Gypsy parents they would never meet, already had three healthy children. There was a notable distinction to the coincidence. Where Robert and Pauline Stevenson had three girls and longed for a son, the Senzes had a small trio of boys and yearned for a daughter. An engaging, modest, and intelligent couple, they were preoccupied during their latest pregnancy. They had just moved to a new home in Newbury, Oregon, a quiet rural community twenty-five miles south of Portland. The Senzes' new house was on a ten-acre plot, with a beautiful large barn, surrounded by farms— but Richard was not a farmer. He was responsible for the management of any modifications to the medical instruments his company designed and manufactured. His division specialized in oscilloscopes and heart monitors.

Rhoda worked as a supervisor at one of AT&T's regional outlets. She thrived in pregnancy and did not pay undue attention to the fact that her doctors had been strangely vague throughout the preceding six months. Drs. Ivan Langley and David Moore, a respectable local partnership, had attended to all three of her births. They had then been particularly exact about each new stage of those pregnancies, but this time was different. They were more hesitant and had much less to say. Rhoda also asked fewer questions. The priorities of parenting were different with three little boys racing around.

As the birth approached, Rhoda and a few of the experienced older mothers in her own extended family decided to give her baby a reminder that it was time for him, or her, to make an appearance. They still called them "old wives' remedies." She tried them all before reaching for the definitive "baby-shifter." The castor oil, again, did its magic.

Richard drove her to the hospital in Portland. As was customary then, he was not allowed to be with his wife at the birth and so, in a familiar routine, he waited for the good news in the fathers' waiting room. Like Rhoda, he felt relaxed and ready.

Rhoda, who had not needed more than an occasional sniff of gas to help her through her first three births, was immediately oblivious to her fate. Rather than being offered the chance to give birth naturally, she was anesthetized.

Richard Senz's life changed forever in the moment the door to his wife's delivery suite opened. He looked up to see Dr. Langley walking slowly toward him. He knew they were in trouble. The shock made him feel as if his own heart had turned over. He waited for the words. Langley eased him down into the darkness, step by step, line by line. Rhoda was okay. Rhoda was going to be fine. He could see her soon. And then the "but" came, and the doctor's altered tone of voice spoke volumes.

This strange new word, "anencephalic," jammed in the back of Richard's throat. But Langley was also a father accustomed to pain in his own family. Richard knew that one of Langley's children needed constant medical attention. That human link enabled him to absorb the doctor's words.

Langley explained why they had waited to impart the shattering news. The doctors had felt it best for the couple to discover the fate of their fourth boy as late as possible. Richard understood. They would have been lesser parents to their other children if they had been told months before. Then, more strange words fell from Langley's mouth: *"Maimonides . . . Kantrowitz . . . transplant . . ."*

Unlike the Maimonides committeemen, Langley had not needed much persuasion when the Portland obstetricians had passed on the letter requesting an anencephalic donor. Reports of Kantrowitz's work on the heart had spread across America. Yet this concerned more than surgical renown. Miller Stevenson's need for a donor was now desperate.

Langley revealed Kantrowitz's desire to create a new life from the wreckage of two tragic births. Richard soon nodded. Yes. And again, another nod. Yes.

Before he could face his wife, Richard talked to his brother, Robert, in California. He also spoke to his sister-in-law, Barbara, who was in the midst of taking a master's degree in administrative nursing. She was familiar with the promise of transplantation and the finality of anencephaly. Barbara knew another clinching truth. Yes, Richard should follow his instinct and donate their baby's heart, but he should not allow himself or Rhoda to see their son. It might seem unspeakably cruel that they would never get to hold, let alone see, their baby; but it would be worse if their eyes rested for a moment on their headless baby. They had to release him.

Rhoda slowly regained consciousness. She wondered, between his and her blinking, whether her husband had been crying. There was no sign of the baby. Richard told Rhoda what had happened to their fourth son. Then he spoke of their "three R's," little Richard, Randall, and Ronald. He and Rhoda had to go on for their sake. She held him tight. It was only when he mentioned Langley's suggestion that they consider allowing their baby to be used as a donor patient that Rhoda cried out. She wanted to see her baby. She wanted to cradle him. She wanted to keep him close to her for as many days, or hours, as he might live.

Richard knew his wife was not easily deterred. But she sank deeper into his arms, and he knew that, as always with her, pragmatism and generosity would defeat anger and despair.

Langley was called into the room, and he again went through the procedure methodically, stressing the thread of trust that ran from them to him to the obstetricians and cardiologists in Portland to Kantrowitz and his team. Their baby would be escorted to JFK, where he would be met by Dr. Neches. The people at Maimonides had been emphatic that the treatment of their son would be dignified and respectful.

Rhoda lifted her head and nodded. Even though her baby's heart maintained its regular beating, she had the courage to understand he was already lost to the world. She could sense the plain "rightness" of the transplant. They looked at each other; and then Rhoda turned to Langley.

"All right," she said.

They did not even ask the question as to when Kantrowitz might take the heart. If it was to save the life of another baby, they assumed it would be removed while it was still beating. In less than an hour their baby would be rushed to the airport. Richard arranged the baptism and chose his son's name—Ralph Edward Senz.

Maimonides Hospital, Brooklyn, New York, June 29, 1966

That next night, down in the sweltering depths of the scrub room, Kantrowitz moved slowly and carefully as he hunched over the gushing taps. Soapsuds poured down his right arm. He repeated the same procedure with his left arm before returning to the methodical washing of his hands. Those brawny hands would try to save Miller Stevenson.

The travelers who had swept down on Maimonides had made it plain to the young resident doctors on Kantrowitz's team that they would regard failure to save the boy as a slight on their Hungarian Gypsy heritage. None, however, had dared confront Kantrowitz. Even the Gypsies realized that the massive surgeon should be left to his work while they maintained their vigil.

Kantrowitz knew that an anencephalic baby could not sustain a heartbeat for more than a few days, even with the aid of a ventilator and IV fluids. Yet as long as the heart pumped blood around a senseless shell, Kantrowitz believed it might be taken to restore life in another. At eleven-thirty on that steamy summer night in Brooklyn there was little time left. As the surgeon scrubbed, the donor baby was wheeled down the maze of corridors linking the hospital's nursery station to the operating room.

Once he had wiped his scrubbed hands dry with a blue towel, Kantrowitz felt ready. The surgeon faced the plain swing-doors leading to the OR and took in another slow and deep breath. Lost in the moment, Kantrowitz felt strangely serene.

"Okay," he said, "let's go . . ."

The white doors swung open with a sigh and then, making a hiss and scrape, they closed behind him. There was a deep and sudden silence in the scrub room. The big man had crossed over to the other side. He had stepped into the wild and secret darkness of the unknown.

At exactly 11:45 p.m., he stood silently over the small anencephalic body. A bath of ice water had been prepared to begin the process of lowering the baby's temperature in the operating room. Kantrowitz planned to carry out the transplant using just hypothermia rather than a heart-lung machine. It was a radical decision—and the first of many for which he would have to find vindication through a long night.

Kantrowitz had other battles he needed to win first. His own personal preference to remove the beating heart had suddenly been opposed in the OR by members of his own team. They had again chosen to drape the baby's ruined head with a towel. The surgeon knew why they kept it in place. Even if the towel changed nothing, it allowed his colleagues around the operating table to see the perfect body of a new baby. Yet Kantrowitz was sure that Richard and Rhoda Senz would not have wished to have a towel placed over their baby's face.

In the hushed OR he reached out and pulled back the towel. Kantrowitz wanted them to bear witness to the incomplete skull, to the empty oblivion of a body born with only half a head. He needed them to recognize that, without a brain, there was no life. He wanted them to realize that this body had never really been alive. He made them look.

His brutality was driven by compassion. Kantrowitz had moved beyond the race to transplant the human heart as soon as he saw Miller Stevenson that night. The Gypsy prince had literally only half a heart but, unlike a body trapped in an anencephalic shell, life poured out of him. He had a fully functioning brain and a chance of survival if he could be given a new heart. Life resided in the brain and, for that reason, Miller Stevenson needed all the help they could give him.

For Kantrowitz there was no choice. They had to open up the chest and transplant the donor heart. Jordan Haller, his first assistant, stood at his side. He knew Kantrowitz was right. If they waited for the heart to stop they would almost certainly fail. It was a conviction shared by most of the younger members of the team that night—especially Bill Neches, who had invested something of himself in both babies. Yet Haller knew, too, that most of the senior figures were ranged against Kantrowitz. They were led by Howard Joos, the senior pediatrician, and Harry Weiss, the silver-haired anesthesiologist who would soon help ensure the birth of Haller's own son. Both were good men, but they were ready to dig in. The hospital board had inserted a crucial clause into the application for a donor. It made the surgical promise that the heart would be removed only *"after the clinical death of a donor (absence of heartbeat by auscultation and absence of regular coordinated respiratory activity)."*

Weiss shook his head. He looked at Kantrowitz—the team leader, but a man twenty years his junior. Weiss took the towel from the surgeon's hand. He cloaked the head.

The operating room was quiet as they looked at each other over the infant's body. Joos moved closer to Weiss, reaffirming his allegiance to the older man. Kantrowitz stared at them. Their masks concealed their faces but everything could be seen in their eyes. Haller was transfixed by the contrasting emotions flaring so intensely between their masks and caps. Even their glasses could not soften the flaming passion of Kantrowitz or the bleak determination of Weiss and Joos.

At the first objection to the start of the transplant, Kantrowitz had spoken of the need to set aside thousands of years of mythology and linguistic confusion. In the OR he reiterated that every subtle human emotion, every miraculous thought, flowed from the brain. Only blood spurted from the muscle that pumped mechanically in the middle of the chest. No one but a blind romantic could cling to the belief that life was defined by a heartbeat. They had seen too much blood, and far too many deaths, to hesitate now. They had to remove the beating heart from this anencephalic baby so that they could complete the transplant and save another life. The force of his words was doubled by the softness of his voice.

Once more he stretched out his gloved hand and withdrew the towel. "There is no brain," he repeated. "There is no life."

Haller felt the horror of the moment as Joos again used the towel to protect the brainless body.

"You cannot take the heart, Adrian," Joos said. "This baby is alive . . ."

"Yes," Kantrowitz said, "the heart beats and the liver and the lungs function. But where's the brain? Where's the human life?"

As if arranging a stretch of cellophane over a funeral bouquet, Weiss smoothed the towel so that it sheltered the missing upper part of the head.

"Harry," Kantrowitz said, the exasperation lending an edge to his voice, "the parents gave us their blessing."

"Only God can decide," Joos said. "Not you, Adrian, only God."

Kantrowitz had dreaded this supposedly spiritual, but ultimately melodramatic, confrontation. He had been told earlier that such caution was prompted by the highest regard for medical ethics. Kantrowitz cared more about life than ethics. He always knew he would be ready to bend the rules, and even break them, if it gave him a better chance of success.

He turned away to monitor the electrocardiogram. The EKG readings were worsening. He could see the small heart entering the last stretch of its journey. It only managed to keep up its wayward beating because of Weiss's ventilator and the IV line Neches had set up. The heart would soon wither to the point of stillness. Even Weiss and Joos agreed. The heart would not survive another hour.

Kantrowitz needed to remove it from the chest and place the heart in the protective cradle of cold saline while they prepared the recipient. As soon as he gave them the signal they would lower Miller Stevenson into his own icy tub and monitor the gradual drop in his body temperature. His sick heart would slow in time with the gathering cold. When it was time, his chest would be opened and the diseased organ removed.

The surgeon was tempted to tear the towel away one last time but, facing the glare of Joos and the silence of Weiss, he knew there was no point. He could not attempt the first human heart transplant until he had the backing of his whole team. Haller slumped a little. Without the authority of the older men, there was nothing he could do to help Kantrowitz.

"I'm sorry," Weiss said.

Kantrowitz walked out of the operating room and down the corridor. In the adjoining room the second surgical team looked up expectantly from the anesthetized body of Miller Stevenson and the small white basin packed with ice.

"Not yet," Kantrowitz said.

A hushed vigil was maintained in the OR. Kantrowitz eventually rejoined them. He tried to curb his despair as they followed the slow and irregular beep of the EKG. It was excruciating. He had never just stood around and watched a heart die. Not long after midnight, at 12:21, it stopped beating.

Kantrowitz did not have to give the command. Haller had already begun to saw his way into the donor baby's chest. He could cut fast and hard, without even thinking of the need to cauterize or tie off the blood vessels. He concentrated on reaching the heart.

"How does it look?" Kantrowitz asked.

"Not good," Haller murmured. He pulled away to let Kantrowitz replace him at the head of the table.

Kantrowitz stared down into the cavity of the small chest. He saw a tiny heart, blue and inert. Its color and stillness chilled him.

"C'mon, let's move."

The machine began to whir and pump. They stood and waited. Kantrowitz knew from his work on hundreds of dogs that the little heart should almost immediately turn a beautiful shade of pink as the muscle tensed and firmed with an infusion of blood. This cyanotic heart, however, only altered its shade from blue to purple.

He knew he could remove the heart and store it in a basin of ice-cold saline solution. And then, more carefully than anything he had ever done before, he would carry the heart-filled basin the short walk that separated the two operating rooms.

The tiny muscle, however, did not turn pink. Kantrowitz tried to stimulate it, but still it only contracted spasmodically. He knew that, after completing the cutting and the removal, they could try again while the second team opened up Miller Stevenson. They could still proceed with the transplant, in the hope that they could shock the unpromising heart back to life. They would have achieved at least one objective then—and transplanted a human heart. Kantrowitz controlled his own craving. He knew it would take another thirty minutes to implant the barely twitching heart.

The sense of futility was overwhelming. Kantrowitz covered his face with his hands. The hope drained out of him.

"I'm sorry," Harry Weiss repeated.

Kantrowitz turned away. He had to face the parents of Miller Stevenson. They would understand that the aborted transplant amounted to a death sentence for their own baby. He needed to be the one who gave them the awful truth.

As Kantrowitz walked down the hospital corridor he did not know that, in Oregon, Richard and Rhoda Senz wanted him to take the heart of their baby before it stopped beating. He could only guess what Shumway or Lower would have done in such a moment. All he knew then was that he had failed. Miller Stevenson would be dead within weeks. The families of the two boys would suffer most of all. But Kantrowitz, Joos, Weiss, Haller, and Neches, and everyone else in the OR that night, would never shake that image of the towel and the head from their minds, no matter how long they lived.

Kantrowitz pushed open a set of hospital doors and, stepping out of the emergency corridor, turned left toward the room where the Stevensons waited. He tore off his cap and mask and gloves because he knew he would want to hold out his hands to them before he spoke. And they would want to see his face.

After he had stopped and spoken and taken all the time the Stevensons needed to accept the news, Kantrowitz started walking again. He climbed on his motorbike, the old Indian, kicked it into life, and wove slowly through Brooklyn to his wife. Jeannie would understand. She would tell him to keep moving.

Kantrowitz felt a cool dampness on his cheeks as he rode through the blackness. He felt as if he was traveling, like the Gypsies, into the unknown. The faces of the baby's parents still reeled through his head. Kantrowitz wished, with sudden and piercing yearning, that he had been able to tell them something different.

Nine

THE STEAL

Early on Saturday, July 2, 1966, the start of a long Fourth of July weekend, a weary and disconsolate Adrian Kantrowitz was suddenly galvanized. It looked like the Gypsy prince would be given one last chance. The St. Francis General Hospital in Pittsburgh—one of the five hundred medical centers cabled with a request for an anencephalic baby—telephoned with the startling news. Two of their doctors had spoken to the parents of a baby that had been born anencephalic the night before. Like Richard and Rhoda Senz, the Smiths of Pittsburgh had agreed to give up their son to help Kantrowitz try to save Miller Stevenson.

Kantrowitz sucked in a deep breath. You just never knew what might happen next. He was down, and now, incredibly, he was up and racing again. Speed was everything. They needed the donor baby desperately. Kantrowitz stressed that his team would hire a charter plane from Pittsburgh. Within another two hours a twin-engine Apache left Allegheny County Airport carrying Baby Smith, accompanied by Ronald Hamaty, a twenty-seven-year-old resident of Johnstown, Pennsylvania.

Hamaty had never been out of the state before, let alone flown in a plane. It was also the first time he had seen an anencephalic baby. He looked down at the troubling sight of the flawless body born without a brain. Hamaty lifted the baby gently into his arms. He felt unusually reverent toward his tiny patient.

Bill Neches was waiting with an ambulance at La Guardia, and as they screamed toward Brooklyn, Hamaty began to feel queasy. The enormity of the transplant threatened to overwhelm him. He was relieved that Neches, who had been through the same trial only four days before with Ralph Senz, took care of the baby.

Inside Maimonides the atmosphere was strained. Kantrowitz was ready to face down Joos and Weiss this time. Joos assessed the heart of the Pittsburgh baby and confirmed Kantrowitz's claim that it seemed relatively strong. Hamaty watched Kantrowitz with awe. The surgeon was a huge and striking figure. His intensity made him still more compelling as he strode impatiently around the room, only stopping to check the electrocardiogram or to underscore his argument with a clenched fist. Kantrowitz seemed to be winning the battle. Hamaty kept hearing the words "*It's looking good!*" and "*We're ready to go!*" Joos and Weiss were about to concede, while Kantrowitz and Haller prepared for the scrub.

And then more trouble descended. The mood darkened as they hunched over the readings. Baby Smith's heart had begun to falter. Kantrowitz's silence deepened as he stood over the small body. This time they would not even make it into the OR.

"Fuck it," he said softly as he closed his eyes. When he opened them again, he knew the truth. They had lost again. And soon the Gypsy prince would be dead.

Two days later, on July 4, 1966, Marius Barnard arrived in America. The next morning, after forty hours in transit, he would be expected to begin work in Michael DeBakey's operating room. It would have been bad enough if he was meant to assist his hysterical brother, Chris—but *DeBakey*? Black Mike had been known to humiliate visiting surgeons to the point that they broke down and wept.

A familiar feeling of inferiority swept across Marius. He had long been dismissed as Chris's younger brother. Even when the Afrikaans newspapers reported that he was on his way to America to study surgery with the legendary DeBakey, they described him as *"die broer van die bekende hartspesialis prof. Chris Barnard"* (the brother of the renowned heart specialist Professor Chris Barnard). America was meant to change everything. There was a secret degree, acknowledged quietly among South African surgeons as the BTA. Unless you had done your BTA (been to America), you were doomed to obscurity.

Marius, unlike Chris, did not exude the typical swagger of the cardiac surgeon. But he now yearned to make his mark as one of South Africa's leading vascular surgeons. Nine months alongside Michael DeBakey and Denton Cooley would propel him beyond the long shadow of Chris. His plan had at least begun well. DeBakey offered him a place as a fellow in cardiovascular surgery on an annual salary of $4,200.

The following morning, DeBakey's OR felt like hell. "You're two days late," snapped the first nurse to whom he introduced himself. "Get out of my light," Black Mike snarled an hour later when Marius, holding the retractor, leaned forward to obtain a better view. The pattern was set. The maestro operated and Marius and the rest watched blankly. DeBakey understood the futility of their presence. He once looked up at Marius and said, "Do you know, Dr. Barnard, a man can watch another play a piano for twenty years and not learn a single note?"

DeBakey was the star; and yet he was troubled by his protégé. Denton Cooley was a conjurer at the table, a man with hands that moved so quickly and smoothly it seemed as if he opened and closed his patients with a kind of alchemy. Cooley was everything DeBakey had never been—a tall blond athlete who had always been the most charismatic and popular kid in class. DeBakey's Lebanese parents ran a Louisiana drugstore, while Cooley was the son of a rich society dentist whose family owned a large chunk of north Houston. The pain he caused DeBakey was captured by another Texas surgeon who described Cooley as "the handsomest son of a bitch to ever pick up a scalpel. How'd you like to shave Mike DeBakey's face every morning and then have to look across the table at Denton Cooley?"

When Marius switched from DeBakey's service to Cooley's, the mood changed. He did not do much more work, or learn anything, while he watched the Texan's hands flash and cut and stitch with blinding speed, but at least Cooley cracked a few jokes while being charmingly obnoxious. "Just call me G.O.D.," he told Marius, "Good Old Denton."

Cooley stirred the pot constantly. "So, Marius," he said one afternoon, while zipping through one of the sixteen operations he considered his daily minimum, "how does it feel watching me do so many cases when your little old unit back in Africa might do only two or three a day?"

Marius was ready. "Dr. Cooley," he said, "you remind me of a story I heard. During the Second World War a big American battleship came through a tremendous storm and then cut across a small British destroyer being tossed on the waves. A cry rang out from the great American battleship—'Hi, how's the second-biggest navy in the world?' And the answer came back: 'Fine—how's the world's second-best navy?'"

Cooley stopped cutting for ten seconds—a surgical eternity for him. He stared at Marius as if wondering whether he should kick his butt straight out of Texas. Eventually, Cooley lowered his head and resumed his lightning slicing and stitching.

"You son of a bitch," he said quietly.

Chris Barnard soon followed his brother to America. The thought of Marius, seven years younger, learning new techniques in Houston with DeBakey and Cooley unsettled him. He was too far ahead of Marius to fear he might be overtaken by his brother, but their spiky and complex relationship, fueled by arrogance on one side and resentment on the other, meant that Chris felt increasingly restless when he imagined what he might be missing in Houston. He was the one meant to thrive in America, not Marius.

Chris considered Cooley the greatest technical wizard in American surgery. Of Cooley's cutting he wrote: "It was the most beautiful surgery I had ever seen in my life. Every movement had a purpose and achieved its aim. Where most surgeons would take three hours he could do the same operation in one hour. . . . Some surgeons drove themselves, their hands groping for a solution to the imbalance before them. Dr. Cooley's hands moved effortlessly, as though he was simply putting everything back in place. This allowed him to make direct and often dramatic entries which would seem daring if done by anyone else. In dissecting the femoral artery, for example, one normally would make a small cut, then another, and another, until it was exposed. Dr. Cooley simply made one slit, and the femoral artery lay open. No one in the world, I knew, could equal it."

Just as the spacemen of Houston were shooting for the moon, so Cooley and the Texan surgeons in cowboy boots were out to conquer the heart. Yet Barnard was not tempted by a return visit to Houston. Apart from not wanting to jostle alongside his little brother, he would learn little from DeBakey and Cooley. Black Mike would never be willing to share any of his research findings, while Good Old Denton did not believe in anything as mundane as laboratory experiments. Barnard knew that he had to look elsewhere for inspiration as he prepared to haul himself to the forefront of transplant surgery.

He wrote to David Hume in Virginia to ask for help in studying rejection—as a precursor to beginning kidney transplantation in Cape Town. Hume, having met Barnard on numerous occasions, immediately responded with an invitation to attend a course on rejection at MCV in Richmond from August to October 1966. Barnard's desire for Deirdre to win the world waterskiing championships the following year would once have made those dates impossible to fulfill. Three months of missed training at such a crucial stage in her training would have been catastrophic—had he still believed she could win.

As merciless as he once was in driving her on the lake, Barnard prepared himself for an even more ruthless act. Having spent so much time coaching her, he was now ready to abruptly shut her out from all but the periphery of his life. Twenty years later he would reflect, in an unsettling insight, "I think in her unconscious mind I was more than a father; I was virtually a boyfriend. I mean, we were everything in each other's lives because I didn't find all that satisfaction in my married life. We were always together then, even at parties."

Deirdre's feelings echoed her father's. "He suddenly became non-existent. Before that we had been so close and we were so fond of each other—he was everything to me—that being dropped like a hot potato felt ten times worse. It hurt me terribly."

Barnard made the decision. "I knew it was over between us. The time had come to cease using my daughter to satisfy my own ambitions. . . . No longer compelled to transfer myself into my daughter's career, I could concentrate on a far larger transplant."

He also contacted Tom Starzl at the Veterans Administration Hospital in Denver, again asking for advice in fighting rejection. Starzl, having done great work on the kidney graft, was about to try again with the liver—an organ so difficult to transplant it usually took eight hours to complete the protracted dissection of so many intricate veins and arteries. He had failed in his first five attempts in 1963 and declared a moratorium on the liver transplant for the next three years. Yet consumed as he was by his enormous workload in kidney grafting and liver research, Starzl invited Barnard to spend as long as he wished in Denver. Among most American surgeons, then, the mood toward Barnard was one of generosity and encouragement.

Although he would visit Starzl, Barnard resolved to spend the bulk of his time in Richmond. He felt an affinity for Hume, a deeply motivated but hedonistic man whose personal life always seemed about to career out of control. There were two additional reasons behind his choice of Richmond. He was intrigued by the possibility of meeting Lower—Barnard's request to visit Shumway at Stanford had been met with a predictably cool response. Even more pressing than the chance to watch Lower work, Barnard was desperate to see his former perfusionist, Carl Goosen, in the hope he might persuade him to return to Groote Schuur to run the heart-lung machine.

Weary of Barnard's abuse, Goosen had been keen to start a new life in America. He had worked more closely with Barnard than anyone since 1958, but Goosen loathed his fellow Afrikaner. Where he'd once experienced stress, he eventually came to feel cold anger whenever the surgeon screamed at him. Barnard, suddenly anxious to win him back, reminded Goosen of how much they had been through together—from the technical stunt of a two-headed dog to their more significant work in carrying out the first open-heart surgery in Africa, developing bypass procedures, and designing heart valves. Goosen could not forget how much he had suffered. And so he left South Africa and began working in Lewis Bosher's lab in Richmond in early July 1966, just when Marius arrived in Houston, making Chris feel even more isolated in Cape Town.

Goosen discovered that life at MCV was only marginally smoother than at Groote Schuur. Bosher had fallen out with Hume and been demoted after the appointment of Lower, who now worked in an adjoining lab. For all Lower's deft interpersonal skills, the atmosphere at MCV could be prickly. Yet Goosen enjoyed the comparative peace of life without the Barnard brothers.

And then, to his flesh-crawling horror, the moment came in August 1966. Working quietly in Bosher's lab, he heard the loud braying that had haunted him for so many years. Goosen thought he had gone suddenly insane. He had been in Richmond for a month, and it now sounded as if an especially convincing impressionist had come to town. He soon discovered an even worse reality. The nightmare voice belonged to the real Chris Barnard.

"Howzit, Carl?" Barnard said as Goosen stared at him in shocked despair. "I thought I'd find you here. Listen, man, when are you coming home?"

After David Hume died, in 1973, inadvertently flying his plane into a mountain, one of his colleagues in Richmond murmured an epitaph for a transplant surgeon of almost inextinguishable conviction: "Hume obviously believed the mountain would just move out of his way."

In 1966, however, Barnard was thrilled to be working so closely with Hume. The American crackled with bravado and purpose—and, like Barnard, he loved women and a sense of risk in everything he did. Serious work, however, dominated his life. In Hume's hothouse of inspired research and surgery, Barnard thrived again. He thought rarely of Deirdre, Andre, or Louwtjie. The waterskiing fantasy was erased from his mind by the exhilaration he felt in racing alongside Hume. He knew that this was where he truly belonged, in an American laboratory or operating room, striving to keep up with doctors of flair and imagination—rather than out on a boat, pulling his reluctant daughter across a lake. Richmond saw his rebirth as a surgeon.

"There was a spirit of open scientific inquiry at Richmond which was stimulating," he wrote. "The staff included Dr. Richard Lower who had worked with Dr. Norman Shumway on the technique of heart transplantation. Prodded by Dr. Hume, we never slept, and the drama never ceased."

Barnard chose not to write about the private drama of his encounters with Lower, preferring to focus instead on his work with Hume. During their ward rounds, Hume had pointed out a jaundiced young man suffering from acute liver failure. Hume had introduced a technique called "exchange trans-fusion," in which the patient was given fifteen pints of fresh blood, one pint at a time, while the same amount was gradually withdrawn from his body in an effort to dilute the poison in his system and allow the liver time to repair itself.

Hume knew the possibilities of success were limited. Even a more radical approach, hooking up an excised pig liver to the man's body, could only be used for a maximum of eight hours. Hume was intrigued when Barnard sug-gested that a baboon's liver might be more suited to the task. His assistant, Mel Williams, was skeptical, reminding Barnard that the baboon's natural antibodies in its blood would attack a human patient.

"I'll get rid of them," Barnard said.

"How?" Hume asked.

Barnard proposed cooling down the baboon, washing out his blood with water and then filling him with human blood of the same type as that of the terminally ill young man.

"You believe you can do that?" Hume asked while Williams shook his head.

"*Ja*," Barnard shrugged, feeling the old confidence surging through him, "I can do it."

When they finally obtained a baboon Barnard was surrounded by a crowd of doctors and students, several of whom recorded his work with amateur movie cameras. He used three heart-lung machines. The first circulated the baboon's blood through the machine with a heat-exchanger attached for cooling. When the temperature dropped to 5 degrees centigrade (41° F) and the baboon reached a state of profound hypothermia that protected its brain and heart, Barnard cut the pump and drained all the blood from its body.

The second machine, containing Ringer's lactate solution, washed through the baboon's system, the liquid eventually emerging without a trace of blood. Barnard had by now hooked up the third machine, containing human blood, to the animal. The baboon's heart began to fibrillate. Yet, after Barnard warmed and shocked it, the heart pumped human blood through its cham-bers and out into the arterial system.

The following morning, Barnard went back to the laboratory. His baboon was sitting up in a cage, human blood pulsing through him as he ate an orange. The movie cameras were still rolling to record the successful culmination of a blood transplant. Hume was impressed. He assured Barnard that they would eventually use the technique in a human.

By the time Marius arrived in Richmond, on Saturday, September 3, 1966, during the Labor Day weekend, Chris was so immersed in his work that he paid only minimal attention to his brother. Marius had hitched a lift from Houston with a student named Ken Johnson, who had managed to get himself arrested in New Orleans for speeding. They were taken to the local prison for a formal charge to be lodged against Johnson. While Marius waited outside, the policemen watched him suspiciously. They knew he wasn't an American and so they began to question him. When they learned that he was a South African their mood changed abruptly. Marius was told his people sure knew how to deal with "niggers." He was offered a Coke and treated like a visiting dignitary. Johnson was given an easy ride as soon as the police inside the jail realized he was "a buddy of the South African."

Chris was more interested in hanging out in the lab than listening to Marius's anecdotes. He did nothing to make his brother feel part of the intellectually vibrant Richmond set. They would have time to talk properly, he told Marius, once they were back in Cape Town, the following year. Marius was chilled again by Chris's ability to detach himself from his family and devote himself to a more private quest.

He returned to the loneliness of Houston on September 6—to be greeted by DeBakey's news that the South African prime minister had been assassinated earlier that day. Hendrik Verwoerd had been stabbed by a parliamentary messenger, Dimitri Tsafendas, a Greek South African who was later certified as mentally unbalanced. A week later, John Vorster, the minister of justice, who had led the crackdown that imprisoned Mandela and so many other black leaders, succeeded Verwoerd. South Africa would not shift from its course. "Apartheid is cast in stone," Vorster promised.

Chris Barnard's plans, meanwhile, were about to change radically. One afternoon, while talking to Goosen, and failing to convince him to return home, Barnard watched idly as his former perfusionist cleaned the dog lab. "What are they doing next door?" he asked.

"Richard Lower's about to do another heart transplant," Goosen said quietly.

Barnard had skimmed most of Lower and Shumway's papers over the last six years without seriously considering anything more than the cursory transplant attempts he and John Terblanche had made in 1964. Those few operations had failed hopelessly. "How does Lower do it?" Barnard asked.

Goosen had observed the procedure on numerous occasions after he had been invited into the lab by Lower's technician, Lanier Allen. And so, as he washed and sterilized the bottles and tubes in Bosher's lab, Goosen repeated the basics of Lower's operation. He could tell that Barnard was absorbed, and, as it was a change from his old boss badgering him to fly back home, he suggested that they watch the next experiment as it happened.

"Lower's a good guy," Goosen promised. "He won't mind."

Lower knew that Barnard was a heart surgeon from South Africa, and that he had done some decent valve work, but he was oblivious to the Minnesota connection. Shumway was not in the habit of talking about people he didn't like, and so Barnard's name had not been one he and Lower had ever discussed. Lower allowed the two South Africans into his lab with a cheery wave. Sure, he said, of course it was fine for them to watch him work.

Lower was assisted by Allen, whose black beard and unkempt hair were in stark contrast to Barnard's short-back-and-sides and close-shaven face. Barnard looked a gaunt and aloof man, leaning against the wall with his intense stare absorbing every detail of the transplant. Lower went back to his work. He and Allen repeated the procedure they had done so many times over the past year in Richmond. Using hypothermia and the same surgical technique Lower had developed with Shumway, they switched a heart from one dog to the other with the minimum of fuss and drama.

"*My God, is dit al wat dit is?*" Barnard said softly to Goosen. My God, is that all it is?

Lower listened to the strangely guttural Afrikaans, a language he had never heard before, as he completed his perfect suturing. He soon forgot his visitors as he closed the chest of the recipient dog. They now had another dog to monitor over the coming weeks, months, and even years it might stay alive with a new heart.

Barnard returned the following afternoon. Lower didn't mind. Allen and Goosen were buddies, and Barnard didn't get in the way. Lower concentrated on his work, oblivious to the scrutiny of the South African. The sight of an actual transplant transfixed Barnard, and the simplicity and precision of Lower's surgery encouraged him to believe he could carry out the same operation in Cape Town. Barnard resolved to steal every moment he could in Lower's lab so that he might familiarize himself even more completely with the task of switching hearts.

The sheer power of the heart struck him with renewed force each time he stared down into the empty chest of a dog in that compelling moment just before Lower sutured a new heart in place. The world, Barnard suddenly knew, would be fascinated by a cardiac transplant—for the heart, far more than the liver or kidney, exuded a primal force of life that could not be ignored. A fevered excitement surged through him at the thought that he might actually beat the cautious Lower and Shumway in replicating the technique in a human. He had worked with enough dog hearts to know that they were more difficult to handle than their human equivalent. Barnard could barely believe that Lower and Shumway had not already attempted a transplant in man. He knew that he would be far less cautious than they, for the transplant of a human heart would give him the status for which he had yearned so long.

Hume allowed Barnard to visit Starzl in Denver. Barnard was equally thoughtful as he watched Starzl at work on the kidney and the liver. When he asked him about the heart, Starzl was candid. Shumway and Lower had done outstanding work, and the time for a clinical attempt was near. Starzl had already decided that once he'd cracked the liver transplant in Denver, his unit would turn to the heart. He told Barnard they had recruited a thoracic surgeon, George Pappas, with the intention of following Shumway and Lower into heart transplantation. Barnard did not mention his own sudden interest in the cardiac graft and reiterated his focus on a new renal unit in Cape Town. Starzl welcomed him to the world of kidney transplantation and wished him luck—offering any further help that he might need.

Barnard went back to Richmond for his last few weeks. He maintained the kidney story with Hume, and quizzed him hard about rejection. He also spent a few more afternoons in the lab. While Lower transplanted his dog hearts, Barnard watched keenly and silently.

He was more garrulous with Goosen. Barnard had given up hope of getting his old perfusionist back, but he yearned to return home with his latest idea. "I'm telling you, Carl," he said, "I'm going to bloody do it. . . ."

"What?" Goosen said suspiciously.

"A heart transplant."

"In dogs?"

"*Ja*, I'll do a couple of dogs," Barnard said, "but I'm going to do it in a human."

Goosen looked steadily at Barnard. He believed him. He knew the extent of Barnard's capabilities and the depth of his ambition. Once he made up his mind, there was no stopping him.

The next morning, Goosen told Allen about Barnard's new aim. It was a warning that Barnard was determined to be first. Allen duly relayed the message to Lower. "You're crazy!" Lower laughed as he hunched over one of his dogs. He looked up at Allen and shook his head. "How can he?"

Barnard had done no research, while Lower and Shumway would soon enter their eighth year of preparation. Goosen didn't care who got there first, but he knew the Americans had better watch their backs. Barnard was on his way.

A few days later, Barnard was even more certain. In London to see Donald Ross, his old University of Cape Town classmate who had since become Britain's leading cardiac surgeon, he could not contain his exhilaration. Barnard told Ross that observing Lower so closely at work had opened up his mind to the enormity of cardiac transplantation.

"Christ, Donny," Barnard exclaimed as he gripped Ross tightly by the arm, "I'm going to do it!"

O n January 27, 1967, the first Apollo spacecraft shimmered on launch pad 34 at Kennedy Space Center. A little over three years had passed since JFK's assassination. America had changed, but the old Kennedy fire still burned in the country's consciousness—for an American to be the first man to walk on the moon. The first two stages of the NASA program had been completed successfully. From May 1961 to May 1963, six Mercury craft, each containing a single astronaut, had orbited the earth safely. Ten Gemini flights, blasting twenty men into space, had stretched from March 1965 to November 1966. Each Gemini mission had lasted for a minimum of two weeks and had included a docking with an unmanned craft in space. Apollo would be the third and final leg, culminating in three men landing on the moon.

By 6:30 that evening a trio of silver-suited astronauts—Gus Grissom, Edward White, and Roger Chaffee—had been locked in *Apollo 1* for five and a half hours. They were in training for their upcoming launch on February 21. It had been a long and fraught Friday afternoon with numerous failures in command-center communication. At 6:31 there was another crackle on the radio and the terrible sound of Chaffee's shout: "Fire! I smell fire!"

Two seconds later, White's cry could be heard. "Fire in the cockpit. . . . Get us out of here!"

They were about to be burned alive. Ground staff raced toward the capsule.

The last screams were heard seventeen seconds after Chaffee's warning. *Apollo 1*'s hatch, which opened inward, was fixed tight by latches and an interior pressure far higher than the atmospheric pressure outside. Under ideal conditions it usually took a crew, carrying ratchets, at least ninety seconds to bust open the hatch. This time the intense heat kept driving them back until, five minutes later, they forced a way into a blazing craft. The astronauts had almost certainly perished within thirty seconds of the fire's start.

The New York Times, beneath an "Apollo Program Dealt Hard Blow" front-page headline the following morning, reminded its readers that "last March, President Lyndon Johnson reaffirmed the goal laid down by President Kennedy when he announced the Apollo program in May 1961. The United States, Mr. Johnson said, still intends 'to land the first man on the surface of the moon' by 1970. Less than a week later, the President sounded a note of caution. . . . Apollo, he said, 'has more elements of as yet unproven capability. The months ahead will not be easy as we reach toward the moon.'"

While Secretary of Defense Robert S. McNamara claimed, "Our brave men in uniform, whether in Vietnam or seeking the frontiers of the future, mourn with all of us the tragic loss of three gallant and dedicated American airmen," NASA imposed an immediate four-month suspension of its program.

The Soviet press, having anxiously watched the Americans close the yawning gap between the superpowers in space, was emphatic. "The astronauts fell victim to the space race which the men in charge of the U.S. program launched," insisted *Trud,* an official state newspaper. "Recently, the hurry, the haste in space flights, has continued to grow. There were a number of flaws in the Apollo system. We can say with assurance that this tragedy is far from being a pure accident."

The space race had grown darker and more somber. In a similar way, the cardiac-transplant race would soon turn more fierce, and deadly.

In late May 1967, the *Los Angeles Times* reported, Norman Shumway "disclosed that Stanford surgeons almost attempted a human-heart transplant a few weeks ago, but the proposed surgery was not quite right. Dr. Shumway thinks that replacing a faulty human heart with a heart taken from a cadaver is preferable to implantation of a mechanical heart . . . and it may happen any day." Shumway, as usual, was dead right. They were very near.

Dick Lower had also come close to a human heart transplant eight months earlier. A few weeks after Barnard raced away from Richmond, in the fall of 1966, Lower and Hume were locked in passionate debate. They had a patient in desperate need of a new heart, and they seemed to have found a donor. Hume was ecstatic. The recipient was anesthetized and wheeled into a room where he was lined up alongside a brain-dead man who had the potential to give him a new heart. Virginia's chief medical examiner, who had worked closely with Hume on the examination of kidney donors, was sympathetic to the prospect of the procedure. The donor heart was also on the verge of stopping. Lower knew that as soon it halted, he could cut it out, store it in cold saline, revive it, and then transplant it in less than thirty minutes.

"C'mon," Hume urged, *"do it!"* Lower, however, was less impulsive. He pored over their only obvious problem: ABO blood-type incompatibility between the donor and the recipient. Hume tried to dismiss it as an irrelevance. *"Do it!"* he repeated. They were set up for the transplant and everything made for a perfect match—except, as Lower coolly reminded him, for the different blood types. A person with one blood type automatically forms antibodies against another blood type. In a transfusion there is usually an immune reaction and different symptoms occur—from fever and jaundice to blood in the urine. With full supportive care, a full recovery can still be made after an ABO-incompatible transfusion. Death can also result.

Hume argued that the recipient was going to die anyway. What did they have to lose? He encouraged Lower to begin the world's first human heart transplant. Lower was tempted, but he resisted. He and Shumway had worked carefully for so long. Perhaps Hume was right and they would get away with it. But this was not how he had imagined the first transplant—marching in despite a blood mismatch. It didn't feel right. Lower refused to proceed.

He still felt he had made the right decision even when Hume lamented the fact that they might not have another chance for a year or two. There was an alternative. Since leaving Stanford, Lower had worked on the idea of using a cadaver heart. All scientific and medical logic pointed to the necessity of removing a heart from a brain-dead patient as soon as possible to give the recipient the best chance of survival; and yet it was illegal to take a beating heart from a body. Lower knew that the law and public opinion had yet to catch up with him, Shumway, and Kantrowitz. Even Hume, who had endured his first kidney failures, seemed unsure about pushing the concept of brain death. He had been so positive about their near transplant because the donor heart looked likely to stop just when they needed it most. It had been a coincidence, spoiled only by the blood-match issue.

Lower was not a man to rely on coincidence. He set out to prove, instead, that it was possible to remove a heart from a dead body and bring it back to life. Time was a crucial factor but the tests he ran in dogs had shown that if you removed a heart within fifteen to thirty minutes after it stopped beating, stored it in cold saline, and then perfused and nourished it with oxygen-rich blood from a pump-oxygenator, it would begin to pulse again. Sometimes, Lower said, it would beat so hard you could hear it in the hall outside.

Shumway had run his own tests at Stanford. During his first trials, in October 1966, he managed to revive and transplant ten cadaver dog hearts into animals who survived between ten and thirty-eight hours. Shumway and a Stanford research fellow, William Angell, extended the life of a recipient dog with a revived cadaver heart for thirty-three days. They explored different techniques—sometimes storing the cadaver heart in the neck of another dog, or else helping it recover by means of cross-circulation before the actual transplant. The *L.A. Times* speculated that, in a human case, Shumway might "put a healthy volunteer subject in a hospital intensive-care unit where his blood would be used in a cross-circulation set-up to nourish the donor heart until time for transplantation."

Dick Lower would soon try something simpler, if hardly less outrageous.

Medical College of Virginia, Richmond, Virginia, May 28, 1967

It was a hell of a way to spend a Sunday night in Richmond. Lower had his warm corpse. The kidneys had already been taken from the body so that David Hume could graft them into a patient dying of renal failure. Lower could now have the heart. He closed the doors so that, in the cutting room, he and his research colleague Richard Cleveland would not be disturbed. The recipient was a big and ominously silent bruiser who looked as if he could knock your head off with a right hook. They would need to be careful when they put him under. He was a baboon.

Cleveland imagined the worst. Rather than delighting in the idea that he would witness his fellow surgeon become the first man to transplant a human heart, he was paranoid that both their careers might be ruined by the attempt. Yet Lower had been researching cardiac transplantation for seven and a half years. He was ready to work with a human heart.

Lower and Cleveland worked secretly that night. It was best to keep even Hume out of the room. Lower removed the heart from his fresh cadaver and prepared for the transplant by placing it in the familiar icy saline solution that would lower its temperature to four degrees centigrade (39.2° F). Cleveland, meanwhile, had opened up the chest of the baboon so that Lower could excise its heart and begin his transplant. The human heart was easy to manipulate and suture. It soon began to beat vigorously inside the baboon's chest. Lower had done it. He had transplanted a human heart.

"I know what we should call this," Lower said. "A reverse Hardy!"

They stared down at the baboon stretched out on the laboratory table. It was hard to lift their eyes from the sight of the human heart beating inside the animal.

Lower had never intended it to be anything more than a Sunday-night experiment, simply to prove that a cadaver's heart would actually resume functioning after a transplant. It was another measured step toward the first full-scale clinical attempt between a human donor and a human recipient. By restoring a "dead" heart to life in a different body Lower could now, in an extreme set of circumstances, consider using the morgue as a potential donor pool for future transplants. Although his description of a "reverse Hardy" was a little joke that Shumway would have appreciated, Lower decided not to publish the results of his work that night. He could already tell that the size of the human heart precluded their closing the baboon's chest. And so, after an hour, with the heart still beating, Lower decided to terminate the experiment.

Cleveland let slip a thankful sigh. Only he and Lower had seen the surreal transplant. Their careers, at least for a little while longer, were safe from scandal.

A bleak and rainy winter settled over Cape Town that June while Marius Barnard transplanted hearts between thin, worm-ridden dogs from the pound. Table Mountain rose majestically into the dense gray clouds, and Robben Island could be seen faintly through the gloom. The third anniversary of Nelson Mandela's imprisonment on the island passed on June 12, 1967. He was mourned in the townships of Langa and Gugulutu and ignored in suburbs like Gardens and Pinelands.

Two months earlier, Marius had been rescued from the Texas purgatory where he had wilted beneath the scorn of DeBakey and Cooley. In a rare gesture of brotherly compassion, Chris had offered Marius a position as a cardiac surgeon on his service. He went against his chief, Jannie Louw, who could hardly bear the thought of both Barnards brooding at his hospital. Chris was building his heart-transplant team and he knew Marius would be a diligent addition.

While their work with kidney grafts in the lab was successful, Marius and his "non-white" assistants, Victor Pick and Hamilton Naki, struggled to record a heart transplant survivor. As Lower had discovered in 1958, the aortic tissues in their dogs bled terribly. Chris showed typical irritation at their failure and set aside a day to rescue the situation. His own work was little better. Another few dogs bled to death.

They soon improved. By the end of June, both Chris and Marius had emulated Lower's simple technique, but they made no effort to fight rejection. Chris Barnard was much more specific in his desire to transplant a human heart at the earliest opportunity. He planned on using a human kidney transplant as a test run—for he wanted to confront the patterns of rejection in a human rather than spend years studying immunological problems in dogs. Barnard was convinced the benefits of a thorough preparation for a kidney graft would affect his heart transplant bid. They were still about to leap into the unknown depths with only a fraction of the research knowledge gleaned in Palo Alto, Richmond, and Brooklyn.

In early September 1967 Barnard carefully selected his patient—a middle-aged white woman called Edith Black. Her kidneys were riddled with disease, and so, two weeks later, Barnard and Jannie Louw carried out a bilateral nephrectomy—the complete removal of both kidneys. Barnard inserted a plastic shunt in her arm by which she was attached twice a week to an artificial kidney to clean her blood. They could keep her alive, using the dialysis machine, as long as it took to find a donor.

Realizing that South African law offered them a unique opportunity, as it only required the agreement of two doctors to declare a patient "legally dead," Barnard drew up a set of criteria that would offset any accusations that he was pirating organs from a "living body." He agreed with Lionel Smith, professor of forensic medicine at Groote Schuur, that the donor patient would be examined by a separate neurological unit.

Yet Barnard's greatest contribution to transplantation focused attention on, and obtained clearance for, a simple definition of brain death. He forced through legislation that decreed that a neurosurgeon could confirm brain death if the patient showed no response to light or pain. Once family consent had been obtained, the neurosurgeon would be at liberty to hand over the patient to a transplant team. Those procedures, if handled effectively, could be carried out within thirty minutes—the maximum time Barnard believed they could risk leaving the donor organs in their host body.

He was scrupulous in his assessment of each potential new kidney donor, and the first six candidates were considered incompatible. And then, just before five a.m. on Sunday October 8, 1967, Barnard decided they had found a perfect match. A young colored man involved in a car crash had been declared brain dead and compatible with the recipient. The man's distraught family gave their assent to the transplant.

Barnard was typically nervous as he began Africa's first human kidney graft, screaming at one of his favorite nurses when she was slow to pass him his scalpel. "Oh you are stupid," he yelled at Pittie Rautenbach. "You should work with the baboons in the laboratory." Accustomed to his hysterical outbursts, the transplant team remained calm. Their head nurse, the opera-loving Peggy Jordaan, had always joked among them that Barnard was an even more temperamental diva than Maria Callas. Eventually, he completed a painstaking and exemplary graft.

"The South African newspapers hailed it as a major surgical event," Barnard later reflected on that stressful operation, "and the foreign press gave it overtones of racial integration in a limited physiological arena: 'Mrs Black Gets Black Kidney.' Three weeks later Mrs Black—with a kidney whose potentials of rejection or tolerance did not depend on the color of skin—left the hospital to begin a normal life."

Edith Black, her new kidney making her "feel like a million dollars," would live for another twenty years. In the transplant lab, however, Chris and Marius could not produce a single dog that survived longer than a week with a new heart. Yet the jubilation of the kidney transplant persuaded Chris that "The machinery of the transplant team had functioned perfectly. . . . We [are] ready to undertake a heart transplant."

Chris Barnard wanted the prize of a world first. He wanted medical immortality.

Three days before Barnard transplanted his first kidney, Shumway once again addressed the issue of cardiac transplantation. On October 5, 1967, at a convention of the American College of Surgeons in Chicago, Shumway followed Dick Lower onto the podium. Lower had ended his own lecture with a short film featuring a large brown-and-white mongrel running around and wagging her tail. She was one of two dogs that had been alive for more than fifteen months since receiving new hearts in Virginia. Lower emphasized that "after eight years of laboratory experience we are now quite convinced that cardiac transplantation is a perfectly feasible procedure from the technical as well as the physiological standpoint."

A big man sat near the front of that packed gathering. Adrian Kantrowitz was an expert analyst of the typical Shumway lecture. He'd heard enough of them in the past. But Jordan Haller, his director of cardiovascular surgery, noticed how Kantrowitz leaned forward as Shumway began talking that October afternoon.

"The time has come," Shumway said at the climax of his speech, "for clinical application . . ."

Kantrowitz's elbow slammed into Haller. "Get going." Kantrowitz hissed.

"Why?" Haller gasped as he rubbed his ribs.

"Did you hear him?" Kantrowitz asked in exasperation. "Shumway's gonna do it!"

Ten

THE WAIT

Val Schrire, the chief cardiologist at Groote Schuur Hospital in Cape Town, had gained an international reputation for the scientific precision of his work. He was appalled by Barnard's intentions to transplant a heart after such limited and largely ineffective research. If he had not seen in close-up so much of Barnard's open-heart success, and the extraordinary compassion he brought to his postoperative care, Schrire might have sought a way to block his transplant plans permanently. It was as if Barnard was blind to the risk. He tried to convince Schrire that, because any recipient would be close to death and without any other hope of survival, there was no need for caution. Schrire maintained that the reputation of his hospital—of medicine itself—could be endangered by such a cavalier dismissal of responsibility.

He was even more curt in rejecting Barnard's written suggestion that, for a recipient, they should "take a Bantu with cardiomyopathy because it is a disease common to them with no known cure. This will give us a young man with a good body who has only one defect—heart disease."

Barnard's casual description of black South Africans as "Bantu" and "them" revealed the extent of apartheid's grip on his language. "Forget it," Schrire said angrily. He knew that choosing a black patient for the first heart transplant would open up Groote Schuur to accusations of experimenting on an already persecuted majority. Barnard became increasingly anxious in the midst of such resistance. The most he could coerce from Schrire was the grudging agreement that he'd "think about it."

Barnard's disquiet caused his arthritis to worsen dramatically. His hands and feet began to swell until the pain was so intense he feared it would prevent him from operating if and when Schrire finally decided to approve a patient.

Schrire kept Barnard at bay while he considered the possibility of a transplant. He was aware of the surgeon's opportunistic streak, but Schrire was too reasonable to ignore his achievements. He could not forget Barnard's work on the tetralogy of Fallot, which produced results the equal of any surgeon in the world—including Norman Shumway. Schrire was not a man given to gambling, but he understood that Barnard had the talent to compensate for his hustler's mentality. The cardiologist knew that he was weakening when, without informing Barnard, he began to assess the records of some desperately ill patients. One name kept jumping out at him.

Louis Washkansky had been admitted to Groote Schuur on September 14, 1967—the Jewish New Year. Washkansky, a fifty-three-year-old Jew born in Lithuania, had been placed on the critical list. His wife was warned that it would be a miracle if he was still alive before darkness fell that evening. Six weeks later he lay, breathless and dying, in ward A1, his blue and bloated body barely sustained by a heart reduced to a third of its pumping capacity. The remaining two-thirds were literally dead after the second of two massive heart attacks, in 1965, had destroyed most of his left ventricle. He slid away into a diabetic coma in late October.

Washkansky finally regained consciousness. Yet he had also swelled to twice his normal size with edema and, despite barely eating, had put on thirty-five pounds in four days. Washkansky had to be propped in a chair so that, after drilling holes in his legs, they could drain the excess fluid. His eyes had become like slits in a grotesquely bloated face. The pain was almost intolerable. His wife, Ann, leaned over him because he could hardly talk. "Louis," she said, "how are you?"

Louis managed a smile with his whisper: "I'm on top of the world."

On November 10, despite also suffering from kidney and liver failure, Washkansky was put forward by Schrire as a possible recipient for a heart transplant. Barnard recalled that he had turned down Washkansky as a candidate for cardiac surgery in July—and he was reminded why when he again studied the X-rays of the patient's ruined heart. He had never before seen such destruction of a single heart. It seemed inexplicable that Washkansky could still be alive.

Believing that the psychological makeup of his first patient would be crucial, Barnard went to see Washkansky on his own. As he entered the ward he saw that Washkansky was reading a paperback. The cover featured a cowboy holding a smoking gun.

"He was obviously very sick," Barnard remembered later, "but you could see that he had once been quite strong and good-looking. There were also the features of a generous man—a large mouth, with the face folds of one who smiled often. He had big ears and big hands, and his eyes, peering at me over the spectacles, were gray-green—and waiting. So I spoke to him. . . . [Washkansky replied:] 'I'm ready to go ahead.' He said no more. His eyes remained on me, but with no indication that he wanted to know more. . . . As I turned to go he began reading again. How, I wondered, could he return to pulp fiction after being suddenly cast into the greatest drama of his life? What was it about human nature that caused such a reaction? No man in the history of the world had ever met the surgeon who was going to cut out his heart and replace it with a new human one—at least not until this moment, which was now being lost somewhere in a Western novel. What had made him turn away? He was a realist. He carried no false illusions. He lived for the moment, for the hour, for the full living of all of it. And now I had offered him just that—life. For a dying man it is not a difficult decision."

Ann Washkansky found her husband to be oddly buoyant. He told her that the "big noises"—Barnard and Schrire—had been to see him. Barnard wanted to transplant a heart into him. When she asked if he meant a valve, Louis raised his voice to a shout.

"Not a valve! A heart! He's going to put a bloody heart in."

"Don't swear, Louis," Ann chided. She looked anxiously at Louis's sister, Anne Tabiel, before suggesting that he must have misunderstood Barnard.

As Louis became increasingly frustrated, his sister whispered to Ann, advising her not to argue with her terminally ill husband. "Just humor him. If he says a heart, let it be a heart."

Ann turned and saw a handsome man in a white coat. She muttered to her husband in Yiddish—"*Ver iz er?*" Who's he?

"That's him," Louis hissed. "Barnard."

She was horrified and could barely understand Barnard when he explained the techniques and consequences of cardiac transplantation in his thick Afrikaans accent. All that stuck in her head was the answer he gave when she asked what chance Louis had of surviving such an operation.

"An eighty-percent chance," Barnard said without hesitation.

Ann could think only of the twenty-percent risk, and of the eerie operation, when Barnard left them. She was convinced that Louis would shed his own character and absorb the personality of the dead person whose heart they would give him. She hated the idea of waking up next to someone who looked like Louis but, because of his strange new heart, acted like someone she had never met before in her life. And how could he keep on loving her without the heart he had given her, at least symbolically, so many years before?

They took swabs from Washkansky's skin, nose, throat, mouth and rectum to identify the different organisms living either on or inside his body. Ann shuddered and Louis laughed when Barnard explained that each human is estimated to have 60,000 germs on each square inch of his or her skin. With Louis's immune system needing to be stripped of its power to attack a new heart, the transplant team had to identify which antibiotics they would pump into his body to fight the most dangerous of those organisms lurking inside him. He was washed down continually with pHisoHex, an antiseptic solution, while room 270, where he would be nursed after the transplant, was fumigated. Staff assigned to his intensive care were also swabbed to determine if their bodies could spread any threatening disease—despite the sterile caps, masks, gowns, and gloves they would wear whenever they approached him.

As a hot summer enveloped Cape Town, hastening the passing of another year, Louis Washkansky's spirit revived. He was dying but he believed in the transplant. Barnard would save him. Washkansky began to call him "the man with the golden hands."

He had smiled sweetly when Barnard caught him with a half-empty bottle of lemonade that he'd tried to hide behind a stack of James Hadley Chase paperbacks. He lowered his reading glasses from the bridge of his nose to examine the illicit bottle of sugary drink. "Never seen it before," Washkansky declared while one of the nurses, Sister Marie Papendieck, confirmed to Barnard that she had also caught him with a bag of cherries smuggled into his ward by his brother-in-law—the resourceful professional wrestler Solly Sklar.

The nurse laughed as, having shoved a thermometer into his mouth, she ruffled Washkansky's hair. It was true what his wife said about him—everyone loved Washy.

Norman Shumway and Ed Stinson had already earmarked a thirty-five-year-old patient as the likeliest recipient for the world's first transplanted human heart. After intensive radiation for Hodgkin's disease, the man's heart had begun to fail. Nothing, beyond a transplant, could rescue him. Shumway and Stinson were intent on proceeding because they suspected his immune system, similarly diminished by radiation, would be too weak to reject a new heart.

The recent development of antilymphocyte globulin had given them further hope that they might overcome the onset of rejection. In kidney transplants the use of the drug—derived from a serum produced in animals and used to suppress lymphocyte cells that destroy foreign tissue—had significantly improved the long-term survival rate in organ grafting. Shumway obtained the consent of both the patient and his family to attempt a heart transplant.

While he waited for a donor, Norman Shumway went public. In a rare interview with the *Journal of the American Medical Association*, he repeated that the time had come for clinical application of a technique he and Lower had perfected during eight years of laborious research. "We think the way is clear for trial of human heart transplantation," Shumway was quoted in *JAMA* on November 20, 1967.

Early copies had been released to America's leading newspapers a week earlier, and Stanford's media liaison officer, Spyros Andreopoulos, was inundated with requests for further information. Harry Nelson, the science correspondent of the *Los Angeles Times,* was typical in his desire to be kept informed of Shumway's plans:

> *Dear Spyros:*
>
> *The article by Shumway in the current* JAMA *saying that it won't be long before Stanford or someone does a heart transplant triggers this letter. If you are keeping a list of science writers who are to be informed (perhaps ahead of time on a to-be-released basis), please put me on the list. Just want to make sure I hear about it as soon as anybody else. Thanks.*
>
> *Sincerely,*
> *Harry*

Andreopoulos's reply was even more succinct:

> *Dear Harry:*
>
> *We will certainly keep you posted if and when Shumway does a heart transplant. I don't think it will be soon, but again it might occur if the ideal circumstances prevail.*
>
> *Sincerely,*
> *Spyros*

One of the twentieth century's most dramatic stories was about to break. David Perlman, the science correspondent for the *San Francisco Chronicle,* suggested that "A decade ago, if such an operation was in the offing, it would be a medical secret as closely guarded as an atom bomb. No surgeon would talk about it until the first one was a proven success. Now, however, Dr. Norman Shumway of Stanford University Medical School is announcing publicly that his division of cardiovascular surgery has solved the technical problems of heart transplants, and is ready to attempt the operation in its first human patient."

As Shumway had always planned, the world was becoming more accustomed to the once surreal concept of heart transplantation.

Maimonides Medical Center, Brooklyn, New York, November 21, 1967

Adrian Kantrowitz gazed at the baby with the miraculous hair. He knew they were losing Jamie Scudero. Twenty-four hours earlier he had been summoned when a chest X-ray of the baby revealed a cardiothoracic ratio of 60 percent and increased pulmonary vascular markings. The P waves on the EKG were worryingly tall and spiking, measuring four to five millimeters. A cardiology report duly concluded that "The diagnosis at catheterization is Tricuspid Atresia with patency of the interatrial septum. . . . The patient is thought to be in congestive heart failure."

He'd prepared Jamie quickly for surgery. At 8:30 p.m. on November 20, he and Jordan Haller had opened the baby's chest and inserted a four-millimeter shunt that linked the ascending aorta to the right pulmonary artery. The shunt was known as a "modified Potts" and required intricate anastomosis, the sewing together of blood vessels, to increase the oxygenation of the baby's blood from 45 to 80 percent by allowing the mixed blue blood to travel through the lung again. The additional oxygen would help Jamie "pink up" to a more natural color. His sleek black hair, his distraught mother was promised, would look even more gorgeous against his rejuvenated complexion.

Even after the successful insertion of the shunt just before midnight, his breathing had to be assisted by an endotracheal tube. Kantrowitz had confronted something darker than just tricuspid atresia. Ebstein's anomaly, which results in a severe malformation of the tricuspid valve and causes catastrophic damage to the right ventricle, ruined the baby's heart. The chances of survival were negligible.

Kantrowitz felt compelled to take the last dark risk. He turned away from the incubator to find the baby's mother. He would need Anna Scudero's consent before he could make his own attempt at history.

Groote Schuur Hospital, Cape Town, South Africa, November 22, 1967

Barnard knew that Shumway, Lower, and Kantrowitz were ranged against him—and more disturbing news filtered in from Britain. Donald Ross, Barnard's former Cape Town University classmate, had been persuaded to act as chief surgeon on a possible British attempt at the National Heart Hospital in London. Ross had just returned from Chicago, where, sharing the stage with Lower and Shumway, he had announced a successful breakthrough in thirteen human cases where he'd used the patient's pulmonary valve to replace either their damaged aortic or mitral valve. His surgical renown added credibility to this unexpected British bid to win the prize.

Barnard's first chance came late that afternoon. His old friend Fritz Mangold, a doctor in Caledon, a ninety-minute drive from Cape Town, had found a possible donor for Louis Washkansky. A young colored man from one of the neighboring farms in Riversdale had fallen off a truck and suffered seemingly irrevocable brain injuries. His eyes were dead beneath even a penetrating beam of light. The heart, however, continued to beat inside his chest. Barnard knew he'd have to battle Val Schrire, his chief of cardiology, on account of their privately agreed-upon stipulation that both donor and recipient patients should be white. He would take on Schrire later. Barnard urged Mangold to send him the patient by ambulance.

"And Fritz," he said anxiously, "please hurry."

Even if he had still not quite recovered from the distress of thinking the previous afternoon that Shumway might have already won the race—after he half heard a radio news report of a possible Stanford attempt—Barnard was now perhaps only hours away from the first transplant. At least he would not have to face the same struggle as the Americans when it came to declaring brain death. If the trauma was as complete as Mangold implied, a couple of the neurosurgical boys could wrap up confirmation in ten minutes.

Yet the massive advantage he held over Shumway, Lower, and Kantrowitz—in being free from the draconian U.S. legislation, which could technically charge a surgeon with murder for taking the heart of a brain-dead patient—

was offset by the stigma of apartheid. In a country where black life was rendered so cheap, Schrire was adamant that they could not risk following that same narrow path in an operation as portentous as the world's first heart transplant. He reminded Barnard that hundreds of black South Africans were hanged every year. Tens of thousands were jailed while the remaining millions were oppressed and treated as little more than a cut-rate labor pool. The presence of a black heart donor in a momentous transplant would refocus attention on apartheid rather than their medical breakthrough.

Schrire insisted that they should restrict their search for a donor to the white population, which comprised less than twenty percent of South Africans. Ninety percent of patients suffering from heart disease, meanwhile, were white—for they mostly lived with the indulgence of the typical citizen of the Western world. So while the overwhelming number of recipients in need of a new heart would always be white, the largest donor pool remained unsuitably black.

It would help him to be the first, Barnard knew, if they could take the nearest available heart for Washkansky. And so he wished he could make Schrire see that his very life had been mapped out by his father's dedication to a colored congregation. Barnard was sure that none of the colored people who had carried the coffin of his father would begrudge him using one of their own men as a donor to save the life of poor Louis Washkansky. It was as his father had always told both him and them. We are all the same on the inside. We all bleed the same red blood.

He stared at the clock. Only an hour had passed since the call from Caledon. The ambulance would still be speeding toward Cape Town. Barnard looked down at his hands. Amid the stress of waiting they had begun to ache again.

Finally, just after seven that Wednesday evening, the colored patient arrived. His blood pressure was low and his breathing irregular. The neurosurgeons, led by Peter Rose-Innis, placed him on a respirator and his circulation improved rapidly. There was, however, no brain activity. His blood type, A-positive, was found to be the same as Louis Washkansky's. Dr. M.C. Botha confirmed that the tissue-typing between donor and recipient was similarly compatible. They had their donor.

Barnard phoned the police in Riversdale to request help in tracking down the patient's family so that their permission to remove his heart could be

obtained. He then called the rest of his team, starting with Marius and ending with Dene Friedmann, Deirdre's young waterskiing friend, whom he had
just begun to train as a perfusionist. They were all prepared for their role in
that night's transplant—as was Louis Washkansky.

The call came through from Riversdale confirming that the colored family, in shock after they were confronted by a policeman, had agreed that their
son's heart could be given to an unknown white man. That man, meanwhile,
had his chest and belly washed and shaved in preparation for the transplant.
Washkansky was pensive as they removed the hair from his body. His heart
would be next.

The Barnards and two other surgeons—Rodney Hewitson and Terence
O'Donovan—joined Schrire and the colored donor. The cardiologist was the
eldest of the group, and even though they were so close to making medical history, he still resisted. He could already imagine the headlines in New York and
London. Barnard, however, was determined. The more important issue, he
argued, appealing to Schrire's medical instincts, was to save Washkansky's life.

Schrire hesitated and Barnard pushed forward. He reminded the surgeons of their respective duties. Marius and O'Donovan would put the donor
on bypass, cool him down, and then remove the heart within five minutes of
opening his chest. He and Hewitson would open up Washkansky and carry
out the actual transplant. Hewitson was quiet and thoughtful, a brilliant surgeon with the technique and composure Barnard himself often lacked. And
yet Hewitson, the man Barnard depended on most, had never even attempted
a transplant in a dog—their preparation had been that sketchy.

They were about to take a huge risk and plunge headlong into the
unknown—until Schrire made the decisive intervention. The EKG showed
depressed ST segments, indicating that the heart may have been damaged or
was not receiving enough oxygen-rich blood. Schrire, they all knew, wanted
to provide them with a medical reason to bow out. They could use his exper-
tise as a cardiologist as an excuse not to proceed. Both Chris and Marius wa-
vered. It was as if the courage suddenly drained out of them. Perhaps, after
all, they were not quite yet ready to risk the wrath of the world.

Chris finally nodded to Schrire. "Okay," he said. "Not this time."

"You've done the right thing," Schrire murmured.

They would try again to find a white donor.

Even though Washkansky had been painted with iodine in preparation for the OR, they would wait a little while longer.

Barnard spared Washkansky the real political reason, blaming their false start on problems of blood and tissue typing, and promising they would soon find someone more compatible.

"Do you think we might get another one soon?" Washkansky asked.

"Maybe," Barnard murmured. "I hope so . . . yes."

"It was one of those lies you tell," he wrote later, "to keep courage and hope both for yourself and the patient. I had no way of knowing when we might get a heart for him—if ever."

Ann Washkansky saw the despondency in her husband that night. If she was relieved that the transplant had been delayed, he was mortified. He despaired that they would ever find him a donor. Louis ate his favorite meal, which Barnard had ordered in an effort to console him—steak with an egg on top. He chewed with the solemnity of a fifty-three-year-old man facing his last meal on death row.

Two days later, on the cold Friday morning of November 24, 1967, Adrian Kantrowitz and Bill Neches approached Anna Scudero with devastating news. Her son, Jamie, a mere six days old, had only weeks to live. There was a lone chance, she was told, that her baby might be rescued by a heart transplant. Kantrowitz explained the operation, emphasizing that it had so far been limited to the laboratory. Anna nodded mutely. She would try anything that might save her baby.

Kantrowitz moved fast. A telegram was sent that afternoon to the same five hundred hospitals across America that had been contacted by Maimonides in the search for an anencephalic donor. Kantrowitz prepared himself for the wait, unsure whether it would extend days or weeks. He remained composed. No amount of fretting would hasten the arrival of an anencephalic heart. But this time, as had not happened with the fated Gypsy prince, he was determined he would give his little patient a chance to live. When the call finally came, he would be ready.

Norman Shumway complained to *Business Week* in late November that "we can't get donors. We have a small hospital here. It doesn't get the victims of acute accidents. The ideal donor is somebody who died of brain death—a terminal brain tumor patient." In raising the issue of brain death in a nonmedical magazine, Shumway had continued to broaden the transplantation debate. Yet, when it mattered most, he was still forced to wait.

Earlier that week they thought they might have found a potential donor—until Shumway noticed the ethnicity of the brain-dead patient. He was Chinese, and his family, as customary in their mother country, refused to allow his body to be used for medical purposes. They were not even willing to discuss the wild Western concept of heart transplantation. Shumway, respecting their beliefs, resumed his vigil.

Cape Town, South Africa, December 2, 1967

That Saturday afternoon, Edward Darvall and his wife, Myrtle, sat in the backseat of their daughter's new car, a little green Ford Anglia. Behind the wheel, twenty-five-year-old Denise sang the wordless tune to "Lara's Theme," from *Doctor Zhivago*, which she had spent the past hour trying to teach her brother to play on the piano. Keith was fourteen, and his loud humming in the front passenger seat joined his sister's more tuneful singing as the car edged slowly through the traffic toward Milnerton, where they were expected for tea.

They had decided to drive down Main Road rather than take the faster freeway because Myrtle wanted to buy their friends a caramel cake at the Wrensch Town Bakery in Salt River. Joseph Coppenberg's bakery was famous for its doughnuts—"with or without cream"—but Myrtle, watching her weight, resisted her husband's encouragement to buy a half-dozen. "We'll just get the cake," she insisted as she and Denise climbed out of the car, opposite the bakery, at 3:35 p.m.

They hesitated outside the car as they waited for a break in the traffic. It was a section of Main Road known as "The Bronx." Most of the shops and small houses, dwarfed by the surrounding factories and industrial warehouses, belonged to colored families. Some of the older colored children played "chicken" along Main Road, timing the moment they ran in front of a speeding car so there was just enough danger to make the watching *skollies* (delinquents) whoop in admiration. The less fortunate miscalculated their run and joined the 4,000 victims killed in road accidents in Cape Town during the previous two years.

Denise and her mother were more sensible. A conservative and reserved girl, Denise worked at a bank and lived with her parents. Yearning to meet her first serious boyfriend, she was fond of ballet, classical music, and romantic novels. That morning she had asked her only close friend at the bank, Jean Coetzee, to pick up the new Barbara Cartland novel for her. She was similarly struck by the sentimental Christmas decorations all over town— fairy lights depicting scenes of reindeer and snowmen, cascading icicles and shivering robins. Under the glaring African sun, Denise loved the fantasy of a traditional white Christmas from a faraway land.

Even the Jewish bakery had entered into the Christmas spirit. Chocolate log cabins and snow cakes topped with beaming Santas and plastic pine trees dominated the window display. Denise and Myrtle Darvall stood patiently in the long line, waiting for their sticky caramel cake.

Ann Washkansky, meanwhile, drove slowly out of the Groote Schuur parking lot and down the hill toward Main Road. She and her sister-in-law, Grace Sklar, had just been to visit Louis. He was the lowest they had ever seen him. Since the canceled transplant attempt ten days earlier, Barnard had come no closer to producing a donor. While Louis lay in bed that Saturday morning, a couple of the doctors had dropped by to check on him and to reveal that they were heading off for a weekend of fishing. It felt to him as if the world was simply spinning on without him. Doctors were fishing while he was dying.

"They can go to hell," Louis said to his wife. "I'm getting out of here." But with legs too swollen and poisoned for him to walk, and without enough breath in his body, Louis simply wheezed on his back in the cramped bed. His bloated belly and bluish skin made him look like a dying whale washed up on the beach.

"We'll see you tonight, Louis," Ann had promised as she bent down to kiss him.

Denise and Myrtle Darvall left the bakery at 3:40. They could see the green Ford in front of them, but their vision to the right was obscured by a large truck making its last delivery of the week. Driving in the opposite direction from Ann Washkansky, a thirty-six-year-old Afrikaans salesman and police reservist named Frederick Prins kept his foot down on the accelerator. He had been drinking, and with his eyes on the truck rather than the road in front of him, he never even saw the two women.

Keith and Edward Darvall, waiting impatiently in the car, wondering if they would make it in time for tea at four o'clock, had tired of looking across the street at the bakery. And so they heard, rather than saw, the accident. It came with a loud thud and a high screech of tires. Prins's car hit Myrtle hard, killing her instantly, before it knocked Denise into the air. As she fell, her head cracked against the back hubcap of the Zephyr. She rolled as she hit the road, ending up in the gutter. Blood was already streaming from her nose, mouth, and ears. Her mother lay in the middle of Main Road.

Keith Darvall saw the bodies. "Dad!" he screamed. "It's Mom and Denise!"

A crowd had already gathered by the time they ran across the street. Edward could not get near his wife but her absolute stillness terrified him. He turned to his daughter and tried to pick her up but another man, racing toward him, yelled at him. "No," the man shouted, "don't touch her." He was a doctor, Louis Ehrlich, who had just been to a bar mitzvah.

The Groote Schuur ambulance arrived within five minutes of the accident. Fred Munnik, the driver, saw the crumpled posture of the first body and knew that they had at least one fatality. Ehrlich soon confirmed that the younger woman had suffered a compound skull fracture. She was still alive, breathing heavily and turning her head from side to side.

Ann Washkansky's car slowed on the other side of the road. She and Grace Sklar stared out at the carnage. "Oh my God," Ann said. "There's a woman in the road."

"There're two of them," her sister-in-law replied. She then recognized the doctor attending to the thin body in the gutter. "That's Louis Ehrlich . . ."

Ann shuddered, less at the coincidence of seeing a doctor they knew than at the presence of death. At least Louis was still alive. She drove on, unaware that out of such mindless tragedy a possible source of hope had been found for her husband.

Chris Barnard had left the hospital for home around midafternoon. He recalled later that, after an argument about him returning late, Louwtjie had locked herself in their son's bedroom while he listened to his Ink Spots records. Barnard eventually became drowsy and he drifted in and out of sleep. He claimed in subsequent accounts that his subconscious took over, leaving him with the sudden conviction when he woke that he should not follow Lower and Shumway's surgical technique to the letter.

In Richmond, while studying Lower at work, Barnard had watched the American surgeon cut away the back wall of the atrial chambers of the donor heart so that the remaining bulk of the organ could be sutured to the dangling remnants of the recipient heart. This entailed cutting across the septum, or central wall, of both hearts, and could damage the donor organ. Barnard resolved that he would instead allow the septum to remain intact in the donor heart and that, rather than cutting away the entire back wall, he would slice open two small holes—giving him access to the two venae cavae and four pulmonary veins. He would then suture these holes to the dangling lid of Washkansky's old heart. The septum of the donor heart would remain untouched.

It was one more example of Barnard following his instincts—rather than testing his theories laboriously—in a surgical modification that could possibly threaten the life of his patient even as he sought to protect his new heart. Supposedly energized by the innovative twist he planned to add to the Stanford procedure, he made himself dinner and was just about to go back to his bedroom when the phone rang. Coert Venter, the doctor responsible for Washkansky on ward C2 that night, claimed excitedly that they had found a brain-dead donor and detailed the extent of Denise Darvall's injuries.

"Is she colored?" Barnard asked.

"No," Venter said in surprise. "Why?"

Barnard didn't have time to explain the political ramifications of his battle with Val Schrire. He told Venter that Peter Rose-Innis, the hospital's senior neurosurgeon, should call him as soon as he had finished his final examination. A long hour passed. Barnard paced up and down his study, tormenting himself with doubt and longing for a definitive diagnosis.

At Groote Schuur, Rose-Innis studied the X-rays which revealed that Denise Darvall's skull had been fractured in two places. The first break extended across the base, from one ear to the other in a grotesque parody of a smile. A second crack ran deep inside her skull, to the very point of her nose. It was obvious why her eyes were lifeless and why she registered no sign of pain when they poured ice water into her ear. Her brain was devoid of any sign of electrical activity when they ran the scan. Only a blood transfusion and a respirator maintained the beat of her heart.

Barnard shivered when he heard the news. The donor's blood type, O-negative, although not the same as Washkansky's, was considered compatible. While he yelled in exasperation when he heard that they had not yet obtained Edward Darvall's consent, Barnard was exultant on the inside.

He shouted out to Louwtjie that he was racing back to the hospital—"*I'm going to do the transplant tonight!*" His jubilation was greeted only by silence. Barnard did not even try to coax her out of their son's room. He was already running toward his car.

Edward Darvall sat on a hard wooden chair in a hospital office. He had never felt more alone. His wife was dead. His daughter, her skull crushed, lay on a table behind the closed doors across the hall. He thought that the doctors inside were still trying to save her life. Darvall had held himself together just long enough to ensure that his teenage son had been taken away by two of his cousins. The sixty-six-year-old man was an old father. In the last year, part of his stomach had been removed in emergency surgery, and he'd also suffered a coronary thrombosis. He thought he should be the one on the slab—not his fifty-three-year-old wife or his sweet, innocent daughter. His family had been ripped to pieces in an instant, just because they had stopped to buy some caramel cake.

The doctors had sedated him earlier that evening. He was still in a daze when Coert Venter knocked gently and opened the office door. Venter was accompanied by another doctor on the transplant team, Bertie Bosman, who, before speaking, made him rest on the couch. Bosman revealed gently that there was nothing more they could do for Denise. The father stared at the doctor, his eyes wide and unblinking. Bosman, a sensitive man, found his task almost unbearable. But he kept talking, choosing his words with great care as he explained that while Denise could never be brought back to even the most remote semblance of consciousness, her heart continued to beat. But it pumped inside an empty shell—his daughter had already taken leave of her body.

Bosman paused, allowing the terrible impact of his words to be absorbed. Darvall shook his head. First his wife, and now his daughter. "That's pretty hard luck," he said softly.

Darvall saw the kindness in Bosman's eyes. That helped him focus on the next series of shattering words. There was a man in the hospital, Bosman said, whom they could still save. He was desperately ill and in need of a heart transplant. Bosman's voice shook as he suggested that Darvall could do a great favor to the man, and to all humanity, if he would allow them to transplant Denise's heart. Darvall remained quiet. Bosman and Venter withdrew, stressing that he should take as long as he needed to consider their request. They would understand if he declined to give his consent.

Edward Darvall said later that, in the four minutes it took him to reach his decision, he thought only of his daughter. He remembered a birthday cake she had once made for him. She had carved a heart into the icing and written the words "Daddy We Love You" across the top of the cake. He also remembered that, with her first week's salary from the bank, she had bought him a bathrobe. That was Denise, that was his girl. That was how he would always think of her. She was full of love. She always wanted to give rather than take. He knew that the world needed more people like her. And now Denise and her mother were lost to him. He began to cry; and it was in that moment that he knew what needed to be done.

After composing himself, he summoned the doctors back into the small room. Bosman and Venter would never forget his words. "If you can't save my daughter," Edward Darvall said, "you must try and save this man."

They sat on the floor together, Chris and Marius Barnard, enjoying the coolness of the scrub room tiles against their skin. It was almost midnight but the December heat hung over Cape Town. They were about to shower and then scrub their arms and hands with antiseptic solution. Chris's hands, at least, were free from pain. They would apply antiseptic ointment to their nostrils and dress themselves in surgical greens, then cover their heads and faces with caps and masks. They felt more like brothers than they had in years. It was the kind of night, a once-in-a-lifetime night, when they wished they could see their father again. Their mother was now in a nursing home in Cape Town. Her mind was slipping away, and she would never comprehend the scale of what her sons were about to attempt. Yet she had always driven them to be first in anything they did.

Chris had already been to see both Denise Darvall and Louis Washkansky. He noticed how pretty she looked, with her dark hair and soft features not totally obliterated by her caved-in skull and the brain tissue oozing from her right ear. He and Washkansky, meanwhile, had been through the same dance the previous Wednesday, which perhaps helped explain why the ill man lying on his back sounded so wry. Washkansky reminded Barnard that he was a betting man. The doc's prediction of an eighty-percent chance of success translated into bookie's odds of four to one.

"The odds always change at the last minute," Washkansky reminded Barnard. "Are they moving my way—or against me?"

"Your way," Barnard said.

The orderly had begun to shave his stomach. "Tell Ann," Washkansky said to Barnard, "it's in the bag."

In the scrub room with his brother, Chris felt the old doubt rise up. He was so close, but the task suddenly seemed impossibly daunting. He thought of all the dogs he had lost after transplanting their hearts. He was not like Shumway or Lower or Kantrowitz, with their long-term survivors. He was just an Afrikaner from the Karoo, from a country without even a single television set. And now he and his brother were about to attempt the most daring operation in medical history.

Marius calmed him. He began to discuss the surgical practicalities, stressing that he and O'Donovan would open Denise's chest but that Chris should excise her heart. It was essential that he acquaint himself with the size and feel of the donor heart as early as possible.

Chris knew he should thank his brother for his foresight, but the words would not come. He was already lost in the transplant.

Theater A, Groote Schuur Hospital, Cape Town, December 3, 1967

When he saw Louis Washkansky's heart for the first time, after Rodney Hewitson had exposed the huge bloated muscle in the early hours of that Sunday morning, Barnard looked at the "heaving waste and ruin of a ravaged heart . . . rolling and heaving, one beat after another, like a boxer about to collapse in the ring."

Hewitson's brown eyes lifted in amazement over his pale blue mask.

"Did you ever see anything like it?" Barnard asked.

"Hardly," Hewitson replied in his typically clipped manner as he lifted the left ventricle.

Barnard later wrote that the "chamber was bigger than anything I had ever seen—its walls scarred as the humps of ancient whales, bloated and extended from coronary attacks and muscle death." It was almost beyond belief that it had kept Washkansky alive as long as it did.

Instructing Hewitson to prepare Washkansky for bypass, Barnard walked to the adjoining Theater B, linked by a short corridor at the rear of the two green rooms.

Marius and O'Donovan were waiting for him. It was 2:20 a.m. They made a note of the time as Denise's ventilator was silently switched off. Unable to sufficiently oxygenate her heart with her own labored breathing, they knew that it would stop beating naturally from hypoxia, or lack of oxygen in the blood, within ten to twelve minutes. Yet her heart would be unnecessarily damaged while they waited for it to die. O'Donovan insisted, however, that he would not lift a surgical instrument until the EKG line had flattened. They might have the law on their side, but the ancient lore of medicine cast a heavy shadow over the table. It seemed wrong, at least to O'Donovan, that they should cut out a beating heart.

Chris needed Marius, once more, to intervene. Stressing that their responsibility lay with the recipient rather than the brain-dead donor, Marius urged Chris to overrule O'Donovan and take the heart. If he needed it to stop beating, as conventional medical ethics dictated, they should inject it with potassium. And then they could take it and begin the transplant. While a measured dose can help maintain a regular beat, a strongly concentrated infusion of potassium literally paralyzes the heart for a period of time. Once stilled, Marius argued, they could remove the heart quickly and implant it in Washkanksy, offering more hope for success than if they adhered to outdated medical ethics. Chris knew that Marius was right. He nodded his assent. Marius reached for the potassium while O'Donovan watched silently. It was a decision that they swore would always remain secret from the world outside.

"All right," Chris said after the potassium immobilized her heart, "start cutting."

Barnard scrubbed again at the small basin while he listened to the sound of the saw cutting into the chest of Denise Darvall. They worked quickly, and by the time Barnard completed his final scrub, the small heart looked blue and inert. Marius had already inserted the catheters into the right atrium and the ascending aorta.

"Pump on," Marius told Alistair Hope, who switched on the heart-lung machine.

The little heart immediately turned a beautiful shade of pink as cold blood flowed from the machine.

They needed to cool her body to below 28 degrees centigrade (82.4° F). When Hope called out that the temperature had lowered to 32 (89.6° F), Barnard knew that they were close. "Okay, boys," he said, "I'll be back in a minute."

Fourteen people were waiting for him in Theater A—surgeons, perfusionists, and nurses. "Hook onto bypass," Barnard instructed. "All set, Rodney?"

Hewitson nodded, silent behind his mask.

"Pump on," Barnard said.

The room fell silent as the motor began to hum. Blood flowed through the tubes and in and out of Louis Washkansky, bypassing his heart and lungs.

Dene Friedmann, Barnard's young perfusionist, spoke the first alarming words: "Line pressure's just over 200."

It rose to 250, then 275. Ozinsky confirmed the readings and the likelihood that a narrowed artery was blocking the flow of fresh blood. Barnard knew that without the inflow of newly oxygenated blood they would not be able to keep Washkansky alive long enough to attempt the transplant. When the pressure reached 300 and Barnard was convinced that the lines were about to blow, he instructed them to cool Washkansky down as fast as possible so that they could interrupt his circulation and buy themselves some time.

Once his temperature had plummeted to 26 degrees (78.8° F), Barnard made a purse-string stitch in Washkansky's aorta, stabbed a small hole in its center, and plunged in a catheter so that it could be hooked onto the arterial line of the machine.

"Clamp the line," Barnard ordered his senior nurse.

Peggy Jordaan did as she was instructed. Yet she clamped the line before Barnard issued the order to switch off the heart-lung machine. Blood began to spill onto the floor, while air filtered through the pump and up toward Washkansky's brain.

"Cut the pump!" Barnard yelped.

The hum of the machine died away into a terrified hush. They were in desperate trouble. Barnard knew that air, deadly to the brain, was curling up through the pump. As soon as the air hit Washkansky's brain they would be facing certain doom. Their patient would be brain-dead even before they had a chance to give him his new heart.

"Dammit!" Barnard screamed helplessly. "Are you stupid?"

"But you said, 'Clamp the line,'" Jordaan protested.

"I never did," Barnard roared, knowing that everyone had already heard him say those exact words.

Amid his fury, the impossibility of removing the air from the machine was suddenly replaced by an instinctive gesture. Reacting with lifesaving speed, Barnard ripped the leads from Washkansky before the air could hit his brain. He then reconnected them and gave the calmer command: "Turn on the pump."

Barnard knew that his automatic reaction would probably clear the arterial circuit of its lethal air bubbles. Ozzie's voice soothed him further. "Don't worry . . . there's still plenty of time."

Dene Friedmann, meanwhile, used a couple of green towels to mop up the pools of blood. As she wiped the floor clean they waited in silence. It took two minutes before Johan van Heerden, the chief perfusionist, finally said the words that confirmed they had removed the last vestiges of deadly air: "All clear."

Ozinsky revealed that the line pressure had returned to 100. "Maybe you should go get that other heart," he told Barnard, "before someone else claims it."

In Theater B, Barnard made the first two incisions, cutting the superior vena cava and inferior vena cava, before he turned to the aorta and then the pulmonary artery. Four vessels were left—the four pulmonary veins leading into the left atrium. He made sure that he used his modification of the Lower-Shumway technique, and when he had cut each vessel, the heart was free. Marius held out a steel basin filled with ice-cold Ringer's lactate solution.

Chris Barnard lifted the small heart out of Denise Darvall's chest with his gloved hands. He placed the heart in the container.

"Okay," he said, taking the dish from Marius, "here goes . . ."

Slowly and carefully, his eyes never leaving the heart, he walked the thirty-one steps separating one operating room from the other.

In Theater A, at the head of the table, he gave the heart to Peggy Jordaan. He swung back to Washkansky's opened chest.

Barnard cut the aorta close to Washkansky's heart, but, using a technique he had seen Dick Lower apply in Virginia, he left behind more tissue than he needed. He cut the pulmonary artery in the same way and prepared for the six smaller vessels. After a few more minutes, the chambers were at last opened and he cut down through the septum—allowing the heart to fall back into its cavity.

When Barnard lifted Washkansky's bloated heart up and out of him, he looked down into the blasted and empty hole of his chest. It was huge. Barnard felt the enormity of the moment, and wrote later of a chill ripping through him as he stared into the chasm. "I had never seen a chest without a heart or with such a hole—as though the hole itself was fixed and permanent, while the man, with his chest split open, was merely a temporary object, existing briefly around the hole. And, in fact, it was just that—something few men had ever seen: a human being without a heart, yet held in life by a machine eight feet away."

Barnard understood the profundity of what he was about to attempt, but he did not have time to linger. He nodded to Hewitson, who then delicately placed Denise Darvall's heart into the chest of Louis Washkansky.

"For a moment I stared at it, wondering how it would ever work. It seemed so small and insignificant—too tiny to handle all the demands that would be put upon it. The heart of a woman is twenty percent smaller than a man's, and the heart of Washkansky had created a cavity twice the normal size. All alone, in so much space, the little heart looked much too small—and very lonely."

The surgeons began to sew and stitch. They worked mostly in silence, as they attached the heart to its new home. When they reached the aorta, they decided to cut the machine so that they could work without perfusion and remove the catheters and clamps to give them more space. It took nineteen minutes to cut and shape the aorta and then complete the anastomosis. The heart had turned blue.

At 5:43 a.m. that Sunday morning, Barnard released the venous snares and allowed the blood to flow once more. The heart tensed as warm, oxygenated blood flooded into the muscle. Slowly, it turned pink and began to fibrillate. Ozinsky injected 100 mg of suxamethonium, a muscle-relaxant drug, into the heart-lung machine to prevent Washkansky's body from jerking violently when they shocked the heart.

Barnard called for the paddles. Peggy Jordaan passed him the two gray discs, wired up to the defibrillating machine, which he attached to each side of the heart. Hewitson inserted a sucker into the pericardial sac to drain excess blood from around the heart.

"Go ahead," Barnard said quietly, "shock it."

Ozinsky sent a 20-joule charge into the heart. "For a moment," Barnard wrote, "the heart lay paralyzed, without any sign of life. We waited—it seemed like hours—until it slowly began to relax. Then it came, like a bolt of light. There was a sudden contraction of the atria, followed quickly by the ventricles in obedient response—then the atria, and again the ventricles, Little by little it began to roll with the lovely rhythm of life."

As soon as they switched off the machine, the transplanted heart faltered. The blood pressure reading dropped to 70. Barnard ordered them to revert to the pump. They waited for five nervous minutes before they tried again. The same pattern occurred. Barnard remembered grimly how many dogs he had lost when he could not wean them off the machine.

At 6:13 a.m. they made another fretful attempt. "Cut the pump," Barnard said.

There was another hesitation in the heart, as if it was deciding whether or not to live in its huge new body, and then it began to beat more strongly. The pressure soared back up to 90.

"Jesus, dit gaan werk!" Barnard said, reverting to Afrikaans. Jesus, it's going to work!

He looked around the room. "Eyes over masks blinked back," he remembered later, "moist with joy and wonder. In the theater the tension of silence broke with mixed sighs, mumbled words, and even a little laugh. All of us, like the heart itself, were suddenly sure of ourselves."

Barnard had won the race. He had become the first man to transplant a heart from one human being to another. The surgeon watched it beat for another minute more and then, smiling behind his mask, he removed the last catheter and tied the purse-string suture. The heart pulsed steadily and determinedly. A solid echo of its beat resounded from the EKG. The machine lit up with a perfect green pattern on the black screen.

Barnard stretched his right hand across the opened chest of Louis Washkansky. Rodney Hewitson did the same. His glove was also red with blood.

"We made it!" Barnard said as their hands locked across the pumping heart. "Jesus, we did it!"

Eleven

FAME AND HEARTBREAK

At 6:45 that crisp and light December morning, four and a half hours after they had begun the procedure, Chris Barnard gave into ordinary human craving. Suddenly desperate for a cigarette and a cup of tea, he walked out of Theater A and left Rodney Hewitson to close Louis Washkansky's chest. Peeling off his mask and the unusually thin surgical gloves he wore in an effort to spare his arthritic hands during surgery, Barnard walked alone down the corridor toward the tearoom.

Marius and Bertie Bosman were waiting for him. It was typical of their postoperative routine that Chris, notorious for never buying cigarettes himself, would bum a smoke off Bosman. As he took his first long drag and stirred his sweet tea, his brother brought over a plate of avocado sandwiches the hospital caterers had prepared for the surgeons after their night-long ordeal. Smoke snaked from his nose as he rested his cigarette in the ashtray. His eyes were flat with fatigue. Chris bit into a sandwich while he allowed Marius to check his pulse.

Three and a quarter hours earlier, at 3:30 a.m., with his own work done for the night, Marius had joined the small crowd of doctors and nurses who had gathered on the wooden benches in the theater gallery to watch the making of history. As a way of passing the time, for there was little they could see as Chris worked with his back to them, Marius had tried to measure his brother's heart rate. Watching a vein throbbing in his neck with alarming force, Marius counted the beats. While his method was crude, relying on the naked eye, he estimated that Chris's heart pulsed 130 times a minute during the most extreme periods of the operation.

In the tearoom, with his finger on Chris's wrist, in a more traditional and reliable gauge, it reached 140, sixty beats per minute faster than normal. Marius, who had almost cried when Denise Darvall's heart had begun to live again in its new body, understood how the intense drama had affected them all. There was no need for words as Chris took a couple of deep and furious puffs before he drank his tea in three fast swallows. He could not stay out of the OR for long.

Hewitson was in the midst of sealing the chest while Ozinsky confirmed that Washkansky had opened his eyes briefly and responded to light. His brain had evidently not been affected by the transplant and his pulse, in an improvement on the surgeon's own galloping heart, had steadied to 120 beats a minute. While Barnard fretted, reminding Ozinsky of the exact amounts of hydrocortisone and Imuran he needed to administer to prepare for the anti-rejection treatment, Hewitson worked around the tubes they had inserted into Washkansky. Once the stitching had been completed they would carefully lift Washkansky from the table and lay him on the trolley without disconnecting any of the nine bottles and drips feeding fluid and drugs into him. Then they would shroud Washkansky in a sterile plastic tent, tucking it under his mattress to keep him cocooned against infection, and wheel him away to room 240.

Barnard returned to the tearoom, where M. C. Botha, his immunologist, had joined the smokers. Offering Barnard another cigarette, he suggested that they should telephone the hospital's medical superintendent, Jacobus Burger, to inform him of their success. A disgruntled Burger, plainly unhappy to have been woken just after seven on a Sunday morning, took a few minutes to be convinced that Barnard had transplanted a heart between humans rather than dogs. Yet within half an hour, confirmation of the transplant had been delivered to John Vorster, South Africa's bullfrog-faced prime minister, by Lappa Munnik, the Cape provincial director of hospital services.

Vorster immediately saw the opportunity to use the transplant as a publicity coup for white South Africa. "We must take every opportunity for international prestige this breakthrough gives us," he wrote in an internal memo to his cabinet. "We can link a moment of medical history to a positive image for the country after all the propaganda directed against us around the world. We should congratulate and encourage the head surgeon—Professor Christiaan Barnard—at every turn."

The newspapers that morning had devoted most of their front pages to the "Weekend of Suspense for SA," as the Johannesburg *Sunday Times* described it. The tension did not relate to either the previously secret transplant or some profound public concern about apartheid. The white minority were entranced instead by a tense Davis Cup tennis tie between South Africa and Spain at Ellis Park, in Johannesburg. With the campaign for a sports boycott of apartheid South Africa gathering momentum, any international contest featuring the nation's white athletes had assumed a heightened significance. While they would eventually lose 3–2 to the Spanish team of Manuel Santana and Manuel Orantes, on Sunday morning there was still a chance for a home victory. *The Sunday Times* featured a photograph of an anxious Vorster watching the doubles the previous afternoon at Ellis Park before confirming that he was "immensely proud" of the South African players. He also pointed out, in a rare attempt at Nationalist humor, that the drama of the Davis Cup was "not good for the heart." The transplant, however, was about to bring extremely gratifying news for Vorster and his government.

Barnard's concentration that night had been focused solely on the surgical demands of the first transplant. He had not thought to take any photographs of the operation or to tip off any local reporter that a world scoop was set to unfold early that Sunday. While he wanted to beat Shumway, he was even more intent on a successful transplant that would save Washkansky. In the event, after the actual operation, he needed to do little to generate a near-hysterical momentum of interest. By the time he called Burger, news of the transplant had already spread throughout the hospital. An unknown but enterprising hospital employee made the first contact with the *Cape Times*, while Burger was instructed by civil servants in the health department to record details of the transplant for the South African Broadcasting Corporation's national radio news at noon.

Just before eight, having monitored the return of Washkansky to his sterilized room, Barnard anxiously checked the EKG readings, which indicated an occasional atrial flutter. Washkansky was otherwise stable. He had opened his eyes again and been told that he had come through the operation safely. Barnard could not be sure, but he thought that Washkansky nodded in recognition before he slid back into oblivion.

He next saw Ann and Louis's brother, Tevia, who had arrived from special prayers at their synagogue. Barnard offered a guarded sense of hope. The next twenty-four hours, he stressed, were critical.

His exhaustion was mingled with elation as, finally, he changed back into the navy-blue shirt and cream trousers he had pulled on thoughtlessly twelve hours earlier when he'd first heard about Denise Darvall. Barnard hated the shirt, a present from Louwtjie, and usually never wore it. Now, feeling like the luckiest guy in the world, he decided it would become his favorite shirt. He headed for the hospital's front entrance in search of some fresh morning air before driving home for a few hours of rest. Barnard was conscious of how many people seemed to be either beaming or gawking at him. He grinned back, already feeling like a star.

The first face he recognized belonged to Raoul de Villiers, who had worked with both Barnard and Kantrowitz. De Villiers, whose dislike of Barnard had long been obvious, had just met another ecstatic doctor when he arrived for his Sunday-morning rounds. As he parked his car, de Villiers had been greeted effusively by Johan de Klerk, a urologist at Karl Bremer Hospital.

"Hello, Gay," de Villiers said, addressing de Klerk by his customary nickname.

"Raoul! Raoul!" shouted de Klerk, who was literally bouncing up and down with a cooler in either hand. "I've got two kidneys here. I'm going straight from here to do a transplant."

"Good for you," de Villiers said coolly, unaware of developments the night before. Edward Darvall had also consented that his daughter's kidneys be used in a transplant at Karl Bremer. The recipient would be a ten-year-old colored boy, Jonathan van Wyk, who suffered from chronic kidney disease. They could cross the color line with a kidney—but not yet with a heart.

Chris Barnard was one of the last men de Villiers wanted to see next, especially so early on a Sunday morning. But there was no escape. Barnard bore down on him and called out his name.

"I've just done the world's first heart transplant," Barnard exclaimed, knowing that de Villiers, after his Brooklyn sojourn with Kantrowitz, would appreciate the international significance more than most at Groote Schuur.

De Villiers heard the historic claim but made no reply—he did not even lift his eyes. He stalked past his fellow Afrikaner in a determined show of disdain. At the hospital entrance, just as he was about to turn left to the elevators, de Villiers looked back. He saw Barnard staring in amazement at him. It was as if Barnard expected de Villiers to bow down to him. But de Villiers knew a more bitter truth. His head was suddenly filled with the names of the American surgeons who had worked for so many years on transplantation. He remembered hearing how closely Barnard had watched Dick Lower in Virginia. As he turned away from Barnard, the questions roared in his head:

What about Lower? What about Kantrowitz? How would they feel?

And then, despite his affection for Kantrowitz, de Villiers thought even more of another brilliant man on the other side of the world. The question echoed through him until it became a statement of silent outrage:

What about Shumway? What about Shumway? What about Shumway!

546 East Seventeenth Street, Brooklyn, New York, December 3, 1967

The night before that fateful morning, Adrian Kantrowitz had relaxed with a drink at home in Brooklyn. His mind was full of Jamie Scudero and the looming transplant, but he felt good. The telephone, he was sure, would soon ring with the news that they had found him a donor. Shumway was close, but Kantrowitz felt destined to be the first. Only a few days, perhaps even hours, separated him from history. The big man settled down in his chair at the head of the dinner table, surrounded by his family, and gathered himself for the momentous week ahead.

Sleep came easily to Kantrowitz that night as, unknown to him, they transplanted a human heart in Cape Town.

His eldest daughter, sixteen-year-old Niki, was the first to wake on a quiet Sunday morning in New York. She ambled into the kitchen and turned on the radio. The morning news drifted over the slow hiss of the kettle. Niki knew how near her father was to the first heart transplant, and so the sound of those same words transfixed her. She absorbed the full impact and then began to run.

"Dad! Dad!" she shouted as she crashed into her parents' bedroom.

Kantrowitz propped himself up on an elbow and blinked at his daughter.

Niki blurted out the news. "Some joker in Africa has done a heart transplant!"

"Jesus . . ." Kantrowitz groaned. He knew who had beaten him. *"Barnard!"*

Kantrowitz soon stood barefoot in the middle of his kitchen as he tried to grasp the truth. He had lost—but not to Shumway or Lower. He had lost to a strange South African he remembered only from past surgical conventions, the last being seven months previously, in May 1967, when Barnard had attended a conference where Shumway, Lower, and Kantrowitz had all presented papers on their progress in transplantation.

He pulled on his clothes and shoes dazedly. He had to get out. He needed to scour the newspapers to see if he could discover any more details of Barnard's transplant.

Kantrowitz quickly established that news of the transplant had broken after the final edition of the New York papers had been printed. He strode bleakly through Brooklyn without a destination in mind. Kantrowitz walked as a way of trying to find reason amid his distress.

Barnard's name would be enshrined forever in cardiac history. Kantrowitz was honest enough to admit that he would have liked a taste of the glory. But that dream now lay around him in pieces, like the trash lining the streets of Brooklyn. Kantrowitz did not think only of himself. As he walked he remembered Jamie Scudero. The longing to save him rose up again in Kantrowitz with renewed force. What did it matter to Jamie Scudero that Chris Barnard had transplanted a heart early that morning? Barnard could take the full glare of attention and Kantrowitz would move on in the same way that he had always done, following his gut—and to hell with the rest of them.

Little puffs of steam curled out of his mouth as he walked. Just because

Barnard had done it first did not ruin the logic of his own plan. Kantrowitz would carry his disappointment inside him, but for now it mattered more that he should still seek to transplant a new heart into the hapless baby. He turned back toward home, his pace quickening. Kantrowitz might have lost the race, but he would try even harder to beat death and save Jamie Scudero.

Stanford Medical Center, Palo Alto, California, December 3, 1967

They sat in the hospital cafeteria just after eleven that same Sunday morning. Ed Stinson, twirling a plastic spoon aimlessly in his hand, tried to think of something to say. Shumway's chief resident was the most gifted young surgeon and the brightest intellectual in Stanford's glittering program. Stinson was also the most humane of men, a Christian of profound and private belief, a gentle and thoughtful presence in the often brutal and egotistical surgical arena. Yet what would he say to Norm Shumway? What words could he use to express his shock and sorrow that nine years of work seemed to have been wiped away by a man they all considered an opportunist?

Stinson rarely heard Shumway speak ill of anyone, but he knew how much his chief loathed Chris Barnard. It went deep, and way back to Minnesota, to the days when Shumway had first recoiled from Barnard. Stinson believed that the grossest injustice had just been committed. He had begun working with Shumway and Lower in 1961. He had seen everything they had poured of themselves into transplantation. There was no doubt in his mind. No one but Shumway or Lower deserved to claim the first transplant. And yet Barnard had taken it from them. Stinson, locked in silence with Shumway and his three fellow residents, kept twirling his spoon, trying and failing to find the words.

Shumway had many gifts but perhaps his greatest remained his ability to identify and then nurture the most precocious and self-effacing residents. He would sometimes lament privately to an old buddy like Dick Lower that his latest batch of recruits were not in the same league as the old gang. He had yet to unearth another Gene Dong or Ed Hurley. And of course no one would ever compare to Lower himself. Yet, as the months passed and Shumway handed out responsibility with the delight of a man who loved giving more than receiving, the Stanford chief surprised himself once again. He would enthuse that, actually, the new batch was fantastic. It was crammed with prodigies and potential greats. They were probably better than any group he had had the pleasure of molding so far.

There had never been any doubt about Stinson. Shumway had believed in him from the very start. Stinson was always going to be "the guy," the man Shumway had chosen to head Stanford's transplant program. It was still extraordinary that the forty-four-year-old Shumway had planned to lead the first two or three transplants and then, after showing Stinson the way, they would switch roles. Shumway, who had never forgotten how Owen Wangensteen had neglected to offer him a chance in Minnesota, would become Stinson's unofficial first assistant in the OR.

The bond between the two men was already unbreakable. While the rising star assessed the condition of each patient with utter seriousness, Shumway would observe Stinson before, when the mood was right, cracking another joke. Shumway turned Sunday rounds into a social event and at the end of every week's tour he would reward Stinson and his fellow residents with a trip to the cafeteria. The doyen of cardiac transplantation would then rock and laugh in his chair and watch his boys knock back the coffee and scoff up the doughnuts he insisted on buying.

Shumway had, as always, shelled out for the coffee and doughnuts, but this time there were no jokes and little conversation. Stinson was moved by Shumway's unprecedented silence throughout their morning rounds. It evoked the kind of sadness Stinson knew most people would describe, without thinking, as "heartbreaking." He looked away from Shumway.

The doughnuts lay untouched on the table, and the coffee was drunk more as a way of filling up the time than out of any Sunday-morning relaxation. After ten awkward minutes in the cafeteria, they were approached by a lone reporter who had tracked down Shumway. The perky journalist introduced himself and immediately asked Shumway for his reaction to the dramatic news.

Stinson cringed inside as he waited for Shumway to speak. It was an excruciating moment. Stinson looked up. Shumway opened his mouth—but he was drained of words. His face was etched with hurt. Stinson glared at the reporter. The hack tried again, but this time Shumway cut him down and sent him hurrying away with the bleakest of stares and the sharpest of words.

Stinson felt a curious emptiness in his chest. It was the bare feeling of injustice.

Shumway stood up. They could not stay like this forever. It was time to get back to work. Stinson rose to his feet, as did the others. And then, soundlessly, they parted. Each of the residents headed toward his own suddenly solitary set of duties. Norman Shumway, meanwhile, walked slowly away from the cafeteria.

South Africa's largest daily newspaper, *The Star*, reflected the world's awe on December 4, 1967, in a banner headline: "Transplanted Heart Is Beating!" "Cape Town, Monday. Thirty-two hours after his historic heart transplant in Groote Schuur Hospital, Mr Louis Washkansky is maintaining his satisfactory condition. Dr J.G. Burger, Medical Superintendent of the hospital, said this afternoon that the fifty-five-year-old patient's condition was unchanged. Mr Washkansky, whose life expectancy was not longer than a few weeks because of a diseased heart, is isolated in a special ward and under minute-to-minute observation. He has tubes in his throat through which his breathing is assisted. But other than that his life is now dependent on the beating heart of Miss Denise Ann Darvall."

A large photograph, captioned "The First," dominated that front page. Louis Washkansky lay flat on his back, his eyes opened and his hands resting in parallel lines across his chest. A grainy glint of his gold front tooth could be seen as he looked straight into the camera. Georgie Hall, a young nurse, leaned over him. Wearing a cap, gloves, and a sterile gown, she had turned her head toward the camera. Her eyes, staring intently over a mask, also gazed directly into the lens.

The photo had been taken by François Hitchcock, one of Barnard's assistant surgeons, who had simply pressed down on the shutter of a camera that had been preset and equipped with a flash by photographer Jim McLagen, who worked for *The Star*'s sister paper, the *Cape Argus*. While Barnard had listened sympathetically to McLagen's request to photograph Washkansky he had stressed that the shot would have to be taken by one of his own team who were allowed access to the ward. He tapped the protective screens that had been placed at the edge of the corridor leading to room 274 on ward C2. A handwritten sign had been plastered against the first screen: *"No admittance— hospital personal only."* The misspelling of "personnel" was pointed out but Barnard didn't care. If McLagen wanted a photo he would have to hand over his camera.

Hitchcock was a competent surgeon but he was strictly an amateur photographer. He cut off the top of Georgie Hall's head but at least he got Washkansky in the middle of the frame, which allowed the *Argus* and *The Star* to run with it as a world exclusive in their late-afternoon Cape Town and Johannesburg editions. While waiting for that historic shot, earlier editions of Monday's *Argus* had featured a different front-page photograph. A beaming Barnard sat behind the wheel of his speedboat, *Pacemaker*, with his right hand raised in triumph. An adjoining profile of the surgeon gushed: "Professor Barnard has lectured in Russia and America. He is a youthful-looking man with immense energy. . . . The Professor, the father of Springbok water-skier Deirdre Barnard, told a reporter yesterday: 'I thought we could succeed this far. The operation went off very well and I am very happy.'"

Within an hour of arriving home just before lunch on Sunday, Barnard's telephone had begun to ring incessantly. The first call came from London, from a reporter intent on establishing the ethnicity of the donor patient. Barnard assured him that Denise Darvall had indeed been white. Similar calls from Germany and France followed before John Stevenson, the science writer for London's *Daily Sketch*, telephoned Barnard in Zeekoevlei to ask him about a different kind of race. Stevenson was intrigued to hear whether the South African was "jubilant" about "pipping both American and British surgeons at the post?"

Barnard told him that "the truth is that, from a research point of view, we were all at the same stage in this work. It was a classic case of who got the first set of right circumstances."

On Monday morning, as international news teams flocked to Cape Town, the BBC and CBS leading the first requests for exclusive interviews with the star surgeon and his famous patient, Barnard realized the need to augment his claims to a research background—to show something at least vaguely comparable to the years of work done by Kantrowitz and, especially, Shumway and Lower.

A front-page *Argus* article adjoining the photograph of Washkansky was headlined "Three Years' Work on Op." "The heart transplant operation at Groote Schuur hospital was preceded by three years of research in the animal laboratory, Professor Chris Barnard, leader of the team which performed the operation, said today. 'This research was to work out a technique. Once we decided we had this worked out, we felt we could do the transplant on a human.'"

Barnard chose not to mention the huge contribution of his American rivals, specifically ignoring the influence of Lower and Shumway on cardiac transplantation.

Shumway, by contrast, emerged in public as magnanimous in defeat. Having allowed his private anguish to be witnessed by Stinson and a few others, Shumway had bitten down hard on his despair. He had confronted the remaining hordes of reporters who descended on Stanford on Sunday afternoon with grace. Quotes from an Associated Press interview with Shumway were printed in *The Star*: "The Stanford Medical Centre surgeon who thirteen days ago announced plans for transplanting a heart said the operation in Cape Town was 'pretty exciting. . . . It sounds to me like a damn fine job.' He and his team were still awaiting the required combination of patient and heart-donor at Stanford. 'We have a few things cooking . . .' Dr Shumway said."

The New York Times revealed that "Dr. Shumway said he worked with Professor Chris Barnard, head of the Cape Town surgery team, at the University of Minnesota about ten years ago. 'We have had numerous reunions since, the most recent in May,' Dr. Shumway said. 'He is a good man, a well-known, well-respected cardiac surgeon.' Dr. Shumway predicted that the heart transplant would become as frequent as the kidney transplant within ten years."

Lower, like Shumway, had resolved to hide his own piercing anger and disappointment. He and his old buddy preferred dignity to despair. They could not bear the thought of Barnard knowing how much he had hurt them. There were also many others, even old rivals, prepared to speak out on their behalf.

James Hardy, notorious for his transplant of a chimpanzee heart into a man almost four years earlier, expressed his chagrin. "My disappointment is enormous, though not so much for myself personally. I know that Norman Shumway's group at Stanford have done the most extensive and the best work in this field. We have long been waiting for them to transplant a heart from one man to another, following which, after more considered research, my team hoped to emulate them. We were technically ready long before Barnard—but we were burdened by the need to protect our public from the possible failure of such a great experiment. Shumway did everything by the book—only to have history stolen from him."

Barnard, however, had some heavy hitters among his supporters. Michael DeBakey, who had his own personal rivalry with Kantrowitz and Shumway, said of the Cape Town team: "They have a very fine group of people there. I have a very warm feeling for them. They are doing wonderful work—it really is a very great achievement." Walt Lillehei, while privately expressing his regret for Shumway, acclaimed Barnard for his "boldness and determination in a procedure which is the equal of anything we did while carrying out the first open-heart operations in Minnesota."

Most American papers that Monday morning adopted a similar laudatory tone, hailing the operation across their front pages as "Heart-Changing History," "Miracle Heart," "The Ultimate Operation," or, in the words of the Washington *Daily News*, "a frontier no less important and far more immediate than the stars." Quoting Barnard in the operating theater, the Washington paper screamed out its own headline in big black letters: "It's Going to Work!"

Barnard's sudden worldwide fame even penetrated the Iron Curtain, drawing praise from some unexpected sources. In Moscow, *Pravda* gave over its front page to the news and suggested to its readers that "in spite of South

Africa's backward place in the community of nations, positive, creative forces seem to thrive there, as proven by the immense feat of Dr. Chris Barnard. . . . His achievement is to be saluted over and above any barriers that may otherwise exist."

There were still many dissenting voices in the constant babble made by an amazed world. Charlie Bailey, who had lost many patients in his risk-taking compulsion to become the first man to perform a mitral commissurotomy in 1948, dismissed Barnard's surgical bravado. He warned that the transplant was "at least ten years premature." Werner Forssmann, who had shared the Nobel Prize in 1956 for his pulmonary research, also railed against the procedure from Berlin: "Is it not a macabre scene when doctors place a patient on the heart-lung machine in one operating room while, simultaneously, in a similar room next door, a second team waits, forceps in hand, around a young person fighting against death. These people are not there to help the patient. With feverish eagerness they are waiting to open his defenceless body in order to save someone else."

Thirty-eight years before, Forssmann had been dismissed as a "macabre crank" after he'd slipped a tube into a vein in his arm and, watching himself on an X-ray monitor, guided the catheter toward the right atrium. In proving that the heart could withstand catheterization, he had endangered himself. It took years, however, before his daring was acknowledged as being scientifically valid. An acclaimed old man now in 1967, Forssmann could afford to take the moral high ground and point out that he had risked his own life rather than that of a patient. Yet, in his self-righteous simplification of transplant surgery, he had lost the vision and courage that had driven his own medical discovery.

The New York Times struggled to find a measured response in the midst of such outrage and delight. "Whatever the final outcome of this historic experiment," their editorial suggested, "the Cape Town medical team has dramatically extended the range of man's accomplishments. This is one of the peaks of modern scientific achievement, fully comparable to the heights scaled earlier in such fields as space exploration or molecular biology. And, as in all such cases, Professor Chris Barnard and his team stood on the shoulders of giants, the men and women who had pioneered the way by developing the heart-lung machine, by pioneering open-heart surgery and simpler types of transplant operations, and by finding and introducing the chemicals needed to protect against infection, blood clots and other dangers faced by Mr. Washkansky."

B arnard walked the tightrope. Reeling between exhilaration and apprehension, he delighted in Washkansky's stable condition while fretting constantly over the possibility of missing any early signs of deterioration. He had to gauge the correct balance of drugs that would enable him to steer his patient safely through the entwined but contrasting threat of infection and rejection. In breaking down Washkansky's immune system, as a way of negating his body's instinct to destroy Denise Darvall's heart, he had stripped a seriously ill man of his defenses against marauding bacteria.

While Washkansky's temperature, blood pressure, and pulse rate were all normal, Barnard could not allow himself to relax. He was like a general awaiting the outbreak of war. The battleground would be Washkansky's battered body. He was lifted most by the small glimmers of fight he discerned in his prized patient. When he arrived at Groote Schuur early on Monday morning, a masked and gloved Barnard peered down at the motionless body.

"Hello, Louis," Barnard said. "They say you're doing fine."

Washkansky nodded and gestured weakly that he wanted to talk. Barnard and Ozinsky agreed to the hopeful request, but they moved slowly and methodically. They called for an oxygen tent to be placed over the bed before Ozinsky disconnected the respirator. He did not withdraw the tube from Washkansky's windpipe until he had established that he could breathe on his own with a new heart. After an hour of monitoring his steady breathing, Ozinsky finally freed Washkansky's mouth.

"How are you, Louis?" Barnard asked.

"Fine," Washkansky said softly. "I'm feeling okay."

"Do you know what we've done?"

"You promised me a new heart."

"You've got a new heart," Barnard confirmed.

Washkansky nodded and lifted his thumb. Barnard explained that they would be moving him every two hours in his bed to help clear his lungs and assist his breathing. They would also need to wake him regularly to take blood samples and administer new medication.

"Okay," Washkansky said.

At the ensuing press conference Barnard relived the conversation, supplying the simple little bubbles of quotes that would make good copy in newspapers around the world. The hospital corridors were crawling with journalists and television crews who had just flown in from America and Europe. An already epic human saga, chock-full of emotion, was made even more compelling by the photogenic Barnard's charismatic presence.

Fame had taken hold of him with a staggering force. Barnard had catapulted himself out of medical obscurity and become one of the world's most celebrated men. He was initially unprepared for the astonishing transformation. Having expected a few scattered press headlines, he had hoped principally to have his name resound ahead of Shumway and Lower in the competitive medical journals of America. The voracious international interest in the transplant surprised him. Yet he was helplessly flattered and revelled in the attention.

Showing his instinctive ease with the media, Barnard also possessed a showman's touch. He allowed Eddie Steinhardt, a cameraman for CBS News, to film Washkansky from the threshold of his room. Steinhardt passed a cordless electronic microphone to Bertie Bosman, who approached Washkansky's bed so that the sound of his beating heart on the EKG could echo down the corridor outside, which was packed with print journalists, radio reporters, and television anchormen.

"Tonight I heard the beat of a borrowed heart," a writer for *The Times* shouted into a public telephone as he dictated his copy to a secretary in London. A freelancer for the New York *Daily News* wired his own personal account, which asserted that "Louis Washkansky's boom-de-boom sounded all right to me."

The international press corps were no less captivated by Barnard himself, whom they described as "handsome," "boyish," "lean," "tanned," "charming," "candid," "amusing," and "refreshing." They were amazed that he had not taken any photographs or made any recordings of the landmark operation.

"What do we want pictures for?" Barnard asked. "I can explain everything you need to know with a blackboard and chalk. Just ask me."

He was ready to talk about anything. "Sure," he said, "I've got rheumatoid arthritis." He held up his hands and a dozen photographers immediately made a small circle around him. They snapped away at the "golden" but "damaged" hands that had held the world's most famous heart before transplanting it into the chest of Louis Washkansky—another irresistible angle for feature editors. Apart from being brilliant, good-looking, and exotic, the tall and slender heart surgeon was afflicted with a disability himself. The story smacked of Hollywood and gave even more of a zing and zip to the "King of Hearts" profiles.

Barnard spoke with just the right mix of pathos and resolve. "I do have pain sometimes on long operations but in this one I was so wrapped up in the job that I felt nothing. It's no good feeling sorry for myself but I just don't know how long I will be able to go on operating."

"What will you do when you have to stop?" an American voice asked.

"I'm sure I'll think of something," Barnard grinned.

And then, just as he began to look a little too wolfish for mass consumption, Barnard would remember his small-town roots and shrug and protest that he and his brother, Marius, "were just country boys." The sibling link provided another enticing theme to the transplant story, and Marius played his role to perfection.

"Chris is dead right," Marius said, smiling. "We *are* country bumpkins. I cannot believe you're hanging onto the words of two Afrikaans boys from the Karoo. . . ."

Marius also showed emotion amid his self-effacement. "You must remember, you know, that I grew up with my brother. We have known each other a long, long time. And although we don't always agree, there are some things we share that we don't share with other people. I know how much he wanted this operation. . . . I hope they give him the Nobel Prize."

The following morning, on Tuesday, December 6, the Barnard brothers gave Louis Washkansky a boiled egg, in delighted response to his request. Newspapers across the globe had their next headline, epitomized by that afternoon's *Cape Argus,* which captured the naïve wonder of the first transplant: "Heart Man: I'm Hungry."

Ann Washkansky had also been swamped by the media pack. She, too, was now famous. Her name was known from Cape Town to Washington, from London to Moscow. *The Star* revealed that when asked "about her feelings as the wife of a world celebrity, Mrs. Washkansky said: 'This frightens me more than anything else.'"

Everyone wanted to talk to her, this ordinary middle-aged housewife from Cape Town, the daughter of immigrant parents, who had never been to university or "read a big book in my entire life." And yet they clung to her every word as if she was touched by some divine inspiration, as if she was the source of all human feeling, just because her husband, her Washy, had become the world's most celebrated patient. Louis was the hero, she said, not she, and not even Chris Barnard. Ann Washkansky just wanted Louis to come back home. She wanted him to show her that he was still the same rogue who had always charmed her with his line: "Stick with me, kid, and I'll make you famous."

Having retold the story, Barnard suddenly shifted the tone of his press conference. He looked directly at the massed hordes of foreign reporters. "See, we South Africans aren't the bad eggs you overseas people so often describe. Have a look round this hospital yourselves and see if you can notice any difference in the kind of treatment that we give to the European and Colored patients in our wards."

His ethnic references were shaped by the semantics of apartheid, but most of the foreign press in attendance were seduced by the intense Afrikaner. He looked as if he had been waiting for this moment his whole life. Barnard insisted that "if all goes well," he hoped to be able to send Washkansky home in three weeks. And then he paused. "But first we have much danger to overcome."

"When is the real danger period?" an American asked anxiously.

"We don't exactly know," Barnard said, staring out into the audience. "From this point onwards, from the initial success of the actual operation, we are treading in the dark, we are approaching totally new medical territory."

He then picked up his chalk, turned to the blackboard, and began to draw as he spoke. It was as if he were talking aloud to himself, the words flowing in simple and natural sentences as, with startling candor, he drew his listeners into the imminent struggle against rejection—explaining how they were girding themselves for the definitive battle.

Barnard gestured to M. C. Botha for a cigarette. As he lit up, an eager reporter, pen hovering over his notebook, whispered to Marius Barnard. Did his brother always smoke menthol-tipped cigarettes? It was just the sort of intimate detail his readers would relish.

"No," Marius said. "Chris smokes OPs."

The journalist looked at him quizzically, wondering why he had never heard of the surgeon's chosen brand.

"OPs?" he said as he prepared to write down his little exclusive.

"Other people's," Marius said dryly. He had already decided it was time to break up the press conference. It looked to him as if Chris was tiring, and they still had hours of meetings ahead of them to discuss Washkansky's condition with the immunologists, bacteriologists, biochemists, nephrologists, and cardiologists they had called in for twice-daily meetings. Marius was concerned that they were being unnecessarily diverted from their work.

He chose his moment carefully. At the first brief lull in Chris's lecture on rejection, Marius shouted out from the back of the room. "Professor Barnard! There's an urgent telephone call for you."

Chris looked up impatiently at his brother. "*Ag man,* Marius," he said in colloquial Afrikaans, "just take a message for me," then turned back to his real audience and waited for the next question.

Time, Life, and *Newsweek* had all decided that Chris Barnard would grace the covers of their next issue. A Cape Town photographer would supply the stills for both *Time* and *Life.* Cloete Breytenbach, brother of the Afrikaans poet Breyten Breytenbach, condemned to exile in Paris for his opposition to apartheid and an illegal marriage to a Vietnamese woman, went to work that Tuesday morning. He convinced Barnard to allow him to take a single shot of Washkansky—which would bump Audrey Hepburn off the previously planned cover of *Life.*

Chris Barnard knew that he should concentrate on monitoring arterial flutters, enzymes and the urine output of Louis Washkansky. He could, however, no longer help himself. He was dreaming of a new life. He was already dreaming of Audrey Hepburn.

Twelve

THE MAN WITH
THE GOLDEN HANDS

Adrian Kantrowitz had another chance. He was only hours away from the cooling and the cutting. A baby, flown in from the Jefferson Medical College Hospital of Philadelphia, had arrived in Brooklyn soon after six on that evening of December 5, 1967. The word of God swarmed around the one-day-old anencephalic boy who had been given the name of David McIntire Bashaw. He had been born into a professional Philadelphia family who described themselves as religious fundamentalists. His maternal grandfather hurled down fire and brimstone from the pulpit of the Bible Presbyterian Church.

Soon after the baby entered the world at 3:35 the previous afternoon without a functioning brain, or even a rounded casing of flesh to seal the head, the formidable Reverend Carl McIntire had turned to his daughter, Celeste, and son-in-law, Keith. Dressed in an inky-black suit and speaking solemnly in a bare hospital room, he had reached for a quotation from Genesis to blunt their grief: "Dust thou art, and unto dust shalt thou return."

The words from the medical report, written by Mary Louise Soentgen, an assistant professor of clinical pediatrics at Jefferson, were just as stark. Kantrowitz, alone in his office, absorbed the jolting brevity of her medical summary.

Physical exam at time of birth revealed an anencephalic male infant. Complete absence of covering of the brain. The brain was grossly malformed and there was bloody cerebral spinal fluid leaking from the posterior aspect. There was no roof to the orbit. Pupils were equal. Mouth normal except high arched palate. . . . The infant moves all extremities. There is a feeble cry. Moro reflex is poor; there is no suck reflex. Birth weight was 2340 grams.

A tiny body, devoid of sense or feeling, had been stripped down to this: "The infant moves all extremities. There is a feeble cry." Kantrowitz could imagine those reflex actions being attributed all the delicacy of humanity by Howard Joos and Harry Weiss, the two devout doctors who had blocked his attempted transplant eighteen months before.

Joos, the director of pediatrics at Maimonides, remained part of their team. While he still insisted that they wait for the heart to cease beating before starting any transplant, Joos had grown more accustomed to Kantrowitz's view that they owed everything to the recipient baby. Life, and so hope, resided only in Jamie Scudero. This time, Kantrowitz was convinced, he would not be stopped.

Sixty hours since hearing about Barnard and Washkansky he could shrug aside his disappointment and concentrate on the Scudero case. Jamie's complexion was a little less dusky and he no longer struggled to breathe. His condition, Kantrowitz told Anna Scudero, had stabilized. The heart rate remained between 120 and 140 beats per minute, while he fed steadily if sparingly. But there was no escaping the bleak fact that Jamie was dying from congestive heart failure and only a transplant could save him.

The donor's condition was poor but Kantrowitz's team quickly confirmed he had the same blood type and a similar histocompatibility as seventeen-day-old Jamie. Even Joos was convinced. They would operate that night.

Maimonides Medical Center, Brooklyn, New York, December 6, 1967

The cooling began at 3:45 a.m. An anesthetized Jamie Scudero was placed in a small bath of ice water that would lower his body temperature from 36 to

15 degrees centigrade (98.6 to 59° F). His face was covered by an oxygen mask strapped to the back of his head of thick black hair. The same procedure was carried out in an adjoining operating room where the Bashaw baby had begun to show signs of an increasingly irregular heartbeat. The heart was dying, but they would still wait, unlike Barnard, for it to stop before they started cutting. A towel, once more, covered the missing upper head of the anencephalic donor.

During their aborted attempt the previous summer, no one in Brooklyn, besides Kantrowitz, had heard of Chris Barnard. Now it seemed as if the world had gone transplant crazy. The corridors were crowded with reporters and photographers. After news of the imminent transplant leaked, they had invaded the hospital at midnight. Kantrowitz stationed a couple of security guards at the door of the OR. The only men who would get to photograph the transplant were already inside the room—Bill Neches, his young pediatrician, and the official two-man team Kantrowitz used to document his most significant operations.

The hospital photographer scaled a large stepladder right above the bath containing the Bashaw baby. Jordan Haller, Kantrowitz's director of thoracic surgery, raised a brow. "I hope the little patient's not taking up too much room," he said dubiously.

Kantrowitz, however, was in command. He watched the fluttering of the green line on the EKG screen. Suddenly, at 4:25, it flattened. Kantrowitz stepped forward and nodded silently. Haller began to saw his way inside the chest of the Bashaw baby while Kantrowitz headed for the room next door where he would excise Jamie Scudero's diseased heart.

Haller immersed the donor heart in a saline solution chilled to 5 degrees centigrade (41° F) and took it slowly to the OR, where his chief had begun cutting into Jamie's chest. Kantrowitz knew, from Shumway's and his own laboratory experiments, that the cold saline could protect the heart for at least seven hours. But choosing to rely on hypothermia alone, rather than a heart-lung machine, meant that he would have to complete the surgery in less than an hour.

At 4:46, Kantrowitz was ready. He allowed one last series of photos as Bill Neches held the tiny donor heart in his gloved hand. Looking no bigger than a large acorn, it would soon begin to pump blood through Jamie Scudero. After Kantrowitz positioned the heart inside the boy's chest, he and Haller began the suturing. It was 4:48.

Forty minutes later, at 5:28, they were set to shock the heart back to life. Kantrowitz supported the heart with a gentle manual massage. He kneaded the tiny muscle until they reached a temperature of 26 degrees centigrade (78.8° F) and warmed blood pulsed through Jamie. Haller looked up at Alex Faltine, the Jamaican head technician responsible for rewarming the recipient on the table. Sweat gleamed on Faltine's brown forehead, but beneath his mask he seemed to be grinning. They were almost there.

The heart had already begun to fibrillate when Kantrowitz gave the signal. When the shock came, at 5:30, the heart kicked into life and picked up an immediate beat of 80 to 85 beats per minute. The eventual suturing slid smoothly into place and, as the body temperature rose to 32 degrees centigrade (89.6° F), Kantrowitz gave the last order for the chest to be closed.

Jamie's new heart reached a rate of 90 to 110, and his little hands and feet moved spontaneously as the blood flowed. His breathing was still labored, but the oxygen steadied and bolstered him over the next forty-five minutes. Three days after the miracle of Louis Washkansky, the world's second transplant—and the first on a child—was complete. The next twelve hours were crucial, but in that moment, at 6:28 on a winter morning in Brooklyn, relief seeped through Kantrowitz.

The surgeon met first with Anna Scudero, a little after seven a.m., then walked wearily to his office to phone Philadelphia. Kantrowitz felt a basic human urge to communicate with the parents of the baby whose heart kept another child alive. He had tried to speak to them four hours earlier, at around three a.m., but Celeste Bashaw had finally succumbed to sleep, and her husband had returned home to be with their five-year-old girl and seven-year-old boy. It was better this way. Instead of informing them that their son was close to death, he was now able to tell them that their baby's heart was still alive and beating in the chest of another boy. He felt drained, but Kantrowitz could still comfort a mother. Her and her husband's generosity, he told

Celeste Bashaw, had made a monumental difference. Out of the tragedy of two hopeless lives they may have salvaged a child.

His whole team had been quietly heroic. While Kantrowitz spoke with a mother who cried softly into the phone, Jordan Haller stared in horror at the blistered hands of Alex Faltine. During the rewarming of Jamie Scudero, one of the heating connectors had loosened. Faltine had simply held the hot water pipes together with his thinly gloved hands. He laughed and shrugged when Haller asked him how many minutes he had withstood the burning.

Faltine, in his mid-fifties, was renowned at Maimonides for two things: his immaculate sense of style, and the one-arm push-ups he sometimes did in the hospital corridor. That feat of strength never failed to impress. Faltine's hands would recover. The fate of the baby he had warmed back to life was less certain.

Eight hours later, Kantrowitz trudged toward the massed throng that had gathered at the hospital that afternoon. It was like a scene from a bad movie. Even in the depths of his exhaustion he was surprised at the sight of hundreds of reporters and banks of cameras and microphones. The vultures had gathered. Kantrowitz spoke carefully so that no one would misunderstand him.

"The baby seemed to be doing reasonably well during the operative procedure, improving all the time up until seven hours following the procedure, when the heart suddenly stopped. We tried to resuscitate the heart but we were not able to do this. So we lost the child. I think it should be clear to you, and you should convey it clearly to your readers and your listeners and your viewers that we here consider that this procedure was an unequivocal failure."

Kantrowitz's honesty remained unadorned. He simply did not believe in artifice or duplicity. If he was regarded as a showman by those who did not really know him, he faced the world with seemingly unbreakable candor.

The New York Times reported: "Dr. Kantrowitz [said that] 'we do not know at this point why this transplanted heart failed.' Lines of tension and sleeplessness underscored the eyes of the surgeon as he told of the 'heroic attempt' of his 22-member team of doctors, nurses and technicians to 'salvage' the infant's life. The team members were 'disheartened and feel sad,' he said. 'We were trying to make one whole individual out of two individuals who did not have a chance for survival when they were born . . . But we failed.'

"Dr. Kantrowitz said an attempt would be made to determine the cause of death and that this would be 'reported to medical colleagues through the medical literature.' The surgeon said he was disturbed and upset because news of the operation 'had been leaked to a newspaper' which he refused to identify. He added that newspaper headlines were not the place to disclose important operations, but that they should first be reported to the medical authorities."

Now that he had been forced to confront the press, Kantrowitz decided to speak of his rivals. "After reporting his own failure, Dr. Kantrowitz praised the work of Dr. Christiaan N. Barnard, who performed the world's first heart transplant on Sunday. . . . The two operations were remarkably similar [but] Dr. Kantrowitz commented that, 'it was harder technically and emotionally to perform surgery' on infants than adults."

Kantrowitz felt ravaged but, still, he thought of another disconsolate man. He might have regarded Shumway as his fiercest competitor but, unlike Barnard in his euphoria, Kantrowitz could find it in himself to stress the seminal contribution of the Stanford surgeon. "At the news conference," *The New York Times* concluded, "Dr. Kantrowitz credited Dr. Norman Shumway of the Stanford Medical Center, Palo Alto, with developing the procedure used in yesterday's operation."

B arnard Has Praise" ran the headline in *The Star* on December 7 as the Johannesburg newspaper assessed Kantrowitz's failure. "'I think it was a very bold effort,' Professor Chris Barnard said of the world's second human heart transplant on a two-and-a-half-week-old American infant: 'It would have been a much more difficult operation than ours. This is because of the size of the patient. It would have been more of a problem putting a patient that size on the heart-lung machine and the nursing afterwards of a baby would have been more difficult. If they had succeeded, and I am sorry they did not, they would have done better than we have done.'"

Barnard could afford the magnanimous gesture. Washkansky was thriving, and the world was agog. In South Africa itself the newspapers were exultant and the government ecstatic. As *The Star* reported in one of its many adjoining transplant articles that afternoon, "The Minister of Health, Dr. [Albert] Hertzog, today described the first heart transplant as 'a remarkable feat and something South Africans can be very proud of—it has been wonderful propaganda for South Africa.'"

The local press, usually mortified by the country's battered image abroad, was even more thrilled to report the gushing good news that "an American television network has offered to fly Chris Barnard and his wife to the United States for a week." CBS had invited him to appear on a Christmas Eve edition of its prestigious show *Face the Nation*. It would provide Barnard and South Africa the kind of publicity for which they had hungered so long.

The world appeared fascinated by reports that Louis Washkansky had eaten a meal of minced chicken and mashed potato. Delighted by his ability to breathe freely again, he had begun to make some of his familiar wisecracks. Journalists reveled in the snippets Barnard fed them, like juicy sardines tossed to a tank of barking seals. After Barnard had called him "a good guy" during a routine examination, Washkansky had apparently responded with "You're a pretty good guy yourself." According to Barnard, his star patient was "talking about everything under the sun" and telling the nurses that he was "the new Frankenstein. How about that?"

Barnard smiled queasily at a reminder that Mary Shelley's Frankenstein was a doctor who created a monster out of salvaged human parts. Despite his charming media reports, Barnard was haunted by a fear that a nightmare would soon engulf both him and Washkansky. That afternoon, December 7, Barnard noted a rise in Washkansky's white-cell count, from 18,000 to 28,000. He rationalized his anxieties by remembering that in Virginia the year before, David Hume and Dick Lower had explained to him that such an increase often accompanied a kidney transplant. Yet Barnard was unnerved further by Washkansky's racing heart.

All the frivolity of the morning press conference was forgotten when his transplanted heart reached a dangerous 160 beats a minute. Val Schrire's advice, that they should use digoxin to slow the rate, was rejected by Barnard.

He still leaned heavily on Shumway and Lower's experiments and stressed that they had found that canine hearts often reacted badly to the drug. Schrire replied pointedly that they were treating a man here, not a dog, but the influence of the Stanford research was such that Barnard opted for an associated form of medication, strophanthin, which acted more quickly but did not exert the same length of control over the heart as digoxin.

The pulse duly became more measured and Barnard decided to allow the recording of Washkansky's first radio interview for the South Africa Broadcasting Corporation—and then to reward him with a visit from his wife. "Bossie" Bosman, in the role of interviewer, asked Washkansky a series of simple questions at his bedside just before five o'clock that afternoon.

BOSMAN: And how you feeling, Mr. Washkansky?
WASHKANSKY: I am feeling quite fine.
BOSMAN: Are you well?
WASHKANSKY: Yes, quite well.
BOSMAN: What do you want to eat tonight?
WASHKANSKY: Something light.
BOSMAN: How do you feel to be such a famous man?
WASHKANSKY: I'm not famous. The doctor is famous—the man with the golden hands.
BOSMAN: Would you like to see your family?
WASHKANSKY: I would.
BOSMAN: We have a surprise for you at 5 p.m.
WASHKANSKY: Very good.

Ann was brought in for a brief but emotional reunion. Terrified that Louis might have become a different person, or that he would not recognize her, she approached the figure shrouded under the oxygen tent with a tentative step.

"Louis," she said, "it's me."

"Hello, kid," Louis said.

Bosman coaxed Ann closer to the bed, but asked her not to touch her husband, for fear of transmitting pathogens. Ann laughed and relaxed a little when Louis said, "All right, I'll do it—but no kissing."

Although neither of them realized it then, their conversation was being recorded by the SABC microphone. "How are you, Louis?" she asked anxiously.

"I'm on top of the world, kid."

Now Ann knew she had gotten her Louis back. She and her husband continued a tender kind of chitchat that was later relayed to the nation.

"You know," Ann said, "your name is even on the Sanlam Building."

"Are you serious?"

"It's running around the top of the Sanlam with the news—and it's in the papers. Everybody is talking about you."

"You mean it?" Louis said wryly.

"Everybody is listening to every word you say. You're a very famous person now, you know."

"I'm not famous. Barnard is famous. What have I done? Nothing."

"Well," Ann said, "you've been very brave. Anyway, your words came true, hey? You always said, 'Stick around, kid, I'll make you famous.'"

Looking at her with his new heart beating inside his chest, Washkansky said, after a pause, "Ann, I'm so happy to see you."

Bosman gestured that it was time. "Goodbye, kid," Louis said as he weakly raised his hand to her. "Don't start any of your old tricks until I get home."

Ann Washkansky was radiant when she left the hospital that glorious summer evening. The press was waiting, but, for once, she did not mind the attention. "He looks beautiful," she said of her husband. "Just too beautiful. He is so much better than I expected and so beautiful and bright."

Barnard knew again how fortunate he had been in his choice of patient. Apart from showing the spirit of the fighter he had been in the ring years before, Louis and his wife were providing irresistible copy to the world.

T oday Louis Washkansky enters the most critical phase of his new life. The first attempt of his body to reject the heart of Denise Darvall is expected today or tomorrow. . . . Despite this, Professor Barnard and his team have so far detected no sign of rejection, and they hope to have their famous patient out of bed by next week. Meanwhile, Mr. Washkansky, in his first bedside radio interview, has described Professor Barnard as 'the man with the golden hands.' . . ."

Driving into work on December 8, and listening to the news on his car radio, Barnard appreciated the irony in Washkansky's description of him. "I looked at my hands on the wheel of the car and thought: the man with the swollen hands," he wrote later. "The arthritis was leaving its mark but so far they were not deformed. Sometimes I did not have the strength to force the mayon tubing on to the metal connectors. But there was still time left—time to do a few more transplants before it was too late, time to give Washkansky another heart if he rejected this one."

The fear of rejection had begun to bite. Barnard imagined he saw signs wherever he looked—whether in Washkansky's unexpected show of bad temper that morning or in his continuing high pulse rate. They had already decided to wing it and give him digoxin in spite of the Stanford findings. Yet Shumway and Lower's work continued to shape their anxious fumbling through a dark maze. Apart from a beat of 150, Washkansky's new heart also showed an alarming drop in voltage. Bosman dug out the Shumway paper that highlighted a link between a decrease in voltage and rejection. Barnard decided on an immediate start to their antirejection treatment, which, while simultaneously attacking Washkansky's immune system, would leave him defenseless against lethal bacteria already lurking in his body. The road had forked and Barnard had made his choice. He could only hope that he had made the right turn.

The impact seemed immediate. When Washkansky woke the following morning he claimed to be completely rejuvenated. His old cheeriness had returned. "I'll eat anything now," he told his nurse, "even hospital food." He claimed to have never felt better, and a day later he warned that "If I don't get steak and eggs I'm going home."

For the next four days Washkansky flirted with the nurses, listened to the radio and read the papers—while skipping over most of the articles about the transplant and his recovery. "We've had enough of that story," he said.

He was, however, pleased to read speculation that Barnard was reputedly being touted for a Nobel Prize and that a second transplant patient was already being monitored. The man in need of a new heart was rumored to be a Cape Town dentist—Dr. Philip Blaiberg—who told reporters that he thought he was "on the list" but that "nothing definite" had been decided.

"All I know is that I feel lousy at the moment," Blaiberg said. "I hope I can be next."

The press had already swamped the Barnard family. Louwtjie was typically unimpressed. "We're not accustomed to all this fuss," she protested to Roger Williams of the *Cape Times*. "We're not demonstrative people. We never fling our arms in the air and yell with delight on such occasions. I've had it with newspapermen—in a big way. Yesterday a man from *Life* magazine wanted to know the color of my husband's eyes, and whether his hair is starting to go gray yet. Do you know that after all these years of marriage, I couldn't tell him with any certainty. This thing has hit me like a bomb—and it is still difficult to grasp what has happened. I keep on wondering why this has happened to quiet-living people like us. I could understand a certain amount of publicity—but never in my wildest dreams did I think we would be getting calls from all over the world."

In an accompanying photograph the Barnards' colored maid, Lizzie Wagner, held the phone to her ear as she took "an important call from overseas." The *Cape Times* caption suggested that "Lizzie has been answering the telephone day and night since Sunday, and Mrs. Barnard described her yesterday as 'a tower of strength.'" Louwtjie also spoke of her children. Andre was still 1,200 miles away in Pretoria, while Deirdre had just completed her final year of school. "She cycles off each morning to the crèche down the road, where she is working temporarily, as if nothing out of the ordinary has happened. Her sixteen-year-old brother, who is in Standard 9 at Pretoria Boys' High School, is reacting rather differently. 'He was so overcome while speaking to his father on the telephone that all he could say over and over again was, "*Ag nee, Pa!*" [Oh no, Dad!]"' Andre—'a quiet thinker, not like my mad daughter,' says Mrs. Barnard—'wants to study medicine but can't decide whether to concentrate on human beings or animals.'"

Trouble, after a serene spell for Washkansky, descended on the thirteenth day of his new life. On Friday, December 15, he awoke after a disturbed night in which he had suffered severe stomach pains. Edgy and weary, he also complained of discomfort in his left shoulder. Without a single press officer to control the outrageous level of interest in him, Washkansky faced another series of high-profile visitors and interviews. After Carel de Wet, the government's minister of planning, arrived at his bedside, he was to be interviewed over the telephone by the BBC, photographed by *Stern*, and filmed holding his wife's hand for the first time by CBS. While Barnard had restricted local press access to his patient, he could not resist any overture from a powerful international media outlet. He was still flattered by the world's interest in him and his patient. Barnard suggested to Washkansky that they should proceed with the day's schedule but restrict each appointment to the bare minimum.

After a gentle opening to his BBC radio interview—with Washkansky claiming to be "one hundred percent"—he was asked how he felt, as a Jew, about having a Gentile's heart in his chest.

"Well," Washkansky hesitated, "I never thought of it that way. I don't know . . ."

Bossie Bosman, fearing an unsettling rush of political questions, immediately cut the connection to London and turned on the BBC's technicians. "How do you feel working for a company that asks a stupid question like that? Everybody's been so kind and good. Why couldn't we leave it like that?"

Barnard was soon preoccupied by a more menacing problem. Washkansky's white-cell count had risen again to a frightening figure of 29,860. While he believed the increase had been caused by the steroids they were pumping into Washkansky's body, there had been an even more sudden climb in his cardiac enzyme level from 368 to 752. Washkansky had also become very emotional, and, unusual for him, had cried during a family visit the previous afternoon. While they managed to stabilize his white-cell and enzyme count with more drugs, Bosman's exhaustive study of an X-ray late that afternoon detected a slight shadow on the left lung. A chill ran through them. Barnard knew that they were losing control.

Washkansky's breathing worsened during the night, the pain in his shoulder intensified and he had a mild temperature. A new X-ray on the morning of December 16 revealed that the lung shadow had grown significantly larger. It looked like the classic onset of pneumonia but Barnard was more unsettled by the mysteries of rejection. How could he be sure that the shadow was not something more ominous than a pulmonary infection? And even if it was not the start of rejection, Barnard feared that a blood clot might have parted from a suture line in the transplanted heart and entered the lungs to cause a pulmonary embolus. With the circulation obstructed, multiple infarctions, or death of a specific area of lung, would result. Pneumonia, by contrast, seemed a less sinister possibility. Barnard was convinced he should prepare himself for the worst. Rejection still seemed to him the most disturbing, and likely, outcome.

Washkansky's voice the next afternoon was ragged and hoarse. His temperature had soared to 39 degrees centigrade (102.2° F). He now complained of pain in his chest. Barnard filled him with penicillin and promised his patient he would soon feel better. The surgeon, however, could not hide his own sense of foreboding. The mood in the hospital changed and queries from the press became increasingly insistent.

A government employee from the Department of Information had taken charge of the daily media conferences, and as *The New York Times* reported, "The hospital cut off telephone calls to the doctors working on the Washkansky case because of a flood of inquiries since it was disclosed last night that he had pneumonia. . . . Dr Christiaan Barnard was giving an interview to NBC television when he got word that Mr. Washkansky had pneumonia."

By Monday, December 18, as they entered the third postoperative week, Washkansky was struggling for breath and his peripheral circulation had begun to falter. His hands and feet were as cold as a corpse's. Barnard knew that Washkansky was dying, but he could not nail the reason. All the treatments they had administered against both bacterial pneumonia and embolism had failed. Hume had spoken of an immunological pneumonia occasionally setting in after a kidney transplant. It was a mystifying condition in which the lung seemingly attacked itself as if it, rather than the kidney, was the transplanted organ. Hume dubbed the syndrome "transplant lung" and prescribed a concentrated course of powerful immunosuppressive medication. Barnard decided to follow the Hume method, even if it meant that they would be traveling even further down the tangled road of antirejection treatment.

Eighteen hours after Washkansky absorbed heavy dosages of hydrocortisone, actinomycin, Imuran, and prednisone, his white-cell count had retreated from 22,200 to 5,640. His body's ability to fight bacteria, the primary task of the white cells, had effectively been destroyed. In confused desperation Barnard and his team changed his medication again—withdrawing the actinomycin and Imuran while doubling the dosage of prednisone. It did not even feel like detective work to Barnard when they scoured the tests and graphs and samples for clues. He knew they had descended into raw guesswork.

Washkansky went back under the oxygen tent. He looked cold and blue as he still gasped for air. Joe Ozinsky, the anesthetist, inserted an endotracheal tube to assist respiration. Washkansky closed his eyes in relief. Barnard stared down at him. He knew they could only wait, and hope, and guess a little more.

On December 20 a report on the bacterial content of a specimen of sputum indicated that Washkansky had developed growths of klebsiella and pseudomonas. They had infected him after the rejection treatment had attacked his immune system with brutal effectiveness. Double pneumonia, which was killing him fast, resulted from this bacterial invasion of his lungs. Barnard was distraught. It seemed as if his mistaken diagnosis, and determination to fight the inscrutable force of rejection, had resulted in almost certain death for his patient.

He immediately changed the medication again and set about trying to obliterate the klebsiella and pseudomonas. Washkansky, however, was sinking. His lungs had begun to send poorly oxygenated blood back into the arteries. Ozinsky connected the endotracheal tube to a ventilator, which he pumped by hand so that he could deliver pure oxygen into Washkansky—in contrast to the 40 percent oxygen offered by the old Bird respirator.

Ozzie pumped the bag tirelessly—between twenty and twenty-five times a minute. As the hours passed that long night, Ozinsky pumped and talked, talked and pumped, reminding Barnard of Shumway with his constant stream of dry but upbeat humor. Barnard could almost remember some of the cracks Shumway used to make in Minnesota as his anesthetist attempted now to charm the distraught nurses. "What's all this I hear," Ozinsky asked of Nurse Marie Papendieck with mock seriousness, "about you and Mr. Washkansky having a dinner date when he gets out of here?"

Barnard could barely smile, let alone join the painful banter. He knew that Ozinsky, just like Shumway would have done, was attempting to restore their belief. And yet, beneath their shared and desolate gaze, Washkansky was dying from a lack of oxygen. It was like watching a man drown as they stood by helplessly. The more Ozinsky spoke, the harder he pumped. Washkansky's color still worsened. He had turned a colder and deeper blue.

A despairing Barnard concocted a wild plan to place Washkansky on the heart-lung machine. It would be a futile effort to "buy a few more hours" while he tried to work out what he might do next. When he left the room to call Val Schrire, Barnard tried to convince himself that if they could keep Washkansky alive just a little longer, his new course of medication would eventually overcome the pneumonia.

Schrire, even when woken at three in the morning, had too exact a mind to encourage Barnard's muddled thinking. There was no point in prolonging the agony by turning to the heart-lung machine. "Chris," Schrire said, "it's all over."

Barnard sagged and succumbed to the bitter truth. He returned to the room and, in misery, gave the order for Ann Washkansky to be called to her husband's bedside.

She thought Barnard looked demented by grief. He told her that the heart was "perfect" but that there was nothing more he could do for her husband. "Louis kept his word," Barnard said mysteriously. "I'm just ashamed we couldn't keep ours."

"Is he dead?" Ann asked in terror.

"No," Barnard said, "not that."

He may as well have said "not yet," for, as much as she talked, Ann could not raise even a flicker from Louis's half-opened eyes. She eventually forgot about the risk of infection. Ann held him close and told Louis about the wonderful life they had shared together.

Ann and the nurse took turns pumping the bag until, at 4:30 a.m., as more family members arrived and departed, Barnard tried to persuade her that it was time to leave. She was crying as she told the doctor her husband revered, the man with the golden hands, that she wanted to stay until the end. Ann's brother intervened. Her son, Michael, had locked himself in their car.

Inside the sealed doors and windows of Louis's red Zephyr, tears ran down his fourteen-year-old face. Ann was needed more by the living than the dying. She still had a son, if not a husband.

She kissed Louis one last time before being led away. Barnard thought, soon after 4:45 a.m., that he heard the sound of their car coughing into life in the empty hospital parking lot. He could imagine Ann and her son driving through the early-morning darkness, the muffled sound of their crying accompanying each mile they moved further away from Louis. Barnard stared at the distant sight of the Cape Flats, where the colored people, his father's people, would soon awake for a new day.

Ozinsky kept pumping in the surrounding silence. "He looks a little better to me," he said.

"No," Coert Venter insisted, "he's still deteriorating."

"Dr. Venter was a cool clinician," Barnard wrote later. "He could see it coming, and he was not going to turn away amid the wreckage of eighteen days. Occasionally Ozzie or Coert said something to Nurse Papendieck, who worked in silence. And when Ozzie needed a rest she pumped for him, or sometimes Dr. Venter took over. Shortly after 5 a.m. there was a rapid deterioration. The circulation fell off, and we gave intravenous calcium—but it did not help. The lungs began to return an increasing volume of venous blood, and he turned dark blue, almost black."

The transplanted heart, meanwhile, kept on beating steadily. Barnard could not stand still. He drifted in and out of the room. Just after seven a.m., the end, even for Denise Darvall's twenty-five-year-old heart, could be delayed no longer. Venter summoned Barnard to Washkansky's beside. Ozzie, refusing to give in, was still pumping.

"Professor," Venter said softly as he pointed to the heart's last sad flight across the EKG screen, "it's gone into fibrillation."

Barnard looked at the beeping graph of the heart "rolling slowly"—he later wrote—"like an ocean settling after a storm. And then suddenly it shot across the screen: one flat green line. Sister Papendieck began to cry. She was a wonderful woman, and I think it was this which made it more than I could bear. I thanked each and every one of them, and then I went out into the doctor's tea-room and just stood there for a while."

Barnard eventually stepped out onto the hospital balcony. He watched the speckled darkness turn to an orange glow as the sun rose slowly over one of the world's most beautiful cities. He had failed. In eighteen days he had become the most famous doctor on earth, and yet, after everything, he was alone and his patient was dead. Louis Washkansky was dead.

The surgeon could not look any longer at the majesty of that Cape morning. He walked back inside and headed for his office. Barnard lay down on the brown couch and covered his eyes with an arm. His numbed reverie was broken by the appearance of Hamilton Naki, the former gardener whom he had trained to transplant dog kidneys and hearts in the Animal House. If not for the color of his skin, Barnard knew, Naki would have been part of his surgical team eighteen days earlier. He had a touch and a gift which was the equal, if not superior, to that of most of the white surgeons who worked at Groote Schuur. Even that could not spare him from apartheid.

The famous Afrikaner turned his reddened eyes toward the black laboratory assistant. Barnard wanted to say, "Hello, Hami," but he could not get the words out of his mouth. He lay silently on his side.

"Doctor," Hamilton Naki murmured before he closed the door gently behind him to allow Barnard his privacy, "you're working too hard . . ."

Thirteen

DEATH AND AMERICA

 "Well," Marius Barnard consoled his brother a few hours after Washkansky's death, "we climbed Everest. Next time we'll know how to get down."

They walked along a narrow lane that, beneath the shadow of Table Mountain, passed the Animal House and wound down toward the flat, ugly building containing the hospital mortuary. The postmortem theater was crammed with pathologists, physicians, and surgeons. Chris and Marius looked bitterly around the room. Many of the doctors present had ridiculed their transplant plans. The chief pathologist, James Thomson, had been one of the more strident opponents of the procedure. He had refused to discuss the possibilities of such surgery whenever either of the brothers had approached him. And yet Thomson now insisted that he would lead the autopsy on the world's most celebrated patient.

Washkansky's naked body was stretched out on a marble slab, his large head propped against a wooden block. With one long vertical slice from the throat to the gut, Thomson exposed the abdominal and thoracic organs. While both kidneys appeared normal, the pneumonia-ridden lungs had turned solid and blue. It was hard to believe that, only two hours before, Ozinsky had pumped oxygen into them. They looked as if they had been dead for weeks.

When the pathologist parted the pericardial sac, Barnard saw Denise

Darvall's heart. It was the same small and inert muscle he had shocked back to life. He recognized the suture lines he had sewn into her heart. They still looked beautifully precise, a feat even Thomson congratulated him on as he searched for signs of rejection. There were none. The heart seemed to be in fantastic shape. Pneumonia, not rejection, had killed Louis Washkansky.

If Barnard had attacked the infection immediately, as he would have done in a normal patient, it seemed likely that Washkansky would still be alive. The surgeon, instead, had devastated a dangerously ill man's immune system in a misguided attempt to overcome a nonexistent pattern of rejection. Barnard stared down at the terrible consequence of his decision. Washkansky had been reduced to a husk of bone, dead muscle, and severed skin, with doctors crowding around in an attempt to persuade the pathologist to give them each a sliver of the transplanted heart for analysis, or as a souvenir. Thomson guarded the heart carefully as if it belonged to him alone.

Marius clucked in disgust and Chris turned away. Mortified by his mistake, Barnard walked mutely back to ward D1. He was due to fly to America the following afternoon to appear on *Face the Nation* with Adrian Kantrowitz and Michael DeBakey, before meeting President Lyndon Johnson on his Texas ranch. It was meant to be a triumphant trip—both a public celebration of a landmark operation and, privately, an opportunity for him to return to America in the kind of glory he knew would stun his old enemies.

He shuddered at the thought of traveling to America in the wake of Washkansky's death. Barnard imagined arriving in Washington a flustered failure rather than the gleaming hero—a role to which he had just become accustomed. Yet he had no alternative. Barnard would meet Philip Blaiberg, his next transplant patient, before confronting the press at two o'clock that afternoon. And then he would go to America. He would keep fighting.

Barnard had gambled by plunging ahead with the first transplant at such an early stage in his own research. And yet, as he repeatedly told himself that Thursday morning, he had kept Washkansky alive for eighteen days. Kantrowitz's transplant had not even succeeded for eight hours.

Washkansky had also been so close to death before the transplant that the odds against long-term success were astronomical. Philip Blaiberg, though, would provide him with a more realistic hope of survival. Yet whereas in

Washkansky he had had a naïve former boxer, Blaiberg was himself a medical man—a dentist. He seemed unlikely to laud Barnard as "the man with the golden hands" while Washkansky lay cold and stiff on the slab.

Terminal illness, however, can blur the differences between men. When Barnard approached his bed, the fifty-eight-year-old Blaiberg looked at him with the same intent gaze Washkansky had clamped on the surgeon six weeks earlier. Even when he heard of Washkansky's fate, in unflinching detail, Blaiberg's commitment to his own transplant remained emphatic. "Just tell me when you're ready," he instructed Barnard.

Bolstered by such confidence in him, Barnard revealed that he would be in America for the next ten days. In terms of medical protocol, it was a curious decision. Blaiberg was in dire need of surgery, but he believed utterly in Barnard. If the transplant had to be delayed a few more weeks while Barnard raced around America, the tolerant dentist would accept his fate.

"You'll find me here," Blaiberg confirmed, "waiting."

The massed ranks of the media were as captivated when Barnard faced them. His handsome face had acquired a potent gravity, and even the cynical reporters did not revel in his setback. As they watched him reach out for a cigarette, which he smoked dejectedly in front of them, the surgeon seemed more likeable than some hectoring politician or movie star. He was just a man.

There was still something extraordinary about his renewed conviction as, through a cloud of smoke, he insisted that "this wasn't an experiment. It was the corrective treatment for a sick man—and there's no evidence that will convince me to discontinue such treatment for patients with these terminal heart diseases. When the next occasion arises we will definitely transplant again."

Most of Barnard's thwarted rivals endorsed that same belief. Donald Longmore, who with Barnard's old university classmate Donald Ross had hoped to achieve the first transplant at London's National Heart Hospital, appeared quintessentially British in his determination to strike a gracious tone. "The operation was a marvelous achievement. 'Congratulations to Chris Barnard,' is all I can say. South Africans have cause to be very proud indeed. I would like somebody to shake him by the hand and say, 'Jolly good show!' from me."

Adrian Kantrowitz spoke more plainly in Brooklyn. "We were very sorry to learn of the events in South Africa last night. However, we believe that the operation performed by Dr. Barnard represents a great step forward. This is the way progress is made. Man takes one step forward and then falls down. I know that this procedure will prove to be successful."

L ouis Washkansky was buried the following morning, Friday, December 22, 1967. The ceremony was televised around the world—excepting South Africa, of course—and the chief rabbi of Cape Town presented a grand eulogy. "The heart, to the rhythm of whose beat a whole world listened, is stilled," Israel Abrahams told the heaving crowd and glinting cameras. "All mankind stands at this moment in mourning beside the grave of Louis Washkansky . . ."

Marius Barnard and M. C. Botha, both wearing yarmulkes and weeping openly, were among the pallbearers who had lowered the coffin into the earth. Chris Barnard had sent his apologies, explaining that he would be flying to America later that afternoon. Ann Washkansky, who'd never quite trusted the man her husband had venerated, churned angrily at the thought that Barnard should be moving ahead so quickly with his life. Surely he could have come, she complained to her family, for the sake of Louis? Surely he could have delayed his packing just a little longer so that he might have paid one last tribute to the man whose name would forever be entwined with his own? Surely Louis mattered more to him than some American TV show?

Her resentment burned inside her. Chris Barnard, she told herself, was not the great man everyone proclaimed. She knew Louis would have scolded her for such thinking, but she was convinced that he, rather than the absent surgeon, was the real man of nobility and courage. They held her back from the hole as, beneath the sound of her crying, Louis Washkansky was buried in the brown earth.

C hris Barnard could not believe the size of the black stretch limousine that pulled up outside his home in little old Zeekoevlei just after three that afternoon. He was suddenly conscious of wearing a frayed blue suit he had bought fifteen years earlier for Deirdre's baptism. Louwtjie wore a navy-blue dress she had made herself. They had dressed in their very smartest clothes, and yet he could imagine the cool gaze of a line of CBS executives absorbing their appearance. He was sure he and Louwtjie would look pitiful among the rich and the famous in Washington and New York.

The luxurious leather seats of the limo soothed him. He usually traveled to the airport in Louwtjie's little Toyota. A chauffeur-driven limo seemed eminently more suitable. Barnard sank back. What the hell, the surgeon decided, he would enjoy himself—whatever they might make of him in America.

They changed planes in Johannesburg and, for the first time in his life, Barnard flew first class. He was almost beside himself with glee when, having kicked off his shoes and eased into his reclining seat, a sweetly smiling stewardess presented him with a glass of "the finest French champagne." Barnard had never tasted champagne before, and the menu was a more confusing treat, full of strange new words like "canapés" and "foie gras." This was the life he had always been meant to live.

"We were to catch a TWA flight from London to Washington," Barnard remembered later, "but we didn't have to go through the airport. They took us by car from the South African Airways flight to the TWA plane. I only then learned that, because the SAA flight was late, the TWA plane had been delayed by several hours so that I could make it. Just for Me! I suddenly felt very important. When we boarded the TWA plane I laughed when the pretty stewardess asked me to autograph that week's edition of *Time* magazine— there was a picture of me on the cover. Three short weeks previously I couldn't even afford to *buy* a copy, I reflected wryly. Instant fame is an intoxicating experience.

"The flight from Johannesburg to London had been overnight but now, to Washington, it was daylight. I felt refreshed and ready to enjoy every minute. Louwtjie was reading a monthly publication, *Path of Truth,* to which she subscribed, so I made my way to the galley and chatted with the two stewardesses. I had always enjoyed the company of American girls. They usually oozed self-confidence and took great pride in their appearance and were almost always friendly and vivacious. . . . Julie was a blonde from Florida and Anne a brunette from Washington. They kept telling me how much they admired my work and what a wonderful man I must be, which was very flatter-ing, and, better still, they made it clear that they were willing to take care of *any* of my needs. The call-bell rang and it was the captain inviting me to the flight deck. Anne showed me the way and I followed her undulating bottom down the aisle to the front of the plane. We passed Louwtjie, who looked up from her *Path of Truth* without any expression."

Even Louwtjie was mesmerized by the sheer opulence of their presidential suite at the Washington Hilton. She and Chris were convinced that, with its two huge bedrooms, two bathrooms, and gigantic lounge it was actually larger than their modest home in Cape Town. Wherever they looked, there were vases overflowing with ornate arrangements of flowers, or yet more bottles of champagne supplied as a welcome from the hotel.

Glossy television people milled around them, ensuring their comfort and explaining a detailed itinerary that centered around Barnard's appearance on *Face the Nation* and his meeting with President Johnson. The surgeon nod-ded casually, as if he was accustomed to such encounters—although, on the inside, he "recognized the first feelings of panic when someone on the CBS staff reminded me that the program was America's biggest by far and that millions of people would be closely watching me."

Barnard feared exposure as a small-town fraud, a raw Afrikaner lost amid the giants of America. Twenty-four hours later, on Christmas Eve, he would face Michael DeBakey, Adrian Kantrowitz, and a vast and frightening coun-try. DeBakey, the notoriously acerbic "Black Mike," had responded positively, at least on the surface, to the first transplant having been carried out in Cape Town. Barnard was certain DeBakey would be less gracious in person. On their last occasion together in an OR, with DeBakey the surgical master and Barnard the humble observer, the famous American had roared at the obscure South African: "Get out! You're contaminating my operating area!" Barnard now contaminated DeBakey's kingdom of medical celebrity. He could imag-ine the Texas-based surgeon grinding his teeth in fury.

Kantrowitz, meanwhile, might still be fuming from the shock of losing the race in the very last days of a long slog that had consumed years of his life. The tough and imposing surgeon from Brooklyn could shred Barnard if he chose to compare his own copious transplant research with the paltry experiments they had carried out in Cape Town. And what would Barnard say if they asked him about Shumway and Lower and his appropriation of their ideas? He shuddered at the thought that he might wither beneath the searing glare of television. DeBakey and Kantrowitz, he knew, could yet shame him.

C BS had extended the program from its usual thirty-minute format to a full hour for the occasion. Twenty minutes before the "live recording" was begun, with actual transmission to occur four hours later, a beaming producer told Barnard that CBS was expecting a television audience in excess of twenty million to watch the program at six p.m. "That's more than the entire population of your country," the man helpfully reminded the anxious surgeon. Barnard was disconcerted further by the novelty of at the same time having his eyebrows combed in the makeup room. He had already been through the ordeal—more like trauma for an Afrikaner from the *platteland* (flatland)—of having his face patted and powdered before, scandalously, pale-pink lipstick was applied by a beautician. Barnard was too shocked to flirt with her, even when she complimented him on his movie-star looks. He nodded dumbly, unsure whether he would be able to speak when the cameras rolled.

Outside the studio Barnard was surprised again. DeBakey's and Kantrowitz's congratulations seemed as sincere as they were generous. He found it easy to pose for publicity photographs around a plastic heart. As the cameras snapped and whirred, Barnard and Kantrowitz sat on either side of the model, while DeBakey crouched between them. Barnard enjoyed the thought that he would appear more photogenic than either the bald and burly Kantrowitz or the bespectacled and much older and shorter DeBakey.

Barnard felt less assured when they were summoned for filming. The stage was hot and glaring while the floor around them resembled a snake-pit of wires and cables. Barnard felt his stomach tighten while he watched the grim anchorman, Martin Agronsky, check once more that the zipper on his trousers had been pulled shut. It never pays to look a fool on national television. Coming from a country that banned TV, Barnard was suddenly terrified. DeBakey and Kantrowitz, by contrast, seemed commanding as they waited quietly next to him. Barnard wriggled a little more and inadvertently loosened his microphone connection. As the countdown began ("Ten, nine, eight . . ."), a furious producer rectified the technical hitch.

She disappeared miraculously at the count of "one." The room descended into an eerie hush, and then a definitively American voice boomed out: "*Face the Nation* proudly presents a special one-hour interview with the South African heart surgeon Professor Christiaan Barnard, who, three weeks ago tonight, made medical history while transplanting the first human heart in Cape Town, South Africa . . ."

Barnard feared he might be on the verge of a more disastrous kind of legacy—as the worst performer in the history of American television. He watched in fascinated horror as Agronsky earned his money by switching his unsmiling face into a radiant mask. Agronsky talked smoothly about heart transplants while Barnard peered into the darkness surrounding the blazing lights. Kantrowitz was invited to ask the first question.

He helped Barnard settle by asking at what stage of the transplant had he begun to believe it might work? "Well," Barnard said coolly, suddenly realizing he was not about to be sandbagged or derided as a medical hustler, "I think we knew all along it was going to work. We've had nine years of experience with open-heart surgery, having performed well over a thousand open-heart operations. It wasn't as if we were operating on the heart for the first time."

Kantrowitz nodded encouragingly. Renewed confidence coursed through Barnard. "We perfected the surgical technique by doing transplants in dogs in the laboratory. I feel these two aspects ensured that the operation would be a success. But, to answer your question, I only thought it would work when, finally, I had stopped the circulatory support of the heart-lung machine and the transplanted heart maintained a good circulation according to the readings of the blood pressure, the venous pressure, and the urine output."

DeBakey suggested that, in terms of surgical technique, Barnard could have carried out the procedure a year earlier. And so he posed a simple query: "Why did you decide at this time to do it?"

Barnard was gratified that DeBakey had highlighted his readiness to proceed earlier. It gave his work a scientific legitimacy that allowed him to make the outrageous claim that "in my mind there was never a race to be first." Barnard already knew that to admit failure with Washkansky, rather than acknowledge the ferocious ambition that had driven him past Shumway and Kantrowitz, would make him appear a far more sympathetic figure. He also understood the need to stress his own South African context, as a way of distinguishing him from Kantrowitz and DeBakey. And so he mentioned the kidney transplant he had done on Edith Black in October as the defining moment when he had gained "experience in human donation of a vital organ, under South African law, and also in the use of immunosuppressive drugs."

Barnard revealed that political sensitivities had actually delayed Washkansky's transplant. He spoke of his and Val Schrire's decision not to accept a colored donor in November because of a wish not to be seen as "experimenting" on a black South African. In doing so, he appeared more socially conscious and sensitive toward the racial turmoil that affected both America and his own country. Barnard was in the swing. He shimmered even when he lied. After he had explained South Africa's unique legislation, which allowed two doctors to declare a patient brain-dead, Barnard insisted that he had waited for Denise Darvall's heart to stop beating naturally before he opened her chest. He knew that the truth would have been too shocking in a country that still defined life by the heartbeat.

He sailed through the rest of the hour with a measured style that encouraged the Washington correspondent for South Africa's largest newspaper, *The Star*, to delight in the fact that "Professor Chris Barnard scored a great personal success on American television's most influential program. Judging from the comments of American journalists, with whom I watched the earlier filming of the program, his quiet, self-assured manner, complete frankness and photogenic good-looks cannot have failed to impress and charm the many millions who later saw the show on their screens."

The Washington Post was more impressed by "the grave and somber mien" Barnard brought to his reflections on Washkansky's death. Seeming as compassionate as he was bold, Barnard stole many more American hearts that night. *The Washington Star* described him as "South Africa's winning answer to Dr. Kildare," while the New York tabloids were even more gushing in their descriptions of him as "Dr. Charisma" and "A Real Heart-Throb!"

By the time the newspapers hit the streets on Christmas morning, the Barnards had already landed in New York, having flown in from Washington on CBS's executive jet. They spent the day at the home of the company's president, Gordon Manning, while rival networks fumed at the news that Barnard's next television appearance would again be on CBS the following morning—when he would be interviewed in depth by Walter Cronkite. As much as he relished such exalted exposure, Barnard was thrilled most by a chance to renew contact with Walt Lillehei, his Minnesota mentor, who had moved to New York six weeks before.

In contrast, Lillehei's arrival in New York had been framed by disappointment. Earlier that year, despite leading Minnesota's revolutionary open-heart program for almost a quarter of a century, while transforming cardiac surgery around the world, Lillehei had been passed over as Owen Wangensteen's successor as chief of surgery. Lillehei, whose playboy demeanor and casual attitude toward the hospital's administration had cost him his rightful promotion, had accepted a similar position at the New York Hospital–Cornell Medical Center's Department of Surgery. He left Minnesota in mid-November, refusing to obey an instruction that the bulk of his laboratory equipment and materials belonged to the university. Lillehei waited until darkness fell one Saturday night and then he and his closest colleagues loaded up three rented trucks. They stripped the Minnesota lab of everything and left a single red rose on the floor of an empty room.

Barnard met up with him again in New York on December 27, 1967. He was impressed to discover that his old hero now rented an apartment on the Upper East Side that offered a stunning view of the Manhattan skyline. Lillehei had begun to sample the slick life of the fastest city on earth and was already accepted as a raucous regular at hip bars like the Recovery Room and the chic La Chansonette. Barnard was inspired once more by Lillehei—not, this time, by his extraordinary surgical innovations, but by his enduring ability, even at the age of forty-nine, to surround himself with uniformly young and beautiful women. His wife, Kaye, who suffered even more than Louwtjie from her husband's philandering, remained in St. Paul. She believed that Walt had "gone berserk" in New York, and waited for him to come home to her.

Lillehei, in his quieter moments, was mildly amused that his own considerable renown had suddenly been dwarfed by that of one of his more gauche residents. He remembered saving Barnard's career after the South African had inadvertently opened a hole in a patient's heart and lost him on the table in Minnesota because he did not have the wit to use his finger to stanch the bleeding. He remembered all the letters he had written to Barnard in Cape Town, bolstering his flagging confidence and encouraging him to continue. He remembered marveling at Shumway's meticulous research in cardiac transplantation and feeling strangely disappointed that the brightest of all his residents had not made history first out at Stanford.

Yet Lillehei merely shrugged at an obvious defect in Barnard's character: he would have preferred Barnard to acknowledge the debt he owed Shumway—but he was not going to beg one former resident to praise another. Shumway would survive his private catastrophe. The Stanford surgeon, Lillehei believed, would almost certainly go on to produce the greater legacy of work. But for now it was Barnard's moment, and Lillehei, in one of his best party moods, agreed to hang out with him for a few days in New York. They made a dashing team. If Lillehei loved a drink far more than Barnard did, they were a match in their seemingly insatiable appetite for women and good times.

They were also both still intensely curious about work, and so an invitation from Kantrowitz to visit him in his animal lab in Brooklyn seemed an excellent reason to suspend the festivities, briefly. Indeed, Lillehei saw something of himself in Kantrowitz—in his gunslinger personality and relentless quest for new ideas. He regarded Shumway as a better researcher and a far more accomplished surgeon than both Barnard and Kantrowitz, but he appreciated that the South African and the New Yorker brought verve and daring to their work, something akin to the qualities he had drawn upon in his cross-circulation and open-heart experiments. Lillehei was certain that his own breakthrough in the mid-1950s was still more significant than the simple mechanical surgery of the transplant—but he understood why the world was in thrall to Barnard.

In the laboratory, however, Barnard stood in awe of Kantrowitz. While the trio of audacious surgeons ambled around the huge room at Maimonides where Kantrowitz had worked for so long, transplanting hundreds of puppy hearts, Barnard would stare in amazement whenever another long-term survivor was brought in on a lead. He would shake his head in disbelief when Kantrowitz told him how many months or years each of these growing and tail-wagging dogs had been alive with a new heart.

"Hell, Adrian," Barnard finally said as Lillehei burst out laughing, "how do you get these bloody dogs to live so long?"

"Practice," Kantrowitz said with a wry grin as he thought of all the years he and Shumway had toiled while Barnard had been out waterskiing with his daughter. "Years of practice . . ."

White South Africans were more fascinated by the news that Barnard had received a personal call from Dean Martin, who had invited him to his home in Hollywood during his next American visit. An unusually star-struck Louwtjie confirmed that "Chris always loved the Dean Martin TV show when we were living in the United States." The South African press, however, was notably cool to some of Barnard's nocturnal activities. In the company of Lillehei he had shown that, as a Reuters correspondent reported, "He knows exactly how to unbend at a New York nightspot while listening to some authentic Dixieland music."

Some of the English papers in Johannesburg and Cape Town printed a photograph of Barnard "shaking hands with an unknown Negro Dixieland musician" in Greenwich Village. *Die Vaderland* (The Fatherland) refused to print the shot and warned instead "that Professor Barnard should not let his deserved fame turn his head. It is not expected that our premier surgeon, an Afrikaner who has done so much brilliant work, should now taint his achievement by appearing in a Negro jazz club. We can only trust that he accepted this dubious invitation out of politeness rather than actual choice."

The South African government exhibited a little more sophistication in their use of Barnard as a force for propaganda. Lillehei was once more a grinning accomplice when Barnard was summoned to a beautiful stone mansion on Park Avenue, where he met Pik Botha, the South African consul in New York and a future minister of foreign affairs. Lillehei recalled the surreal encounter years later. "[Botha] said to Chris, 'Dr. Barnard, you have done a great thing for South Africa. Most people in this country and around the world think South Africans are living in mud huts and wearing grass skirts—in a very primitive society. So I encourage you.' Later Chris told me that the government paid some of his expenses to travel. The consul said to him, 'Talk to as many people, meet as many people and spread the message—not only of the heart transplant but of the cosmopolitan society in our country.' Chris took that very literally."

John Lindsay, the mayor of New York, was an immediate convert. "I have to say," Lindsay insisted, "that Chris Barnard is a great doctor, a great surgeon, a great professional, and, as I have discovered in a very short time, a great guy, too."

He did not have a lock on everyone's heart. Louwtjie had become increasingly disenchanted with the charade of fame. She reminded him that they were just ordinary Afrikaners who should not be seduced by oily praise or fancy living. Barnard was indignant. He had worked, choosing his phrase carefully, as he remembered all the hours he had spent in the lab, "like a bloody dog" to get this far. It was time to enjoy his reward. He didn't care if she wanted to sulk and go home. There were lots of women out there who were dying to meet him. Louwtjie looked at him scornfully. She was not fooled by his arrogance. She knew his every crack and flaw.

Harold M. Schmeck of *The New York Times* gave Barnard an equally rough ride over the bumpy contours of his astonishing rise to fame. Barnard recalled their encounter with vitriol: "It was soon clear that this so-called science writer was not interested in the medical aspects of our work—I suspect he was keener to get something sensational or controversial. 'Dr. Dwight E. Harken from Boston claims you stole the technique from Dr. Shumway,' Schmeck said with a sardonic smile. It was a statement rather than a question. [Barnard replied:] 'I know Dr. Harken. I have great respect for his work and he's entitled to his own opinion.' The reporter wouldn't give up. 'Dr. Shumway said in an interview, and I quote, "The surgical technique used was based on the work done by Doctors Lower and Hurley at Stanford."'"

Barnard tried to suggest he had been influenced more by British experiments discussed by Cass and Brock in a 1959 Guy's Hospital report. In 1960, in *Surgical Forum,* Barnard told Schmeck, "'Lower and Shumway reported their results in canine transplantation using the same technique. I'll leave it to you to decide whose technique I used.' [Schmeck persisted:] 'Dr. Barnard, are you implying that Dr. Shumway made no contributions in this field?'

"Now I was really beginning to lose my temper. 'No, I'm not saying that at all,' I sighed. 'Dr. Shumway and his colleagues did excellent research in this field and I have never hesitated to give them full credit. What I don't understand is why some American doctors feel that I stole his ideas and that *he* should have done the first heart transplant. I'm the first to admit that I made use of a lot of his findings. Surely he published them in medical journals so that other doctors could learn from his experience? That's what I did because, as you should know, doctors share information—which incidentally, is why I'm in America right now.' The reporter finally gave up. He switched off his tape recorder and, with a half-hearted goodbye, he left."

Shumway had endured a deep and private hurt that, in its true density, was known only to Lower and himself. Yet Shumway was determined to erect a ring around that dark place so that he could move ahead with work that mattered even more to him. He and Lower had seen each other on December 28 at Chicago's O'Hare Airport, where, with twelve other eminent surgeons, including Kantrowitz, they had met the National Heart Institute's director, Donald Frederickson, and six of his lieutenants. Each of the fourteen surgeons was in receipt of a National Institutes of Health grant to investigate the clinical opportunities of human heart transplantation. The purpose of the three-hour conference was to discuss the state of their specialist field and to assess ways in which they might proceed in the wake of the voracious transplant fever that now gripped the world.

Although his presence in America was being broadcast across every front page in the country, Chris Barnard had not been invited to attend. He was neither an American nor a beneficiary of NIH funding. But there was another reason. The bulk of American surgeons disliked Barnard intensely and believed, overwhelmingly, that the ultimate prestige should have been accorded, if not to them individually, to Shumway.

CBS nevertheless decided to fly Barnard from New York to Chicago in order that he might make a surprise appearance. They asked Kantrowitz if he would be willing to sign Barnard in as his guest at the airport conference. Kantrowitz, typically, was not about to get bogged down in political niceties. He belonged neither to the CBS gang nor to the Shumway group. Kantrowitz knew Barnard was a surgical hustler, but one part of him admired the South African's bravado. Of course Barnard could come as his guest. Hell, Kantrowitz would have been just as happy to sign in Norm Shumway as his guest. They'd all been racing together.

A furious disbelief settled over the conference. Was it not enough for Barnard to sneak by with the first transplant? Did he have to hijack their meeting as well? They allowed him to join them, but only out of the chilliest form of courtesy. Shumway, of course, shook him by the hand, but the division between Barnard and the rest was plain.

The South African stressed that, despite the death of Washkansky, transplantation could prolong the life of a patient by a significant period of time. Barnard purposely sidestepped the unresolved issue of rejection, for he was already growing impatient with calls for him to curb his transplant surgery. In the full rush of fame Barnard did not want to be detained by caution. He now knew that he far preferred the television studio to the research laboratory. Who would want to work silently and obscurely for years in devising an immunological cocktail that would overcome the rejection of an organ graft, when he could reflect instead on his surgical feat of being the first to transplant the heart?

Shumway and the others, Kantrowitz included, urged a public acknowledgment that their obviously limited understanding of rejection militated against future transplants in any other context than that of a clinical trial. While a patient might have his immediate life span extended by weeks and possibly even months, it was far too early to promise anything further. They needed to work methodically for years and conquer rejection before they could endorse Barnard's claim that transplantation was about to become a routine procedure.

It was an unglamorous and medically driven point of dissension, and CBS chose to skip over the frosty conference in most of their reports. The animosity toward Barnard among his American contemporaries, meanwhile, had deepened. Shumway himself preferred to simply stay out of Barnard's way—just as he had done when he'd flatly rejected invitations to appear alongside him on *Face the Nation* and the *Today* show. Shumway hoped he would never have to meet the South African again.

Barnard's final encounter on his American excursion was similarly loaded with disillusionment. He and Louwtjie spent much of December 29 at President Johnson's ranch north of San Antonio. After lunch and five hours in his company, in which Johnson had shown scant interest in the heart transplant, Barnard was privately scathing. "So that was the President of the United States," he wrote later. "What a disappointment! Perhaps it's unfair to judge a man after such a short time, but I have to say that he was far from the formidable leader I expected. His size and height were impressive—his intellect wasn't."

At the ensuing press conference Barnard suggested that the president looked tired, then dutifully added: "I admire him. I think he's a great man."

B arnard flew back into Cape Town just after three p.m. on New Year's Day. He went home for two hours of sleep before he was roused by a call from Groote Schuur. Barnard had another life to save, and so he sped toward the hospital. Philip Blaiberg's condition had worsened markedly. The dentist had been stricken by a pulmonary embolus while Barnard had been in New York. And yet, late on the first afternoon of a new year, there was suddenly a rejuvenated sense of hope for him.

A twenty-four-year-old man, Clive Haupt, had suffered a brain hemorrhage on the beach that afternoon. Haupt had stretched out on the sand, and his buddies, who had been kidding him about his recent marriage, laughed at the sight. He was either being worn out by Dorothy, his wife of three months, they joked, or he was simply getting lazy. "Then someone tried to shake him," recalled his brother-in-law, Alfred Snyders. "They found that he was unconscious and that his tongue and mouth were swollen. What a fright we got."

Haupt, until his collapse, had been in perfect health. Snyders told the *Cape Argus* that "Clive was a practical joker, a fun-loving fellow. We are all deeply upset. His mother is shocked and his wife just cannot be consoled."

Remembering that Clive had followed the Washkansky transplant with fascination, his mother gave Barnard permission to consider him as a potential donor. His heart was strong and his blood tissue matched that of Blaiberg. He seemed the ideal donor—except for two politically striking facts: Haupt was a colored man, and he was being examined by Raymond Hoffenberg, a neurologist at Groote Schuur who was about to be subjected to a government banning order that would come into effect the following day.

Barnard insisted that, as Blaiberg had again underlined his willingness to accept a "nonwhite" heart, he would not be deterred by the irrelevance of a donor's skin color. Hoffenberg's position was more complex. His compassionate and outspoken opposition to apartheid had resulted in him being charged under the Suppression of Communism Act. A banning order would prevent him from working or teaching in any hospital or educational institution.

The government was so anxious to be rid of Hoffenberg, whose persecution had been followed for months by the liberal press, that they announced themselves ready to cut a deal with the doctor of conscience. They would return his passport, which had been seized in June of 1966, and allow him to travel to Britain for ten days early in 1968 in order to discuss terms for a position he had been offered in London. Hoffenberg's choice was stark—he could either accept his draconian banning order or opt for voluntarily exile in Britain.

He had already agreed to the latter route and, in another bleak irony, Haupt would be the last patient he would examine at Groote Schuur. The pressure on Hoffenberg was immense. Apart from the trauma of his ban and preparing to leave a hospital that he had loved, he was expected to make a quick conclusion of brain death so that Barnard could continue down his blazing path of transplantation. While Hoffenberg had seen the government exploit the first transplant as ruthless propaganda, he was too principled a doctor to allow his political misgivings to affect his medical judgment. He assured Chris Barnard and Jannie Louw, the chief of surgery, that if he found a complete absence of cerebral activity he would be willing to declare the death of Clive Haupt and allow the removal of his heart.

While Chris had refused to speak out in defense of Hoffenberg during the preceding months, Marius Barnard had regularly expressed his support and joined the long line of Groote Schuur doctors who had petitioned the government to drop its harassment of their eminent colleague. Hoffenberg had noted the difference between the political outlook and character of the brothers. Yet even if he felt scant kinship with the swaggering Chris Barnard, Hoffenberg carried out the usual tests. They produced troubling results. While the overwhelming evidence pointed toward brain death, Hoffenberg detected some random neurological reflexes. He was certain that there would be no improvement, but he could not sanction the transplant while there were occasional glimmers of life amid the otherwise total oblivion that had overcome Haupt's brain.

As Barnard paced the room in agitation, Jannie Louw turned to Hoffenberg and addressed him by the nickname—Bill—his physician friends always used. "God, Bill," Louw said in his guttural Afrikaans accent, "what sort of heart are you going to give us?"

Hoffenberg suggested that it would be best if they returned early the following morning to reassess the cerebral function. He would at least be allowed to pay one last visit to Groote Schuur before his banning order took effect at noon.

Reporters, oblivious of the drama unfolding inside the hospital, crowded around a frazzled Barnard as he left Groote Schuur at 9:55 p.m. Asked what he had been doing the past five hours, Barnard snapped: "Working—of course!" Their headlines would have to wait, like him, just a little longer.

Barnard, exhausted by his American trip, slept more deeply that night than Hoffenberg, who tormented himself with doubts that he was "being unnecessarily obstructive."

Early the next morning Hoffenberg arrived for the last time at Groote Schuur. He soon concluded that Clive Haupt had suffered absolute brain death during the night. Hoffenberg could no longer elicit even the slightest reflex cerebral activity. In his final act as a South African physician he made the call, at 9:07, informing Barnard that he could proceed with his second, and the world's third, cardiac transplant.

Hoffenberg signed the death certificate at 10:42 that Tuesday morning, January 2, 1968. Barnard and his team entered the Charles Saint theater on the stroke of eleven. Exactly an hour later their brilliant colleague "Bill" Hoffenberg was banned by the South African government and declared an enemy of the state.

Jet-lagged and complaining of terrible pain in his hands, Barnard made a near-disastrous mistake at the outset of the operation. As he struggled to place an aortic catheter over a metal connector, his arthritic hands began to shake. The connector slipped and Barnard inadvertently pulled an arterial catheter out of Blaiberg's aorta. There was instantaneous and profuse bleeding, which Barnard, remembering the old lesson he had learned from Lillehei, stanched with his finger. Blaiberg was still in desperate trouble and in danger of brain death. Barnard had to compose himself before he successfully slipped the catheter back into the aorta. He was sufficiently distressed to ask his first assistant, Rodney Hewitson, to restore the connection.

There was a further crisis just as Barnard prepared to insert the final stitch in Blaiberg's new heart. A power cut engulfed the entire hospital, casting the theater into darkness.

"Who switched off the fucking lights?" Barnard yelled. "I can't see!"

The heart-lung machine also ceased pumping. Blaiberg had neither a heart nor a machine to keep him alive. In the surrounding blackness, Johan van Heerden, the chief perfusionist responsible for the heart-lung oxygenator, could not even see the crank that would enable him to pump the machine by hand.

On the verge of panic again, Barnard managed to think clearly enough to order van Heerden to remove the tubing from the venous pump so that blood would drain freely into the venous well. He could then, by feel if nothing else, crank the arterial pump.

Barnard decided to try to start the heart. It began fibrillating immediately and then, almost miraculously, picked up a spontaneous and steady beat. As if on cue, the lights came back on a moment later and they could see that the transplanted heart had tautened and turned a deep shade of pink.

"It's beating," someone said in astonishment. "It's beating."

The following afternoon the *Cape Argus* reported in its triumphant front-page story that "Dr. Philip Blaiberg, the second man in the world to have another person's heart beating in his body, is fully conscious in his sterilized ward at Groote Schuur Hospital. He spoke his first words since the operation. According to the official hospital bulletin, Dr. Blaiberg said: 'I am thirsty,' and then, 'please give my regards to my wife.' The fifty-eight-year-old retired dentist is making good progress."

Exultant reportage, which rang around the world, made no mention of the difficulties Barnard had experienced during the four-hour operation. Rather, as the *Argus* confirmed, the successful transplant "was front page news in British newspapers today. Many newspapers emphasized the irony of a white man receiving a non-white heart in the land of apartheid."

While *The Daily Sketch* suggested that Barnard "reveals the temperament of a pioneer and is prepared to gamble with his own reputation," *The Guardian* was more politically caustic. Under the headline "Brothers Under the Skin," their lead editorial writer observed that "in South Africa blood is not transfused from the non-white to the white races, yet Dr. Blaiberg is a white man who owes his continuance among us to the heart of a colored man. Prime Minister Vorster has decisions of his own to make. If a white man can use a colored man's heart after death, can he sit on the same park bench with him when both are living? Probably not. The surgeon should know that he faces grave charges. There is no provision under the Group Areas Act for black hearts to beat in white neighborhoods. Mitigating circumstances may be pleaded for him, but there can be no doubt that Mr. Haupt is committing a posthumous offence."

Two days later, with Blaiberg continuing to rally and appearing far stronger than Washkansky had at a similar postoperative stage, Barnard entered a colored area in Salt River for the funeral of Clive Haupt. He would not repeat the mistake he had made in excusing himself from the burial of Louis Washkansky. The colored funeral, for him, also resonated deeply with the memory of his father.

"When he entered St. Luke's Anglican Church shortly before 3 p.m., thousands waiting outside clapped and whistled," the *Argus* rejoiced, as if covering the arrival of a divine presence. "As he walked through the mass of people, Professor Barnard was almost in danger of losing his jacket as the crowd jostled to get close to him. Most were intent on touching him. Once they had done so, they were satisfied. The scene was the same at the Woltemade Cemetery. Scores of people crowded around the mayor's car in which Professor Barnard and Dr. M.C. Botha left Woltemade. One colored boy came away from the car clutching a copy of the New Testament. On the blank page at the back was the signature of Professor Barnard. A colored girl sprang away from the crowd, screaming with joy. 'I touched his heart,' she shouted. 'Oh, he's just wonderful.'"

Fourteen

THE TRIAL

Stanford Medical Center, Palo Alto, California,
January 6, 1968

Norman Shumway made the call just before noon that bright but cold Saturday morning. The man lived in a neat, modest family home in the neighboring town of Mountain View, in the Santa Clara Valley. There was something reassuringly solid and sensible about his name—Bill White—but Shumway would have understood if he had collapsed amid his wild grief.

At six o'clock the previous evening, Bill White's forty-three-year-old wife, Virginia, had suffered a brain hemorrhage. She had been happy, for she and her husband had just celebrated their twenty-second wedding anniversary. Virginia and Bill had been high school sweethearts and now had an eighteen-year-old daughter and a twelve-year-old son. And then there she suddenly lay, looking swollen and lifeless on the living room floor. At nearby El Camino Hospital it was confirmed that Virginia-Mae White was brain-dead by the time they placed her on the respirator that would maintain her breathing through the night.

Four hours before Virginia's terrible seizure, at exactly 2:00 p.m. on Friday, January 5, a fifty-four-year-old retired steel worker, Mike Kasperak, had had a massive heart attack at his home in East Palo Alto. He was admitted to Stanford, where his physician, Martin Robinson, told Shumway that Kasperak had suffered from chronic cardiac failure for the past two years and, with his heart enlarged and scarred and fibrous, had almost died a few weeks earlier. Kasperak, an obvious candidate for a transplant, listened to Robinson's advice that nothing else would save him. He was sufficiently lucid to ask his wife, Ferne, whether he should submit to such a dramatic operation. "Go ahead," she said, "I want you alive with me."

If he had not been such a coolly pragmatic man, who had already endured a futile eight-week wait for a donor, Shumway might have shivered at the coincidence that the separate fates of two distinct families should collide in this new way, leaving only the hope that one life might be salvaged. All it needed now was for him to speak to Bill White and to obtain his permission to remove his wife's heart.

Shumway always said that he was not the man best equipped to handle such a raw situation. For all his compassion, he liked to keep his everyday conversations light and breezy. This was hardly a wise-cracking opportunity. Yet Bill White, possessed by a strange calm, helped him. Once Shumway had explained the mechanics of transplantation and discussed the concept of brain death, White revealed that his wife had been fascinated by the South African transplant. She and Bill had recently talked to friends about Edward Darvall—who had allowed his daughter's heart to be used for the Washkansky transplant. "How marvelous," Virginia White said, "to give someone else a chance to live."

White needed only thirty minutes to discuss the transplant with his children. His answer to Shumway was decisive. They wanted him to proceed.

"I've got two of the proudest children you ever knew," he said later to reporters. "They think it's great. Knowing that she is helping another is easing our grief."

Virginia-Mae White's body, with her heart still beating, arrived at Stanford at 3:30 p.m. on January 6, 1968. Ninety minutes later, Shumway having obtained a private neurosurgeon's confirmation of her brain death, they were scrubbed and ready. Shumway led the way. Ed Stinson and a team of sixteen followed him into the operating room to begin Stanford's first, and the world's fourth, human heart transplant.

For Ed Stinson, the emotional trauma was as taxing as the physical demands. As Shumway's first assistant, and his brilliant protégé, he assumed the greatest burden. It was Stinson, after all, who had collected Virginia White in an ambulance and accompanied her on the short trip back to Stanford. He and Shumway had also shared the existential moment when, together, they had stood over Kasperak's anesthetized body in the OR. After connecting him to the machine and removing his heart, they had stared into the abyss of a huge pericardial cavity. Stinson admitted later that he had wondered "what on earth have we done?"

In the ensuing hours, and even through the first few days after the transplant, Stinson thought Shumway was exuberant. It was as if he could finally admit to jubilation. He had fulfilled his dream. Shumway was also plainly thrilled at the work done by Stinson, a young surgeon who, without any help from cardiologists or immunologists, led the postoperative fight to save Kasperak.

Shumway, meanwhile, set out to quell the frenzy surrounding his hospital. The first hundred journalists had arrived at Stanford even before he and Stinson had entered the OR. Reporters had since been caught impersonating doctors in an attempt to catch a glimpse or snapshot of Mike Kasperak. Shumway, much as he loathed the task, went out to face the heaving pack at regular press conferences. The surgeon was too astute not to appear amiable, and he always spoke calmly while reminding the zealous horde that the transplant was "the logical culmination of approximately nine years of laboratory work, here at Stanford." He also stressed that "We have reached first base, perhaps, but the work is now just beginning. What will be done in the next several days and weeks in the management of this patient will determine whether the result is truly successful. There is no way at this time that the episode can be termed an actual success."

Most journalists were intrigued by his relationship with Barnard. "Did you go to school in the East with Dr. Barnard?" someone asked.

Shumway nodded. "Dr. Barnard and I were at the University of Minnesota for two years as surgical fellows."

"At the same time?"

"The same time," Shumway said quietly. He folded his arms across his chest as if in self-defense.

"Doctor, this is probably a personal question," another reporter interjected. Shumway turned his gaze on his next interrogator, who hesitated a moment before pressing ahead. "You said on November 20 that you and your team were ready to do this operation, and yet Dr. Barnard went ahead and was the first to do it. Do you feel any personal enmity or bitterness about this?"

There was a sudden hush around the room. But Shumway was ready. Shumway was strong.

"No," he said lightly, "I thought it was a marvelous thing. I admired him greatly for moving ahead in this direction. I thought he did, you may remember me saying, a very good job."

"Have you been in further contact with Dr. Barnard since the transplant?"

"No," Shumway said with a mysterious smile, "but I saw him on television last week."

He returned to Stinson's side and they tried valiantly to stabilize Kasperak. During the first five postoperative days Stinson rarely slept as he struggled against the monumental odds of attempting to save a patient who, it had since emerged, suffered multiple organ failure. In addition to the liver, his kidneys and lungs had begun progressively to fail. Moreover, Kasperak was a heavy smoker who had worked for decades in a fume-filled steel mill, and his lungs were notably leathery. He also bled constantly. With the liver's rapid deterioration, there were attendant clotting abnormalities. On January 11, Stinson attempted to remove the impurities in Kasperak's blood.

Two days later, exactly a week since they had transplanted Virginia White's heart into Mike Kasperak, Stinson and Shumway confronted the latest grave setback. Kasperak had slumped into a semi-comatose state. Stinson quickly identified the cause as an excessive accumulation of bilirubin—a degradation product of hemoglobin, the oxygen-carrying protein in the blood. The crisis had nothing to do with rejection or any blip in the steady beating of his new heart. It was a direct result of liver dysfunction.

Amid the steady deterioration of their patient, Stinson and Shumway salvaged moments of pathos and beauty. They managed to prop up Kasperak in a chair so that, at least for fifteen minutes, he could accept a visit from his wife in a more dignified manner. Although he still could not speak, with tubes running into his mouth, the old steelworker managed to reach for a pen. After looking at his wife he wrote down some words—"I love you"—and then stretched out and gave the note to her.

Ferne Kasperak met the press for the first time, on January 16, shortly after a reporter had been caught scaling a hospital wall in an attempt to take a photograph of her husband in his second-floor ICU ward. Even though his gallbladder had just been removed, in a second operation meant to alleviate the danger to his liver, Mrs. Kasperak was convinced that with the "wonderful support of Dr. Shumway and Dr. Stinson, Mike's going to make it."

Shumway and Stinson already knew. They could not hold back death from a man who seemed to be dying from a dozen different causes. There was little they could do to stop the bleeding and the inexorable decline of his lungs, kidneys, and liver.

Kasperak began to bleed uncontrollably on the morning of January 19. They took him back to the OR for a third time and opened him up once more to find a bleeding ulcer high up in the stomach. Shumway sutured the ulcer and then removed the spleen. Kasperak had moved a little further up the critical list.

Finally, at 1:43 a.m. on January 21, Kasperak died of a massive hemorrhage of the stomach. Ferne was at his bedside with both Shumway and Stinson. Fourteen days and five hours had passed since they had inserted his new heart.

When Shumway faced the press at eleven o'clock that morning, he was weary but composed. He would take no questions but he would make a statement. "Mr. Kasperak, as you know, was a terminal patient who had less than fifteen days of life after heart transplantation—but what should be emphasized is that during this time he survived a fantastic galaxy of complications which we have seen in other kinds of cardiac patients but never in such profusion.

We think that because of his normal cardiac action he was able to survive, first of all, renal failure and then hepatic and liver failure and then three major operations—all of which were done, of course, during the time that his circulation was moved by the transplanted heart. So this gives us some hope. . . ."

Ed Stinson, who had already crawled into bed in an attempt to catch up on over two weeks of minimal sleep, knew an even more emphatic truth. Kasperak's new heart had worked and pumped strongly. A long clinical program of human heart transplantation that would run for decades under Shumway and Stinson at Stanford had just begun. "Where there is death," as the slogan on Shumway's office wall promised, "there is hope."

Adrian Kantrowitz was one of the first to cable Shumway immediately after the Stanford transplant. On January 7, these sincere words came from the heart of a big man: *"Congratulations on wonderful surgical achievement and important further education regarding nature of clinical trial. My best wishes to you, your associates and your patient. Adrian Kantrowitz, M.D."*

Two days earlier, on January 5, he had chaired a meeting at Maimonides in preparation for his own next transplant. With the mania escalating around them, they focused on their key strategies. The minutes from that meeting summarized their battle plan: "We will make no announcement. If things go well, Dr. Sherman should handle all publicity. If things do not go well, Dr. Kantrowitz will handle the press." It was decided further that, apart from medical staff assigned to the two operating rooms, "No one else will be allowed to enter. Guards will be at the door of both OR 5 and OR 6."

A retired fifty-eight-year-old fireman, Louis Block, was in urgent need of a transplant. After a succession of heart attacks, which had begun nine years earlier, his ability to breathe had become increasingly restricted. As his heart grew larger but weaker, a corresponding deterioration in his lungs occurred. Block had been admitted to Maimonides in late December, but Kantrowitz had warned the former fireman of a potentially long wait. His blood type, AB-positive, was found in less than 5 percent of Americans.

While they waited, newspapers thrilled to the daily drama of various transplant sagas and made grand promises that heart disease would soon be conquered. Surgeons on every continent announced their desire to join the dangerous race to carry out the next series of heart transplants. None had engaged in any of the necessary research or preparation. The still inscrutable beast of rejection was conveniently forgotten in the rush to follow Barnard down the path of fame and glory.

Kantrowitz, having been at work in transplantation research for six long years, was more mindful of the terrible medical hazards they all faced. Yet he also knew that chance could not always be denied by caution. When the opportunity rose up you had to take it—even if you risked failure again.

On January 8, 1968, Helen Krouch, a petite and radiant health worker from New Jersey, had read the latest newspaper reports on transplantation. "If I could save someone's life with my heart," the twenty-nine-year-old told her parents, "I would do it. If I knew I was going to die, I'd like to die that way."

Her wish now sounded like an eerie premonition. She collapsed in a parking lot in Paterson the very next morning. The pressure from a previously unidentified tumor on her brain caused her to fall into an irreversible coma. Helen's father, remembering her words, asked the attending doctor to call Adrian Kantrowitz at Maimonides.

It seemed more miraculous than coincidental when it was established that Helen Krouch also shared the same obscure blood type as Louis Block. Kantrowitz felt strongly that, given such an unlikely match, they had to take the risk. Sometimes, he said to the team gathered around him, you just have to ride with fate.

Krouch's heart stopped a few hours after she arrived at Maimonides. And so, at 1:10 on the afternoon of January 9, Kantrowitz began his second, and the world's fifth, human heart transplant.

He swore softly when his eyes locked on the donor heart, which was half the size he had anticipated. The idea of a heart this tiny supporting a large male body seemed unlikely. But when next would they find AB-positive blood compatibility? They had to try.

The anticipated four-hour operation became a bloody marathon in which Kantrowitz turned to the intra-aortic balloon pump he had invented. He would use the helium-driven mechanical device to boost the flagging heart.

Kantrowitz inserted the pump through an artery in Block's groin and advanced it into the aorta. After more than eight hours in surgery, they finally began to stitch the chest shut.

Kantrowitz buried his face in his hands. The surgeon stood there for ten or fifteen seconds, his face hidden, as exhaustion and stress drained through him.

He soon discovered that, after another leak to the press, the hospital was plagued with reporters. Kantrowitz was forced into another impromptu press conference at 9:15 that evening. "The patient is in reasonably satisfactory condition," he said. "But our major problem is that the heart is small and the cardiac output isn't enough to carry the load. We feel we have to be guarded about the outcome until we can stabilize the patient."

"But would you say it's been a success?" a journalist insisted on asking.

Kantrowitz shook his head. "I don't think any heart transplant can be considered a success until the patient goes home."

At 12:40 a.m., Peter Baglio, a hospital administrator, confirmed that Block had "taken a turn for the worse" and his name had been placed on the critical list. "We are having difficulty in maintaining his blood pressure."

Louis Block died at 4:35 that black and snowy morning. Helen Krouch's heart had been beating in his chest for less than ten hours. Kantrowitz was devastated. He would never transplant another heart.

That same morning a report emerged from the briefly forgotten space race. *Surveyor,* the final craft in America's series of unmanned lunar missions, had made a safe landing on the moon, providing a triumphant conclusion to a seven-year program. Within another eighteen months, while surgical teams confronted the failures of transplantation and the terrors of rejection, a man would finally walk on the surface of the moon. One scientific miracle had, at least for a while, taken precedence over another.

Four of the world's first five heart transplant patients—Louis Washkansky, Jamie Scudero, Mike Kasperak, and Louis Block—were already dead. The experimental nature of the procedure meant that their three surgeons— Barnard, Kantrowitz and Shumway—had been forced to accept them as recipient patients when they were already perilously close to death. Until the cardiac surgeon was allowed to face more realistic odds and select a recipient who, apart from a damaged heart, was reasonably healthy, the road ahead looked uncertain. Yet all was not lost. On January 22, 1968, the lone transplant survivor, Philip Blaiberg, passed Washkansky's eighteen-day record and looked set for a full recovery.

Blaiberg, who had been allowed to drink a shandy a few days earlier when his glass of lemonade was topped by a third of beer, had begun to call for the real thing. The dentist demanded a beer, and eventually a "champagne party" to thank the doctors and nurses who had saved his life. He was also, said his wife, Eileen, "eating like a horse."

Barnard, having enjoyed a celebratory dinner with the dour John Vorster and his wife at the prime minister's residence in Cape Town, left for Europe on January 24. "I was glad to get away," he wrote of his latest escape from South Africa. "I had been feeling like a stallion locked up in a stable and only able to look at the distant green pastures and the fillies over the top of the stable door. I needed to get back out into the new, exciting world."

Despite the heady optimism surrounding Blaiberg, Barnard's departure on yet another public relations junket—only three weeks since returning from his previous trip—again seemed a bizarre decision for a dedicated and compassionate doctor. Marius Barnard, who would lead the transplant team in his absence, looked grimly on Chris's apparent preference for fame over bedside duty. He pointed out that rejection could strike at any moment—a reality that Chris tried to deflect by promising that he would telephone Marius every day to monitor Blaiberg's progress and that he could fly back to Cape Town from Europe within twelve hours. During the ensuing bitter row, Chris insisted that he had no choice but to honor his overseas commitments. "Anyway, Marius," he sneered, "I'm leaving Blaiberg in good hands—yours."

Barnard was nearing the apex of his celebrity. He had begun the week by appearing on the cover of *Paris Match* and cutting a long-playing record that featured the beats and cadences of his Afrikaans accent as he talked, rather than sang, about the first human heart transplant. It was a surreal spoken album on shiny black vinyl, the production of which he simply accepted as a natural consequence of his widespread renown. He had penciled in the following week's encounters with the Italian president and the pope as casually as befits a man who had been bored by his recent encounter with the president of the United States. Barnard, of course, was more interested in the sexual conquests available to men of his sudden fame.

In a nightclub on his first evening in Germany, a television producer introduced the surgeon to a beautiful actress, Uta Levka, who whisked him onto the dance floor. Barnard ignored the flaring flash and pop of the paparazzis' cameras as, during the first slow dance, he and Levka ground their bodies together in an impressively candid show of friendliness. They danced together for the next couple of hours and, when they left the club in Baden-Baden, Barnard signed the visitors' book with a flourish: *"An unforgettable evening in the arms of the most beautiful girl in the world!"*

The inscription and seductive photographs were promptly wired to jubilant newspaper editors around the world. They knew that Norman Shumway would never have slipped away on an all-expenses-paid tour of Europe while his second transplant patient remained in intensive care. And Shumway, for all his appreciation of female company, would never have been naïve or dumb enough to canoodle in public with a movie star who, as *Time* magazine suggested, "wears fewer clothes in her new film *Carmen, Baby* than she would on the operating table."

Barnard was soon on his way to Rome. Thousands of cheering and weeping Italians greeted him at the airport. Even Barnard was surprised and asked, in all seriousness, if the Beatles had arrived on a different incoming flight. There were scenes of panic as he was swamped by a large sector of the crowd that seemed obsessed with the idea of touching him—as if even the merest brush against Barnard might transform their lives.

Angelo Litrico, the self-styled "Tailor of Rome," was one of the few Italians not to be wholly impressed by Barnard. Litrico, who had made suits for John F. Kennedy, Richard Burton, Nikita Khrushchev and Jordan's King Hussein, telephoned Barnard soon after he had settled into his sumptuous suite at the Hotel Flora on the Via Veneto. While they had never met before, and Litrico spoke only a fractured English, the tailor did manage to convey the message that Barnard could never meet the pope in a suit as unstylish and ill-fitting as the one seen on his arrival.

Litrico swept over to the hotel, in as imperious a manner as a tailor with an artificial leg could muster, and measured Barnard for a suit that would be tailored for him that evening, free of charge, so that he could wear it the following morning when meeting President Giuseppe Saragat and Pope Paul VI.

Barnard was stunned by "a double-breasted dark blue suit with tie and soft-collared shirt to match. Blue shoes with tapering toes completed the outfit. The suit fitted as if I had been poured into it. Putting these clothes on was one of the most sensual experiences I had ever known—and very new to me. I would never have believed clothes could feel so *good*—almost orgasmic. They were absolutely perfect and I preened in front of the mirror. I was really beginning to feel, and look, important."

While Barnard found another national leader, in the form of Saragat, to be tedious, he was overwhelmed by his audience with the pope. He told reporters that, while he and the pope had "pondered the moral aspects of heart transplantation," he had been moved by the intelligence and empathy shown for his work. "I bless your achievement," Pope Paul told Barnard, "and I invite you to proceed along the same road, doing good, as you have up to now."

His father, a strict Calvinist, had hated the power of the Roman Church and had even included a clause in his will stating that the small sum of money set aside for Deirdre could be inherited only so long as she did not marry a Catholic. Yet after his visit to Vatican City, Barnard "could not believe that I had had a private audience with the Pope, a man who was loved and worshipped by millions of people."

Barnard soon recovered and spent the evening sampling *la dolce vita* among "the beautiful people of the movie industry." He had already signed a deal worth $100,000, which he insisted should be paid into the Groote Schuur transplant fund, from an Italian publisher for world rights to his autobiography. The prospect of turning that story into a movie already appealed to many directors. Barnard simply grinned when he heard that Paul Newman, Gregory Peck, and Warren Beatty were being discussed as candidates to play him in a Hollywood version of the first transplant. The Italian producer Alfredo Bini enticed Barnard away from a small circle of filmmakers, including Roberto Rossellini, Franco Zeffirelli, and the great Michelangelo Antonioni, to suggest an even more intriguing idea. Bini was convinced that even if a master like

Antonioni were to direct the proposed art-house alternative, it should climax in a final scene where the surgeon would play himself. "We'll see," Barnard said with surprising cool.

Yet on the inside he was, in his own words, "hot to trot" when he escaped the directors and began talking to Gina Lollobrigida—described by some Italian critics as "the Mona Lisa of the Twentieth Century." "She really was beautiful," Barnard gushed years later. "I remembered her in a movie I'd seen called *Trapeze* with Burt Lancaster, and for a boy from the Karoo it was an unbelievable experience to be with such a beautiful actress, discussing the movie she was making at the time in Catania, Sicily—*Buona Sera, Mrs Campbell*. Even more incredible was being fairly sure that she was just as interested in me as I was in her."

The following night, according to Barnard in his panting account, "I heard Gina coming into the room. She was carrying a bottle of champagne and two glasses. Huskily she murmured, 'Now we're going to be alone.'" Barnard delighted in his description of "the heaving swell of her breasts" and her jagged breathing. "We celebrated with champagne several times during the night and I left early the next morning. She drove me back to my hotel in her Jaguar—absolutely naked in her mink coat."

Lunch with Sophia Loren, for the lothario of surgery, came next. Barnard was even more smitten by Loren's beauty. Even if their encounter was innocent, as Barnard and his dazzled colleagues M. C. Botha and Bossie Bosman had been invited by Loren and her husband, Carlo Ponti, to an informal lunch at their villa just outside Rome, press photographs implied a more intimate meeting. A resourceful snapper cropped his picture in such a way that Ponti disappeared from a shot that featured the gorgeous Loren cupping the hand of a smarmy and beaming Barnard as he lit her cigarette. The fact that her dress had risen above the thigh to reveal an elegant flash of a black stocking-top as she leaned toward the surgeon only added to the titillation. Barnard, it was wrongly assumed, had conquered yet another.

In London he was less impressed by a different photograph, one that captured the rather more sardonic British reaction to his celebrity lifestyle. Persuaded by a photographer to accept a packet of birdseed so that he could feed the pigeons in Trafalgar Square, Barnard posed dutifully in front of the camera. "Soon the birds were sitting on my head and shitting all over my Litrico suit," Barnard fumed. "A few days later the most ridiculous picture of me and the pigeons made the front page of the *Evening Standard*. I looked like an absolute moron."

He faced more straightforward vitriol on the BBC's *Tomorrow's World*. In a television special titled "Dr. Barnard Faces His Critics," he was confronted by an audience of 150 British physicians, surgeons, and social commentators. Roy Calne, the distinguished British transplant surgeon, and immunologist, argued that "The nauseating publicity that some parts of the press and television and radio adopted for this transplant in Cape Town has done harm to the profession. It's done harm to yourself. Why was it necessary to have the personal details of the donor known to the recipient?"

"If you could have avoided that," Barnard replied acidly, "you're a better man than I am, Gunga Din. If you think that we were asking for publicity, then you must credit us with very little knowledge. First, we never went on television before and said: 'We are ready to do a transplant.' Secondly, we didn't take a single picture during any of these operations."

Malcolm Muggeridge then climbed aboard his soapbox to declare, with due pomposity, that "our human society is being transformed into a vast broiler house or factory farm—such as satirists like Orwell and Aldous Huxley have envisaged. Why was it that this operation was first performed in the Union of South Africa? Was it because in the Union of South Africa there were more brilliant or more audacious surgeons? Was it because in the Union of South Africa there was better equipment, finer facilities? Or was it, I suspect, that, because of the vile doctrine of apartheid, life is held cheaper?"

"I think we have fairly good surgeons in South Africa," Barnard replied calmly. "We have excellent facilities to do this type of surgery. We did this operation with the purpose of treating a sick man and of relieving human suffering," he added, reclaiming the moral high ground, however briefly.

He slipped to a less lofty perch a couple of nights later. After ogling the bare delights of the Crazy Horse in Paris, he and M. C. Botha got caught up in a scuffle with photographers. "Barnard Brawls Outside Strip Saloon," chortled the *Daily Mirror* in London, while in South Africa *Die Vaderland* was suitably scandalized. "For the sake of himself, his family, his people and his country," the voice of Afrikanerdom seethed, "Professor Christiaan Barnard should bring himself to heel. The danger, otherwise, is that all his good work will begin to unravel into humiliation and mockery. We would not wish to see him end up a clown."

L ouwtjie Barnard had been shadowed by the South African press throughout the three weeks Chris had been in Europe. She claimed to be distressed by the media's distortion of "perfectly innocent events." Her own suspicions, however, were not so easily allayed. Barnard reluctantly agreed that she could accompany him on his next inevitable trip, the following month, to Italy and America. Government pressure, exerted by Lappa Munnik and Nico Malan, had also encouraged Barnard to include his wife in his future travels. While Blaiberg continued his steady recovery under the watchful gaze of Marius and the rest of the Groote Schuur team, Barnard prepared the lecture that he would deliver to the American College of Cardiology in San Francisco—in "the domain of Norman Shumway," as he noted anxiously.

But first he would travel alone to Portugal before meeting up with Louwtjie in Italy. In Lisbon he received a passionate letter from Gina Lollobrigida, who invited him to join her on location in Sicily. Barnard declined, reluctantly, though he apparently slept with the pretty young woman who had delivered the note to him—"It's only polite to tip the postman," he reasoned.

Barnard was soon preoccupied by his imminent clash with Shumway. They had been paired on a panel that would face 3,000 cardiologists during a conference to assess the troubled progress of heart transplantation. The world's sixth transplant, performed by the respected Indian surgeon P. K. Sen, had ended disastrously within a few hours. Yet, as long as he could parade the triumphant survival of Philip Blaiberg, Barnard was convinced he would not wilt before his most exacting American rival.

Barnard readily accepted an invitation from the American College of Cardiologists to tour Stanford's laboratories a few days before the conference. Shumway, however, in the elusive style that defined his real character, had already decided to withdraw from the San Francisco panel. He also instructed his Stanford colleagues that he wished to avoid Barnard during his trawl through their medical center. Gene Dong, his staunch ally in the research lab, and Spyros Andreopoulos, the media liaison officer, resolved to spare Shumway the trauma of an encounter with a man who had cost him so much. They steered a bewildered Barnard away from Shumway throughout the course of a long day—only for Donald Harrison, a Stanford cardiologist with a penchant for publicity, to intervene and suggest an impromptu visit to the OR.

Barnard, accompanied by a small group of American cardiologists, interrupted Shumway as he was operating. The response from the Stanford chief was tersely polite. He soon terminated the meeting with the curt observation that he was in the middle of surgery. The deeper message was clear. He had no wish to spend any time with Chris Barnard.

"Two of the world's four heart transplant surgeons—Dr. Norman E. Shumway of Stanford University and Dr. Christiaan N. Barnard of South Africa—met briefly at Stanford," the *Palo Alto Times* reported on February 29. "Their meeting place was singularly appropriate. It was an operating room, where Dr. Shumway was performing surgery. Hospital officials said that because of the operation, the two physicians could talk only briefly. They said there was a possibility that the two men, who were researchers together at the University of Minnesota, might get together again while Dr. Barnard is in the area to attend the annual meeting of the American College of Cardiology in San Francisco."

The word "possibility" was a euphemism, for Shumway had responded, with charming bluntness, to the invitation to meet Chris Barnard again with a winning "no" and "never."

Hilton Hotel, San Francisco, March 2, 1968

Barnard flicked apprehensively through the slides for his lecture. Even the title of the subject they had asked him to address—"Is Human Cardiac Transplantation Premature?"—seemed unnecessarily provocative. He could sense the resentment and animosity as soon as he entered the auditorium. With cardiologists and surgeons spilling over into the aisles, it looked to Barnard as if they had come to crucify him. As Denton Cooley entertained the masses with the lecture immediately preceding his own, Barnard was horrified to discover that he was missing a couple of important slides that demonstrated the hemo-dynamic rejuvenation achieved by Philip Blaiberg's transplanted heart.

He slipped out of the ballroom and, using an internal hotel phone, called Louwtjie in their suite to ask if she could find the misplaced slides. By the time he joined her on the twenty-third floor, he was shocked to see her poised on the ledge of an open window. While searching through his briefcase she had found a love letter from Gina Lollobrigida, one that lingered over the night they had spent together in Rome. "I'm going to end it now," Louwtjie threatened.

Barnard, years later, wrote of the scene: "My heart lurched as she edged herself closer to oblivion. Would she really jump? She was in a strange country, with no friends to turn to—and now she'd found proof of what she had suspected a long time. Where did my priorities lie? In this bedroom on the 23rd floor with a wife who had borne two beautiful children or in the lecture room on the second floor—with strangers who couldn't care less about what happened to me or my family?"

The celebrated surgeon chose the second group. "I looked at the pathetic figure sitting in the open window and made up my mind. My presence in the room could, I decided, accomplish nothing—she was best left alone and I prayed that she'd either lose her nerve or realize that this wasn't the answer."

Barnard, mumbling an apology to his suicidal wife, raced back down to the second floor. He was on the podium within another five minutes. Not surprisingly he forgot his introduction and instead peered nervously into a crowd seething with intelligence, envy, and resentment. He could tell they smelled blood. Barnard could not get any words out of his dry mouth. In an effort to compose himself, he sipped water from a glass held with a shaking hand.

He tried again, and this time the first few words came in halting fashion. He thanked the American College of Cardiology for his invitation, then hesitated again. In desperation, he decided to resort to a joke. "A few weeks ago I had a hair-raising experience," he said as he began one of the apocryphal anecdotes that usually enthralled his South African audiences. Barnard told the story of his chauffeur, a man called Van der Merwe, an Afrikaans every-man who always wore a white coat and cap when he drove the surgeon to his various lectures. Each night they would discuss various aspects of heart transplantation while, at every lecture, Van der Merwe sat at the back of the hall and absorbed the finer points of Barnard's presentation.

"I realized after a few weeks," Barnard said, "that my chauffeur had learned quite a lot about heart transplantation. One night we were driving to this little town where I was sure they didn't even know what I looked like. I was very tired and wanted to relax. I asked him, 'Van, do you think you could impersonate me and give the lecture tonight?' Without hesitation he said, 'Sure, Professor, I know your lecture by heart.'"

They swapped an Italian suit for a chauffeur's uniform and entered the town hall in their changed personas. "I found Van's lecture so interesting," Barnard said enthusiastically, "that I sat open-mouthed in admiration as I listened to him. When he was finished there was tremendous applause and he was asked by the chairman if he would be prepared to answer questions from the audience—and he immediately agreed. He was a little weak on the medical questions but much better on the political questions. Then catastrophe struck. A gentleman in the audience stood up. I recognized him even from the back and went cold. It was Michael DeBakey."

The doctors at the San Francisco conference rocked with laughter. DeBakey, a surgeon most of them feared or loathed, sat among them in the front row. He smiled thinly at Barnard, but it did not look as if he enjoyed being made part of the joke. Barnard grinned back at him and, turning to the rest of his audience, continued his story, saying that DeBakey, in the South African anecdote, had asked his suddenly hapless chauffeur a convoluted question about immunology and rejection.

"I was just about to jump up," Barnard said, "and admit everything when Van smiled. I waited with bated breath to hear what he would say. He cleared his throat and, pulling himself up to his full height, asked, 'Excuse me, sir, but aren't you Dr. DeBakey from Houston?' DeBakey acknowledged that he was. 'Well, Dr. DeBakey, I'm surprised that a man with your knowledge and experience could ask such a *stupid* question.'"

Barnard waited for the roar in San Francisco to subside and then he reached for the punchline. "So Van said, 'To show you how stupid your question really is, my chauffeur at the back of the hall will answer it for you.'"

Three thousand cardiologists and surgeons exploded with laughter, and in that delirious moment Barnard knew that he had triumphed again.

He got down to business and spoke with renewed determination. Cardiac transplantation, he insisted, was far from premature. In fact, he was so convinced of its success he predicted that he and other surgeons would eventually turn to the use of animal hearts to cope with the demand from potential recipients around the world. He saw a possible source of hearts in pigs, although a chimpanzee or gorilla would provide the ideal animal match—but they would need to be bred in "quantity." For a country so disturbed by Jim Hardy's use of a chimp heart in the first failed attempt at cardiac transplantation in man, Barnard's gumption seemed perversely admirable.

He spoke even more cogently when he argued that he and his fellow transplant surgeons had been forced to choose recipient patients who were already close to death. He called for a more open selection policy to favor patients who would be generally healthier and more suitable candidates. "It is not just how long a patient is going to live that should be the doctor's concern," he said as he closed in on his ringing conclusion, "but how is he going to live and how much more improved quality of life we can offer him." The final slide—of Blaiberg shaving himself while he flashed a V for victory sign at the camera—filled the screen above him.

"You will appreciate the significance of this photograph much more than the press. Before the transplant this man couldn't shave himself because the exertion was just too much and he would quickly run out of breath. So, for my patient, and our cardiac team in Cape Town, this was a major milestone and, in our opinion, proves conclusively that heart transplantation *does* cure because it improves the quality of life of terminally ill patients—which is, I'm sure, the goal of all of us here today."

As Walter Sullivan of *The New York Times* noted, "He was greeted by a standing ovation remarkable for a scientific meeting. It was clear that he had won over at least most of his listeners."

In the ensuing panel discussion, Barnard was more muted. Although he claimed later to have missed the presence of Shumway, one can assume he was upset by the thought of his wife on the ledge of a hotel room on the twenty-third floor. Barnard was also taken aback by the American surgeons' repeated concerns about possible lawsuits and unresolved legislation surrounding the definition of death. He remembered, when visiting Kantrowitz in New York, telling the startled Brooklyn surgeon: "You don't understand, Adrian. In South Africa we don't wait for the heart to stop." Barnard suddenly realized, with gloomy introspection, that "I had the legal system of the United States to thank for the honor of being the first surgeon in the world to have done a heart transplant."

When it was concluded unanimously that cardiac transplantation should continue, despite the complexities of the American legal system, Barnard hurried from the stage to his room.

Without a key, he knocked hard and called out Louwtjie's name. Even when hammering his fist on the door he was met only by a chilling silence. He raced back down to the lobby to obtain another key. As soon as he swung open the heavy door he could hear the sound of running water. He burst into the bathroom, fearing that Louwtjie had drowned herself.

She lay in the bath. Her eyes were shut as water gushed from the taps.

Louwtjie was alive—and furious. She could stand no more of either his deceit or rampant ego. Louwtjie told him to get out. It was all over. He had been the first to transplant a human heart, and now he was famous beyond imagination. And yet, alone as he walked back to the conference, he felt as if he were crumbling inside.

Barnard returned to a heaving ballroom. The long break between sessions had not yet ended and doctors spoke animatedly to one another, clutching their now empty cups of coffee. People swerved out of the way as Barnard walked toward them. He kept moving aimlessly forward. When he reached a corner, he found a chair and sat down, then gazed helplessly around the room. As if in deference to the absent master, to Shumway, none of the American surgeons or cardiologists would have any personal contact with Barnard. The South African, the source of so much laughter and applause less than an hour earlier, seemed terribly alone. As the minutes passed, only Dick Lower seemed to feel anything for the lost man. Only Dick Lower felt it necessary to walk over and offer his hand.

"Hello, Chris," Lower said as hundreds of eyes followed him. "Good speech."

Barnard stared numbly at the surgeon from whom he had learned how to transplant a heart. Barnard finally gripped Lower by the hand. "Hell, Dick," Barnard said, "it's good to see you."

Lower, with a light and natural touch, showed kindness and compassion to the surgeon who had literally stolen his and Norm Shumway's invention. Barnard was still a human being, and Dick Lower could not easily have stood the sight of a fellow man, even a man as strange and desperately famous as Chris Barnard, looking so bereft and alone.

Everything had changed. In the months following Chris Barnard's appearance in San Francisco, the surgical world had fully embraced a dark and volatile fever. Surgeons who had never attempted an experimental graft in the animal lab, or given any thought to the most basic questions of rejection, went transplant crazy. They were told that the surgical technique was absurdly straightforward. At the same time they invariably refused to heed any warning that complications still arose in the OR or that rejection was a deadly and mysterious brute.

The race to be next consumed all logic. It turned some doctors into madmen as they strove to be the next famous surgeon to transplant a human heart. They were also propelled into medical mania by a patriotic fervor, as governments demanded to know when their own surgeons would join the transplant revolution. If South Africa can do it, they asked, why not us? And so surgeons, almost always less handsome and competent than the original, dreamed of becoming another Chris Barnard. Which red-blooded cut-master among them would not wish to bed Gina Lollobrigida, lunch with Sophia Loren, and then have Gregory Peck suggested as the perfect actor to play him on the big screen?

Even some of the most talented and renowned surgeons were sucked into the maelstrom. Donald Ross led the first British transplant. He would have been the first in Europe if not for Christian Cabrol, the Parisian surgeon who had been a research fellow in Minnesota alongside Barnard and Shumway. Cabrol, who had remained close to Shumway and prepared himself thoroughly for his first transplant, carried out the world's seventh on April 27, 1968. His twenty-three-year-old male patient, however, died from an embolism on the third day of his new life. Ross, meanwhile, had proven himself an undoubted innovator and pragmatist, and one of the world's most respected surgeons, with a groundbreaking cardiac technique, the "Ross Procedure." He followed Cabrol, on May 2, by implanting the heart of a twenty-five-year-old donor in the chest of a forty-five-year-old milkman. Although Frederick West survived for less than seven weeks, an extraordinary display of chauvinism had immediately followed the operation. Ross and his team had announced the transplant at the National Heart Hospital while waving small Union Jacks and "I'm Backing Britain" placards.

Denton Cooley was already transplanting hearts at a furious rate. On December 3, 1967, Cooley had fired off a cable to Cape Town: "Congratulations on your first transplant, Chris. I will be reporting on my first hundred soon." He was intent on keeping his word. A day before Ross's first British transplant, Cooley made his blistering debut. It took him thirty-five minutes to complete that transplant. His patient, Everett Thomas, recovered from the operation, went home a few weeks later, and resumed work the following month. America was enthralled. People dying of heart disease raced to Texas in the forlorn hope that Cooley could save them.

The Texan loved the adulation and his own dizzying speed in the operating room. He completed a staggering seventeen transplants in the last eight months of 1968—which meant that he had contributed a sixth of the world's transplant total for that year. Yet death stalked his every case. Everett Thomas, died after seven months. Only two other patients among his first seventeen lived for more than six months. Nine were dead less than a month after transplantation. The reason was obvious. Cooley was a surgeon, perhaps the world's best in purely technical terms, but he had scant interest either in laboratory research or in postoperative care—which Shumway insisted were the two prime battlegrounds in transplantation.

Cooley and his team were still fêted in Houston alongside the first astronauts preparing for the moon landing. They were all stars. And so Cooley continued his cutting and his counting. The cheap hotels lining the main freeway running into Houston's medical center were crammed with patients who had traveled across America to beg an audience with the supposed master of transplantation. The death toll climbed as infection and rejection ate up patients remorselessly. Jim Nora, a cardiologist on Cooley's team, would later observe that "Denton realized that we were having problems, but I guess he couldn't let go. We were all caught up in this idea that we can defeat death—and Denton was certainly leading the charge there. I think that he was looking for immortality. He was really not willing to accept that death was a possibility for any of his patients, for any of us. That's what we were trying to do, but we weren't successful. Death comes."

Cooley was finally forced to confront the unanswerable truth. In September 1969, he closed his transplant program at St. Luke's Hospital. The despair had spread far and wide. Its impact could be seen in a simple comparison between annual transplant counts. In 1968 there had been 101 human heart transplants around the world. By December 31, 1969, a mere seventeen transplants had been attempted. Thirteen of those were in America.

Adrian Kantrowitz was sacked, brutally and shockingly, by Maimonides Medical Center in March 1970. His refusal to abandon his revolutionary new intra-aortic balloon pump (IABP), which simply and effectively increased cardiac perfusion in stricken patients, instigated a witch hunt. Kantrowitz had dismissed all the warnings that, after transplantation, he could not take another risky step into the unknown. He refused to buckle. The balloon pump was based on his most original and enduring idea—of "diastolic augmentation," which later became known as "counterpulsation." He knew that coronary flow to the heart muscle occurs mostly when the heart relaxes in diastole, or "between beats," when the aortic valve closes. For twenty years, since 1950, Kantrowitz had been experimenting in the lab with the novel concept of delivering a pressure pulse to the root of the aorta, to enhance coronary flow through even narrowed arteries, at the very moment the heart relaxed. He believed that, by using the balloon pump this goal could be achieved and that, by reducing its workload, an ailing heart would be rejuvenated.

After limited success with his first five balloon-pump patients, he initiated a joint clinical trial. In conjunction with nine medical centers, affiliated with renowned academic institutions like Cornell, Duke, and Harvard, Kantrowitz would study the further use of his pump in eighty-seven patients.

Even though Kantrowitz would coordinate the trial, Maimonides refused to allow him to include his own department in the work. When Kantrowitz ignored them and steamed ahead he was summoned to the office of the president of Maimonides—and advised that it would be "mutually beneficial" for him to leave the hospital.

Kantrowitz shrugged aside the indignity. Where was the shame in being fired? They had fired Galileo! They had called Galileo a maniac when he suggested that perhaps the sun might constitute the heart of the universe. Kantrowitz did not see himself as the Galileo of Brooklyn, but he knew he could make his balloon pump work.

He was offered a post as chief of surgery at Sinai Hospital in Detroit. Maimonides administrators were astonished when twenty-five of their staff—surgeons, researchers, and nurses—immediately resigned and followed Kantrowitz to Detroit. The medical chief at Sinai asked for a cautious pause before they returned to transplantation. Kantrowitz, while insistent that transplantation would eventually prevail, agreed to focus instead on his ventricular assist work. Mechanical assist devices had always been his primary passion, and in August 1971, the viability of Kantrowitz's work was proved in dramatic style when he successfully implanted a ventricular assist device in a man suffering from chronic heart failure. That rejuvenated patient, Haskell Shanks, returned home as the world's first recipient of a left ventricular assist device intended to remain permanently in the body. Kantrowitz was flying again. His ingenious balloon pump, he also knew, would eventually save many more lives around the world than cardiac transplantation.

Barnard, meanwhile, was lost in more personal chaos. He and Louwtjie had divorced in May 1969. The details of his affair with Lollobrigida, and many other women, were revealed in the process. The Italian actress issued an angry public retort: "I cannot blame myself for having had a sincere feeling for a man the whole world loved and admired at the time." Claiming that Barnard had even asked her to marry him, she ridiculed the surgeon as "an idiot, a man seeking unlimited publicity at any cost." Barnard had already fallen for a beautiful nineteen-year-old Cape Town heiress, Barbara Zoellner. They were engaged three months after his divorce and married on Valentine's Day 1970—the day after Louwtjie's forty-fifth birthday. Barnard was forty-seven.

Deirdre and Andre Barnard were dazed and hurt by the divorce and their father's sudden remarriage—to a teenager. Andre, who'd once revered Chris, cut him to the quick when he asked: "What would you have said if *your* father had behaved like this?"

At work, when he was not jetting off on another overseas trip or helping arrange for his new wife to become a model who would make the cover of *Vogue,* Barnard struggled. Val Schrire, his chief cardiologist, regarded him with derision. He would not refer any more patients to the surgeon. Barnard was too distracted by his love life and his own fame to protest much.

And so, between December 1967 and May 1971, he transplanted only six hearts. Four of his patients lived for longer than a year. Philip Blaiberg had left the hospital ten weeks after he had been given Clive Haupt's "colored" heart. He died in August 1969—eighteen months after his transplant. Barnard's two most recent patients, a colored woman named Dorothy Fisher and an Afrikaner policeman, Dirk van Zyl, were both in good health. Both Cooley and Shumway had performed many more transplants (twenty-one and forty-three, respectively), but, calculated as a percentage, the South African's success rate outstripped that of his rivals. Yet Barnard was too self-absorbed to push forward with the new transplant program his brother advocated. Marius despaired at the waste of all their earlier work.

Shumway's more courageous progress meant that sixteen of his patients were still alive. Resisting calls to ban heart transplantation, he was close to proving the long-term validity of the process. Yet, outside Stanford, transplantation had hit a wall. Almost every heart transplant unit around the world was shut down. Only Shumway kept grinding away, refusing to allow a threatened national moratorium on the procedure to persuade him that he should quit. Even if few paid heed to their results, Shumway, Stinson, and an increasingly inspirational team were actually winning the transplant war within the isolated walls of Stanford Medical Center. They would have fought a less solitary battle if Richard Lower had not been put on trial and forced to swap the OR for the courtroom in a distressing case that reached its dramatic culmination in May 1972.

The family of his first transplant donor wanted to see him charged with murder in Richmond, Virginia. In the end they accused Lower, in a civil suit, of causing wrongful death and pursued a million-dollar claim against him. He was said to have ended a man's life by removing his beating heart. For a surgeon as gentle and thoughtful as Lower, it was as if he *had* been accused of murder. He knew that if he lost the case it would all be over. It was not even about the money. Somehow he would raise the cash to stay out of jail. But his career would effectively be ruined. It felt just as cruel that the very premise of heart transplantation seemed to be on trial with him. If Lower was found liable, he and Shumway knew that cardiac transplantation would be pushed back decades.

E xactly four years earlier, on the Friday afternoon of May 25, 1968, Bruce Tucker, a fifty-six-year-old black employee at an egg-packing plant, sat with a friend who pumped gas at an Esso station on Venable Street in Richmond. When Tucker, who had been drinking, finally decided it was time to stagger home for the weekend, he stumbled and fell—and hit his head hard on the station's concrete apron.

He was admitted to the Medical College of Virginia at 6:05 that evening. His condition deteriorated to the point where, at 11:00 p.m., he was operated on in an attempt to relieve the hemorrhage and swelling of his brain. The following morning, at 11:30 a.m., he was attached to a respirator. Fifteen minutes later the attending physician noted that "the prognosis for recovery is nil. Death is imminent."

At 1:00 p.m. the staff neurologist, Dr. Hooshang Hooshmand, ran an electroencephalograph for twenty-five minutes in an attempt to detect cerebral activity. His conclusion was unequivocal. Bruce Tucker was brain-dead. His heart, pulse, blood pressure, and temperature were normal, but he was unable to breathe spontaneously. Three attempts were made to reach his family. At 2:30, the police, who had been contacted by Lower's chief, David Hume, confirmed that the family "could not be located."

Dr. Abdullah Fatteh, the deputy state medical examiner, gave Hume permission to proceed. A more cautious chief of surgery than Hume would have waited longer before instructing Lower that the transplant should begin. But Hume had never forgotten how he and Lower had been prevented from carrying out the first heart transplant two years before by a difference in blood type. He would not allow Lower, or MCV, to be delayed again. "This guy obviously doesn't have any family," Hume insisted.

Lower also knew that his recipient, fifty-three-year-old Joseph Kleet, had been dying for the last three weeks in the hospital. If he did not receive a new heart soon he would be as dead as Tucker.

At 3:30 p.m. the order was given for Tucker's respirator to be turned off. He was pronounced dead, and three minutes later the cutting began. At 3:40, Hume again called Fatteh, who, on behalf of the state of Virginia, gave Dick Lower permission to remove both the heart and the kidneys of the deceased patient.

Lower carried out the world's sixteenth heart transplant—and obtained a more painful first a week later, when Joseph Kleet became the world's first cardiac transplant patient to die as a direct result of rejection.

When Bruce Tucker's family was finally tracked down, his brothers, Grover and William, were sent to the morgue to claim his body. It was only then they were asked: "Did you know they took your brother's heart?"

Dick Lower, in mitigation, could point to the fact that his second, and only other, transplant patient, Louis B. Russell, remained the world's longest survivor with a new heart. On August 24, 1968, Russell had received the heart of a nineteen-year-old male recipient. Twenty-one months later, his full participation in ordinary life was another sign that transplantation could thrive. Lower's own future, however, had dimmed. When the Tucker family filed their lawsuit against him, he was forced to abandon all work in transplantation while he waited for the trial to finally begin—four years later, in May 1972.

The judge's chambers were across the street from the Medical College of Virginia. Whenever Lower left the hospital late at night in the weeks just before the trial, he would look up instinctively at the windows of Judge Christian Compton. They were not dark with foreboding. In their blazing light they looked more quietly terrifying. Compton worked hard, night after night, studying one obscure associated precedent after another in an attempt to negotiate a way through the tangled thicket of a landmark case that, at its very heart, considered the unresolved question of brain death.

Richmond Law and Equity Court, Richmond, Virginia, May 25, 1972

In the somber old granite courthouse the Tucker family was represented by a verbose and ambitious lawyer, Doug Wilder. The first four days of a week-long trial had not gone well for Lower, as Wilder built up an emotional case that seemed to transfix the jury. "It was wrong to take Bruce Tucker's heart from his body," he argued. "They started the operation on Kleet before Bruce Tucker was pronounced dead. They took the most precious thing he had going for him at the time: his heart." Wilder even suggested that Tucker's heart had been removed while there was still a chance that "if they had waited another twenty-four hours he might have started to recover."

Amid the extensive coverage across America, the *National Observer* reported that "midway through the trial Judge Compton stunned the courtroom by ruling that he would 'adopt the legal concept of death and reject the defense's attempt to employ a medical concept of neurological death in establishing a rule of law.'" Compton, in referring to the "legal concept of death," turned to the narrow definition found in *Black's Law Dictionary*: "Death is a total stoppage of the circulation of the blood, and a cessation of the animal and vital functions consequent thereto such as respiration and pulsation." The judge's adherence to this ludicrous Boy Scout definition of death indicated that, as the *National Observer* argued, "the jury would almost certainly be compelled to convict the doctors. Judge Compton reasoned that legal chaos would erupt if the law embraced the concept of brain-death too. He said legislatures, not courts, should resolve the issue."

Lower, struggling to contain his rising anxiety, knew that he was not the only surgeon to have encountered such trouble. Two and a half weeks after Lower had taken Tucker's heart, an esteemed Japanese surgeon, Juro Wada, had carried out his country's first transplant. His patient, eighteen-year-old Miyazaki Nobuo, died three months later from a lung infection. It was only then that Wada was accused by a fellow physician at Sapporo Medical College of not having done enough to save the donor patient, who was declared brain dead after a swimming accident. Wada was charged with murder.

The case against Wada was eventually dropped, the prosecutors conceding there was insufficient evidence to convict the doctor. Yet Japan would not allow another heart transplant for the next thirty-five years. Wada's career remained under a shadow.

Witnesses for Lower pointed to Virginia's Unclaimed Bodies Act, which permitted the state medical examiner to release unclaimed bodies to medical schools and hospitals for educational or scientific purposes. This defense testimony was effective, but largely because Wilder curiously seemed to miss the main point, which was that the MCV doctors had waited less than the statutory twenty-four hours to lay claim to Tucker's heart. Wilder, who would soon be elected state senator and, later, governor, was motivated more by his oratorical battles with Lower's supporters. The attorney was especially captivated by his verbal tussle with Dr. Joseph Fletcher, a nonphysician who was a professor of medical ethics, a theologian, and a philosopher. In the end, the philosopher prevailed: "When cerebral function is lost, nothing remains but biological phenomena at best. The patient is gone even if his body remains and even if some of its vital functions continue. He may be, technically, 'alive.' But he is no longer human. He is, as a human being, undoubtedly dead."

Even if he did not quite feel reborn, Lower was revived. Judge Compton scribbled some detailed notes. And Lower won over some of the jury when he brushed aside Wilder's slur on his character and medical ethics. "You mean to tell me," Wilder spluttered during his sneering cross-examination, "that you actively go out to take hearts from dead folk and put them in your own patients?"

"Now you got it," Lower said dryly.

The jury chuckled appreciatively. Lower felt a little better, but still, his fate looked bleak.

Everything depended on Compton's final instructions to the jury. The judge began by reiterating his reluctance to instruct a jury to overrule the state legislators. Lower hung on. He was waiting for the big "but," a sudden change in Compton's thinking that might swing his way.

Judge Compton pushed ahead determinedly and judiciously. "Death is a cessation of life," he stressed. "Under the law, death occurs at a precise time." The moment, finally, had come. The judge, looking directly at the seven jurors, told them: "You shall determine the time of death in this case by using the following definition of the nature of death. . . . You may consider, among the following elements, the time of complete and irreversible loss of all function of brain. . . ."

The words sank into Dick Lower's own brain. He looked straight ahead but, on the inside, he was doing a little cartwheel, and then a whooping sprint, as if he were a kid again, running free on a spring afternoon. Compton admitted that he had been swayed, in the end, by the consensus among surgeons across America. It was their wish, and even sometimes their secret custom, to move beyond that antiquated "dictionary definition" of death. Compton's implicit advice to the jury was plain: they should exonerate Richard Lower.

The jury returned after seventy-seven minutes. When their foreman was asked for his verdict on the single charge of wrongful death, he spoke not one word but two: "Not liable."

Dick Lower phoned his old friend later that afternoon. He played it cool and simple. "Hey, Norm," he said. "Guess what? I'm a free man."

In the wake of this landmark ruling, the state of Virginia would soon introduce legislation that formalized brain death as a legitimate medical and legal concept. Other states across America would follow suit. Transplantation could continue and flourish. All it needed was for the original pioneers, Shumway and Lower, the last men standing, to slug it out with rejection in the definitive battle of their lives.

After thirteen long years, they were not about to walk away. They were still the same old Dick and Norm, the dog-heart guys. They had lives to save. They had hearts to transplant. They had rejection to conquer. It did not matter that everyone else had failed, or got famous, or simply moved on. Barnard might have won the race. Shumway and Lower would win the war.

Shumway laughed. He would not, after all, get a chance to bust Lower out of jail. They would, instead, with a little luck, stay out of the newspapers forever. All would be quiet. All would be good.

"Okay, Dick," Shumway said, "let's get back to work."

Epilogue: Acceptance

Driving along Main Road in Cape Town, on the last day of my final trip back, I went looking for ghosts. I slowed at the site where Denise Darvall had been struck down. And then, another mile on, drifting past Groote Schuur, I gazed up again at the grand old hospital where her heart had been taken and given to Louis Washkansky in December 1967. I could still remember that blue-skied month in a beautiful city. I was six years old. Apart from the thrill of being on holiday somewhere so new and exciting, and twelve hundred miles from our home in the dry old Transvaal, it was an almost indescribable treat to stay in a small hotel in Fish Hook. How could you not love a part of Cape Town with a name as strangely wonderful as Fish Hook?

Cape Town, that month, felt like the very heart of the universe. The eyes of the world, we kept hearing on our car radio, were on us. Rather than glare down with the usual contempt, they had opened wide with wonder and hope. And when those millions of eyes closed, the world prayed for Louis Washkansky. We were told that he was a good and kind man, though to me he looked more like a ghost lying under a plastic tent. I tried not to think too deeply about what it must feel like to have another person's heart beating inside your chest.

I had to wait for a Friday afternoon in early October 2002 before I next spent a few hours in Fish Hook. I drank a couple of beers and listened to some crackly old Maria Callas records with a confused and emotional seventy-year-old woman, Peggy Jordaan, who had been Chris Barnard's senior OR nurse during all his famous operations. "I'm telling you," she said in her gravelly voice, "it sent chills down you to see a chest cut open without the heart inside it." Peggy began to cry as she thought of poor Louis Washkansky. And then, to compose herself, she said, "What the hell, go on, man, have one more beer." She lit up another cigarette. A cloud of blue smoke hung over her head as she relived the most dramatic night of her life.

"I gave Chris this stainless-steel basin and he went across the theater to the room next door, where old Marius waited with Denise Darvall. We'd heard the saw cutting her open maybe ten minutes before. I just stared at Mr. Washkansky, thinking, 'Hell, pal, what are we going to do to you?' And then Chris brought back Denise's heart. He gave it to me. I looked at it, so small and blue, and I thought, 'For God's sake, Peggy, whatever you do, don't drop it.' If I had done that I think Chris would have bloody killed me with a single scream. But I didn't drop it. I held it, and, I'm telling you, I could also handle Chris. I would always put a pretty nurse across the table from him. He didn't mean it, most of the time, but he could scream down the place if you rubbed him the wrong way. I'd say, 'Chris, you're a bigger diva than Maria Callas.' And because he knew how much I loved opera he took that as a compliment."

While I drank my beer and Peggy coughed and smoked in a tiny apartment in an old block called Coniston Court, across the road from the Fish Hook police station, we observed that Chris Barnard had been dead a little over a year. On September 2, 2001, he had died, in the words of the coroner in Cyprus, of a "bronchial blockage" caused by a violent attack of asthma. I was struck by two facts about his last days: Chris Barnard had died alone; and he had traveled to Cyprus in the bizarre hope of signing a contract to market olive oil. The great South African surgeon of my boyhood—the grinning hustler who danced with Grace Kelly, lunched with Sophia Loren, and slept with Gina Lollobrigida—had suffered a lonely and gasping death. I wanted to know what had happened to him in the intervening years.

Peggy started crying again. The tears rolled down her face as Maria Callas's voice soared with "Casta diva" from Bellini's *Norma*. She told me that she was not only weeping for Chris, but for Louwtjie and Deirdre, too. They had also

lost Andre, their son and brother, when he killed himself in the bath seven
years before his father died.

"The suicide of your son must be a terrible thing," Peggy said, "and I don't
think Chris ever got over that. I think he blamed himself. Maybe everything
started to go wrong when he did that first transplant. I think he was surprised
by how famous he suddenly got. I was amazed. I could never really understand
why the public went so mad about it. Chris understood it better. He told me,
when I complained about all this sentimental reaction to the heart, 'Listen,
Peggy, you can't very well say, "I love you with my two-stroke pump!" which,
after all, sums up the heart' . . ."

The old nurse wiped her eyes. She was also sad for herself. Peggy had suffered a stroke and now forgot "the simplest and stupidest of things." They
had taken her for some tests earlier that week and the doctor had asked her
three questions about herself—she had since forgotten them. All she knew was
that she couldn't answer a single one. Now they were going to move Peggy
from her apartment and put her in a home. "They're transplanting me," she
said, as if to herself.

Peggy walked me to the front door of the home she would soon have to
leave. "It's strange," she said. "I can't remember what I did this morning. But
everything about those transplant years just shines in my head."

I thought of Peggy Jordaan again that sunlit afternoon, two years later,
when I drove down Main Road for the last time. I had always meant to go back
and visit her in her nursing home, but there was always someone else to
see first. The months and years blurred. And I never got around to drinking
another beer or listening to Maria Callas with her again. Instead, I met the
surviving members of the extended Washkansky family, who mostly lived in
Green Point and Sea Point. Ann Washkansky had long since died, but her
son, Michael, could still be seen shuffling around the surrounding streets,
a lost and distraught man who had never quite got over what had happened
to his father. The rest of the Washkansky clan were irresistible. They were
all happy to spend hours showing me photographs of Louis as they retold
stories that confirmed, yet again, that the man who was once the world's
most famous patient had been a "helluva guy"—even when his heart
turned bad.

Chris Barnard was also, in his unique and troubled fashion, a "helluva guy." Yet after my own initial boyish enthusiasm, I had rarely thought much about Barnard. Apart from cocking half an eye at his latest young girlfriend on the front pages, I didn't care about his various marriages, affairs, and divorces. His hustling libido had been mocked by a sly *Private Eye* cover, on June 6, 1969—a photograph of Chris and Louwtjie, smiling between two headlines: "Divorce Shock" and "Mrs Barnard Speaks." In the little speech balloon coming out of her mouth, a grinning Louwtjie said: "Nothing will stop him putting organs into people."

Barnard, of course, was ready to take on the world and tell them how wrong they were—especially about apartheid, or the sports boycott against South Africa. He would huff and puff his little speeches against "the terrorists"—meaning the likes of Robert Sobukwe and Nelson Mandela. He would insist that democracy, as he said in 1978 while supporting the ridiculously far-right campaign of Nationalist politician Connie Mulder, "can only spell ruin for the country and send us down the same horrendous track as the rest of Africa." When I heard reports, or saw snippets, of the angry surgeon on the BBC or NBC, I would understand why Deirdre Barnard used to pretend that she was an Australian rather than a white South African while waterskiing in Europe.

His status among his surgical contemporaries had already disintegrated. The extent of the scorn and jealousy toward him was made obvious in October 1975, when the world's 500 leading cardiac surgeons and cardiologists were invited to Detroit for the Henry Ford Hospital International Symposium on Cardiac Surgery. Only two of the pantheon were excluded—Walt Lillehei, in disgrace after being found guilty of tax evasion, and Chris Barnard. Lillehei would eventually be welcomed back and hailed as the prime innovator in the development of open-heart surgery. Barnard, however, would never be forgiven for "stealing" the work of Shumway and Lower, or for his subsequent arrogance.

Barnard's significant work in tubercular meningitis, intestinal atresia, the development of heart valves, and in helping devise a surgical remedy for the tetralogy of Fallot were all but forgotten. His outstanding results in cardiac transplantation, however, remain indisputable, three of his patients living over twenty years with a transplanted heart. Yet he never again carried out a conventional orthotopic transplant after 1974. Barnard switched instead to his pioneering procedure of heterotopic transplantation, in which a patient's existing heart would work alongside the newly transplanted heart. Dubbed the "piggyback" transplant, its subsequent use by other surgeons eventually dwindled. Yet Barnard continued to transplant "piggyback" hearts through-out the rest of his sporadic career. His retirement in 1983, which he attributed to his arthritis—rather than the simple loss of desire to work—was greeted with little fanfare outside South Africa. A doctor of extraordinary dedication, hunger, and compassion had been smudged and eroded by time and his own vanities.

The next downward phase in his life then unfolded in all its cruel delusion: he became obsessed with age. "Growing old is humanity's greatest tragedy," he averred. Barnard explained that he tried to fight the regrettable process by clinging to the closest beautifully youthful body. The remark was uttered with a laugh, but his seriousness was evident in his ceaseless pursuit of young women. He had already turned sixty when, in 1982, he began to woo Karin Setzkorn, a nineteen-year-old Afrikaner model he had once employed as a waitress at a restaurant he owned in Cape Town. She eventually became his third wife—and, inevitably, even after bearing him two children when he was in his seventies, his third ex-wife.

He seemed a broken old man when he died, at the age of seventy-eight, still mourning the young wife who had abandoned him. Apart from his cracked personal life and soiled fame, he was regarded by most as an eccentric quack flogging ludicrous business schemes rather than a pioneering cardiac surgeon. Barnard brought much of the derision down upon himself.

He had amassed hundreds of thousands of dollars endorsing a "rejuvena-tion centre," Clinique La Prairie, in Basel, Switzerland, where the rich and the ridiculous flocked in the belief they would regain their youth after being "in-jected with aborted lamb fetuses," which Barnard said would revitalize their cells, cure disease, and reverse the aging process. His friendship with Armin Mattli, who owned the clinic, persuaded Barnard to lend his name to the marketing of the center's "miraculous anti-ageing cream," Glycel. While Barnard would privately admit that the claims made on behalf of Glycel were "nonsense," he continued to accept his hefty retainer as $200 tubs of the cream flew off the shelves in stores like Harrods and Bloomingdale's. He was stripped of his membership in both the American College of Surgeons and its cardiology equivalent. Barnard had become a medical embarrassment in America and most of Europe.

But he suffered more from the skin cancer that, in the last years of his life, ate away at his face and left him lamenting the irony that "I now look more like the elephant man than the handsome guy who was once voted one of the world's five greatest lovers by *Paris Match*." He had lost his looks, his three wives, his professional reputation, and all his glory.

And yet the presence of the younger Chris Barnard haunted the four years I spent researching and writing this book. I was compelled to look at him though new eyes and with a more layered understanding. And the people who knew him best affected me the most. They made me look again at a man who had become so disfigured by fame and despair that his real achievements were in danger of being obliterated. As much as I pored over Lillehei's letters to Barnard, and some of the surreal accounts I picked up from yellowing newspaper clippings, or even just wandered around the old Groote Schuur operating room where they had made history in the darkest hours of December 3, 1967, nothing spoke of Barnard with more power than the voices of those who had lived or worked with him. Some revered him, and some loathed him. The largest group, those in the middle, who described the qualities of Barnard as a doctor as cogently as they acknowledged his flaws as a man, clearly influenced me the most.

The people who had lived with him longest, from his daughter, Deirdre, to his brother, Marius, spoke with revealing eloquence. Deirdre told me of his unbearable loneliness toward the end; but at the same time I heard in her voice a humor and compassion that made me warm as much to him as obviously I did to her. "My dad spent those last few years just up the road from here," she said one afternoon at home in a suburb of Cape Town. "He came back to me and said that Karin wanted a divorce and that she wanted him to move out. I found this little place for him which was near to all of us—his original family. It didn't matter what he had or hadn't done anymore. He was just my dad.

"I'd take him to the pool because it helped his arthritis. And afterwards, he loved sitting in the sauna, and I would read *Angela's Ashes* to him. Something in that book stuck with me—the unconditional love one has for a parent . . .

especially a daughter for a father. And things between him and my mother also got so much better toward the end. It was like me and my mom and my own children could give him shelter in his last days. We were like an umbrella for him. It was beautiful in a way.

"But at first, there was so much *snot en trane* [snot and tears]. I was having my own heartache at the time and so *ons het gehuil* [we cried] together. There was this song he used to play over and over again—Kris Kristofferson's 'Lover Please Come Back to Me.' Oh, it was too terrible. It was actually hilarious—we would start laughing. But deep down he was frighteningly lonely. You could count the people who were still there for him on one hand. Yet at the height of his fame, people crawled all over him. He loved it, of course, but in the end it seemed so sad; he was so abandoned. But he had this wonderful sense of humor which saved him from his worst traits.

"I remember he once got a fax from [Mikhail] Gorbachev about this child who needed a heart operation. My dad had to go to a press conference and his office was totally *deurmekaar* [chaotic]. He was ranting: 'Where's this bloody fax?' And I thought this is exactly how he used to treat his nurses in the operating theater. This is how he treats people. I said, 'How dare you talk to me like this? I'm fifty-one years old. And you're a spoilt brat.'

"I went out with a friend of mine for a drink and I started to tell her that I'd just called my father a spoilt brat—but she wasn't really that interested in my soap opera. Her mother had just got Alzheimer's. And I said, 'Don't worry, my dad will have all the answers . . .' So I asked him, and he went through the whole thing and said, 'This is what you can do, go here and there . . . and this is the best medication . . . and these are the alternatives . . .' He was just a wonderful doctor again. And after he'd gone through the whole list of how my friend could help her mother, he suddenly stopped. He gave me a look, with a little smile, and then he said, 'You know what, Deirdre? That's all a spoilt brat knows.' "

If Norman Shumway had come to resemble the J. D. Salinger of surgery, Marius Barnard had reminded me of the reclusive author a couple of years earlier, in October 2002. When he'd leaned down so that he could see me through the open window of my rented car, he'd looked a little like Salinger did in that now famous picture, where, angry and distressed at having his privacy betrayed by a photographer, the writer stared wildly into the unblinking lens of the camera. Barnard had been a part of transplant history sixteen years after Salinger published *The Catcher in the Rye*, in 1951, but they were of the same generation and were tied fast to a single event from the past.

Marius Barnard might have been a few years younger than Salinger, but at seventy-five he had the same stoop, shock of white hair, and blue eyes that flashed with resentment. He was not a hermit like Salinger, for he and his wife, Inez, lived openly in Hermanus, a whale watcher's paradise just over an hour's drive from Cape Town. But Marius was sick of the same old questions about himself and his more famous brother, Chris, and their controversial role in the transplant legacy.

"I don't give interviews," he had bristled with pleasure when I first called him, "and I've never told anyone out there the real story of me and Chris and the whole bloody transplant saga."

He added that he was not about to change his mind just because I had once been a small South African boy back in the days when he and Chris had their photographs plastered across the front pages of, seemingly, every major newspaper around the world. But on a whim, he did agree to my tentative suggestion that I should still drive over to Hermanus to "say hello."

Marius Barnard was an intriguing and contrary man, full of kindness and rage, bitterness and generosity. They might be feelings we all carry inside ourselves but, in Marius, they were striking in the way they existed in such raw tandem. And, in the end, I was fortunate. He eventually spoke of his rage and bitterness while showing kindness and generosity to me.

I learned it was true that Marius had refused for years to grant an interview or to talk in public about his most personal feelings toward Chris—whom he admitted to loathing as much as loving. But believing that we were fated to work together, he decided to tell me "the whole damn story." We settled down for a couple of weeks and spent day after day together, compiling one audiotape after another, as it all poured out of him.

And so, in that moment when, like Salinger, Marius Barnard's face had ducked down through the open window to stare at me with fury and dismay,

I felt acutely for him. His reaction was not caused by my presence. Rather, it was directed at the cancer that, on the inside, was slowly killing him.

The week before, he had learned that there had been a rise in his PSA cell count, which reflected the rate at which the cancer had begun to spread through him again. His long remission had followed a brutal period of "treatment." Marius said that last word so despairingly that I reached out to touch his hand. It seemed a futile gesture.

"Do you know what I can do for this cancer now?" he asked fiercely.

I listened while Marius Barnard, once a famous heart surgeon but now just an ordinary man, looked down silently at me. His eyes were clear and blue.

"Nothing," he finally said. "I can just wait now."

He turned away, and then, still shrugging angrily, he came back and squeezed my arm. "It's okay," he said, "I've had my time."

I murmured a few platitudes and he almost smiled. Marius said I should join him and his wife one afternoon when, at five o'clock most summer days, they went swimming in the sea, a few kilometers from Hermanus. They would then sit down on a large blanket, the water still glistening in their hair, and open a bottle of wine while they watched the sun slip behind the mountains.

"It's not a bad way to end a day," he said.

I liked Marius most of all when, after a typically *Boere* (Afrikaner) lunch at home in Hermanus, he would make me laugh while he told me what it was like to be Chris Barnard's brother. Marius was already planning his own autobiography which he insisted he would call *The Chris I Have to Bear,* or *Heartburn.* He would chuckle darkly when he dredged up some old Afrikaans newspaper clipping in which he was called "The Poor Man's Chris Barnard." He also told me how Robert Kirby, the South African satirist, used to perform a skit during his one-man show in the 1970s. "Kirby would act out the part of Chris, and he depicted all his vanity and paranoia. And Kirby would make Chris turn round and shout: '*Ag man,* Marius! Get out of my shadow!' I was not even allowed to be in the shadow of my brother. I laughed at that one. Chris, of course, hated it. He couldn't stand any criticism.

"But if you really follow our lives after the transplant you will see that Chris did nothing much after that—it was the work he did before that was important. One of the things I resent most is that we had the opportunity to establish the top cardiac unit in the world. Yes, we were the first—but it was more important that the results of our first six patients were easily the best in the world. But Chris blew it. He was too busy racing, chasing young women or yet more overseas glory. I would say, 'You can have all the fame. But let us get on with the work in Cape Town.' Of course he would never relinquish control."

It remains one of the tragic quandaries of this story that it is simply not possible to know for certain what Chris Barnard's legacy might have been had he not succumbed to the seductions that ultimately ruined him. While Marius Barnard is emphatic that their Groote Schuur team was on its way to becoming the "top cardiac unit in the world," it seems unlikely that, without the financial resources or depth of personnel available to Stanford, Barnard's unit would have matched the achievement of Shumway. Yet Barnard's superior early results resonate with a promise that was soon shredded by his own human frailties. His character, crammed full of risk and daring, drove him on in his quest to be the first—and that same intense personality finally destroyed him.

Chris Barnard's life, after he won the race, was framed by sorrow and grief. The suicide of Andre, on February 29, 1984, was the most terrible consequence. "All I knew was that my son was dead," Barnard admitted years later. "I should have given him the love and affection he needed when he was a little boy. It was my fault."

Marius spoke movingly of his nephew, but perhaps his disenchantment with the transplant story that had defined and haunted their lives stemmed from his own resentment toward Chris. He spoke bluntly of the hollow he felt at the very center of their supposed medical "immortality."

"I'm not fooled by the fact that we were first," he said. "I know Kantrowitz and Lower and especially Shumway did all the work. Let them take the credit. But I also have to say that if they had done it first, before Chris, then I don't think it would have been quite such a big deal. Chris drove that story. The heart transplant made him—but he also helped make it this huge story which transcended medicine.

"There are three reasons why the heart transplant became such a massive twentieth-century story. One: Where was it done? In Cape Town, in the days of apartheid. Two: Who did it? We were not Denton Cooley or Michael DeBakey in Houston. We were not Lord Brock in London or Norman Shumway at Stanford. We were just ordinary guys—and some of us, especially Chris, had good personalities in public. We were upfront and we weren't too bad-looking. We were kind of poor—my monthly salary was R600 [$400] then. When people heard we came from this small Afrikaner town in the Karoo where our father preached to the colored people, it was even more romantic. But the biggest thing was number three: the heart. Who were the pioneers of kidney transplantation? [Joseph] Murray? [Tom] Starzl? [Roy] Calne? No ordinary person knows these names. But ask them who did the first heart transplant and they know: 'Chris Barnard.'

"I just think it's sad that the only claim to fame that we have is not scientific—it's just that we did it first. Like Roger Bannister ran the first four-minute mile. So what? Everybody runs it in three minutes something now. The first man on the moon? To hell with him! But people always need a name. And so, with the heart transplant, they got one: Chris Barnard. I think, in the end, the world got what it wanted."

This is another moment. On a plane from Washington, D.C., to Richmond, Virginia, having spent a day crossing a dark-blue ocean to reach America again, the more remarkable reality of surgical risk-taking rose up again in my bleary head. I was 30,000 feet in the air and on my way to meet Richard Lower, a man who had traveled deep into the once unknown wilderness of cardiac transplantation.

The sky outside the smudged plane window was black, and the first yellow dots of light from the most distant edges of town could not yet be seen. Lower was now in his seventies, but I imagined that some of the fire that had fueled his work still crackled inside him. It was hard to guess how he would react to someone as woodenly unscientific as me. I just hoped he would not burn me down. I hoped I could convey my immersion in the extraordinary journey he and Shumway had made.

Shumway himself insisted that Lower was "the greatest experimental surgeon since Alexis Carrel." It was some compliment. At the turn of the twentieth century, the intense young Frenchman had been the first in medical history to perfect the art of anastomosis—the sewing together of blood vessels, which provides the basis of most forms of modern surgery. Carrel had then moved smoothly into his earliest experiments with transplantation, a surgical task utterly dependent on the blood vessels of a newly grafted organ being joined to those of the recipient's circulatory system. In 1902, at the University of Lyon, he removed the kidney from a dog and placed it in the same animal's neck so that he could easily monitor the impact of the transplant. While the dog survived the surgery and the kidney functioned in the neck, infection soon spread.

Carrel was not discouraged by the ensuing death. After moving to America, he continued with his experiments in kidney transplantation and the grafting of legs from one dog to another, before, in 1905, he and his research partner, Claude Guthrie, turned to the most untouchable organ—the heart. They transplanted a dog's heart into its own neck. The animal lived only a few hours.

Some, though not Carrel and Guthrie themselves, regarded it as a medical miracle. Guthrie wrote to Carrel on October 31, 1905, to tell him that "Dr. Miller, the pathologist, has just returned from spending the summer in England and Germany. He says we have a great international reputation in having successfully transplanted the heart! Is it not ridiculous? Newspaper fame again."

I had read one of Shumway's medical lectures in which he relished those derisory phrases—"Newspaper fame again" and "Is it not ridiculous?"—which epitomized his personal contempt for any vaguely journalistic account of his own work which had transcended Carrel and Guthrie's early meanderings in the dark.

It was easy to understand why Shumway had politely resisted all my attempts to persuade him to share his memories of his monumental role in transplantation. I knew he would even be troubled by the choice of a cheap word like "monumental." It was devoid of scientific meaning. So I didn't blame Shumway for his relentless evasions. He had given up on interviews years before. He had always distrusted them, and anyway, he had nothing left to say. The eloquence and the profundity lay in the work itself.

When I made my first cold call to Dick Lower, his wife, Anne, told me he was out shoveling snow. Would I hold on while she went to get him? Of course I said yes, and shortly after received his warm and breezy greeting. Within five minutes he had invited me to Richmond to spend a week reliving those decisive years of cardiac transplantation. He even laughed softly when I offered up my "momentous" adjective.

Lower, in person, turned out to be even more laconic and engaging. He was one of those rare men you imagine you've known all your life after only a couple of days in their company. Lower also explained the development of cardiac transplantation in modest but cogent detail as he took me from the vibrant dog lab to the threatening courthouse, stressing over and over the centrality of Shumway in everything they accomplished together.

One afternoon, as we sat on his large patio, overlooking the green and rolling yard, I told Lower of my failure to pin down his old collaborator. I explained how I had already spent a couple of weeks in Stanford and had spoken to everyone else in their formative transplant story. They all stressed that I had "to get Shumway." He was the master. He was the key to this story.

The master, however, remained resolute in his silence. Lower nodded sagely at a familiar tale. He knew Shumway better than anyone; and so Lower offered me a beer in seeming consolation.

Adrian Kantrowitz, at the age of eighty-six, still sounded indestructible. He was roaring in downtown Detroit. The surrounding streets were blasted and abandoned, but Kantrowitz kept on blazing away in a smart office block on the edge of Lake St. Clair, where he and his wife, Jean, ran L-VAD Technology, their own company, specializing in his cherished left ventricular assist devices.

We spoke often about the fact that, in June 1966, Kantrowitz was prevented from making transplant history only by two elderly members of his own team. "Yeah," he sighed on one occasion, "I could've been famous. I might've been rich. There's no doubt about it. Of course I was disappointed. But what do you do? You don't commit suicide. It's part of the whole deal— nothing works the first time. And you can't always be first. There are some races you lose, and some you win. It just so happened that, the next time we were ready to go, Barnard did his transplant a few days before us. It could have so easily been the other way around. It was horrible when I heard that he had beaten me to it, but I dragged myself up and we proceeded."

And Shumway, I asked, what of Shumway? Kantrowitz rested his big hands on his ample belly and shook his head. "Shumway was devastated—because Shumway had certainly worked as hard, and longer, than we had. I had very good reason to do ours when we did it. So did Shumway. But, for whatever reason, he delayed doing his first transplant. We had been racing against each other, and so he was disturbed by the fact that first Barnard did it, and then I did it, before he did. Looking at it from his point of view, if there was anyone who deserved to do it first, it was Shumway. But you can't wait. If you don't do it, someone else will. So along came Barnard, a big risk-taker. He had no real experience of heart transplants. Barnard tried a few dogs before he did the first transplant, but they didn't survive."

Kantrowitz laughed long and hard, a loud and contagious sound. "Yeah! So good old Chris thought, 'Let's try it in humans instead.' To his credit he felt he could do it. He was absolutely right. He worked out that the surgical procedure was no big deal. And his results, among the few he did, were the best of anyone in the beginning. He was a smart guy. And then of course Shumway kept plugging away, and he turned transplantation into the wonderful success story it is today. Shumway and Ed Stinson made a hell of a team. There's no question about it—it's kinda heroic what they did in beating rejection.

"I, obviously, became absorbed instead in the field of mechanical assist devices, but I remember being part of an NIH transplant review, in the early 1970s, which went to assess Shumway's work after he made a new grant application. Lower was having his courtroom problems, and so Stanford were the only guys still in the transplant game and trying to conquer rejection. It was so obvious they were doing great work, that I came out as Shumway's strongest support and he got all the money he needed. It wasn't because of me—anyone with a modicum of sense could see that Shumway and Stinson would eventually make transplantation work. They had to be supported."

Kantrowitz, by then, had been fired from Maimonides. "They thought you were a madman, didn't they?" I said.

"I was!" he laughed. "From their point of view, I was totally crazy. I did things differently. I started with my implantable pacemaker. And I did the first permanent left ventricular assist device, which, from their viewpoint, didn't work. That was crazy. But the things we're doing now grew out of that U-shape invention. And then we did heart transplants. There was a massive hue and cry. And then I forged ahead with the balloon pump. They said, 'This man is a danger!' They actually said that! They didn't have much difficulty in proving it, because these were wild ideas. To think that you might take a heart from a dead patient and put it into another patient and have that patient live. That is unthinkable. *Wild!*

"A sensitive person would have picked up the signals and done something diplomatic about it. But I was only interested in the work—it was pioneering, and I had the opportunity to do it. That was the great thing—we had the funding and the ideas. To get that opportunity and not do anything, just to protect your job, was unthinkable. I got fired, but so what, here we are, thirty-five years later, and I'm still working. That's the way you've got to do it, because nothing works the first time. Just ask me. Just ask Shumway."

In the spring of 2004, Kantrowitz and Shumway met again in Detroit at an American College of Cardiology meeting. They had once been fierce rivals, but Shumway was gracious toward Kantrowitz, highlighting his massive contribution in developing the balloon pump, which has saved so many hundreds of thousands of lives. Kantrowitz, in turn, paid homage to Shumway as the true leader of cardiac transplantation. They parted on better terms than ever before—two old masters of the heart who, in their eighties, unbowed and unvanquished, had moved beyond rejection and discovered acceptance.

Norman Shumway's reputation in medicine, as the "father of cardiac transplantation," was unsurpassed. Shumway and his Stanford team had proven that immunology and physiology were the cornerstones on which a successful transplant needed to be built. In his quest for scientific knowledge to underpin his clinical ventures, Shumway had transformed cardiac surgery. With associates like Ed Stinson and Eugene Dong, he had obtained long-term survival in the laboratory, refined the operating technique, monitored the denervated heart, and established enduring protocols for the selection of patients and for measuring and treating rejection.

The relentless way in which his Stanford program defeated rejection demands a book of its own. One of his key lieutenants, Philip Caves, invented the bioptome, an instrument that permits the direct sampling of biopsies from the transplanted heart as a way of detecting early signs of rejection. Shumway also oversaw Stanford's revolutionary use of cyclosporine, as well as refining the use of antilymphocyte, during the increasingly successful management of immunosuppression.

"Based on Shumway's work," Stinson wrote in 1984, after cardiac transplantation had resumed in hospitals around the world, "the current level of enthusiasm in the procedure is realistic and the disastrous experience of seventeen years ago is unlikely to be repeated. The results now being reported in a few currently active centers owe much to Shumway's work which has set up standards for cardiac transplantation. They include research, fundamental and clinical, an unusually intensive post-operative management by medical staffs with extraordinary dedication to their patients, and active organ procurement programs."

More than twenty years later, as a direct result of Shumway's intellectual defiance and perseverance in fighting rejection, over four thousand successful heart transplants are carried out annually around the world, with the number of salvaged lives only limited by the availability of donors. In the United States alone, 160 hospitals have their own cardiac transplant units, and 90 percent of patients survive for longer than a year and 75 percent for more than five years. Recipients routinely live for twenty and even thirty years. Their survival owes much to Shumway and Lower.

"Norm and me," Lower grinned one afternoon when we sat out on his patio in Richmond, "had this friendly rivalry going on as to who might do the first transplant. It never really entered our heads that it would be done by anyone else. Most people in cardiac surgery thought the same. I came very close in 1966 and Norm was on the brink in November 1967. So it was a real shock when we got the news about Barnard. I was thinking, 'Who is this guy?' before I suddenly remembered Barnard had watched me in the lab the previous year. It all clicked into place then, and I remembered his old technician telling my lab guy that he was going back to South Africa to do it first. I never believed him. We believed you had to do years of research before you tried this in a human. He was different from us in that respect."

Lower laughed lightly, without bitterness. "Yeah, there was disappointment, of course . . . but after a while, watching the circus around him, I took a more measured view. I said, 'He's welcome to it. I don't need any of this publicity or craziness.' It was kind of ridiculous. Even Norm's first transplant caused a crazy reaction—though they handled it much better at Stanford. I had my own troubles later on, of course, but who could possibly envy Chris Barnard in the end?"

Lower still worked part-time as a GP in a clinic for the poor in downtown Richmond. He looked composed as he spoke softly. "We've had some pain, but if I look at Barnard's life and I look at mine, then I know one thing. I wouldn't trade it for anything. I moved out of cardiac surgery in 1989. I remember Cooley or DeBakey saying, 'Dick Lower? Retiring? But he's just a *kid!*' I was six months short of sixty. DeBakey's still working in his nineties. Cooley's into the eighties. Norm's moved past eighty. And they're still involved—even if they're drifting out at their own pace. I didn't do it slowly. I pulled straight out. I'd done my thing, I was happy. And yeah, there were other factors. . . ."

Like Chris Barnard, Dick Lower had lost a son in the late 1980s. His youngest boy, John, had been killed in an automobile accident, not far from the family home. When the police arrived in the dark, Dick Lower thought they had come to tell him that they had found another transplant donor. He could not have guessed that they were about to inform him of the death of his own son.

"Dick didn't come back to work for at least a month," remembered Sheelah Katz, his transplant coordinator at the Medical College of Virginia, "and on the day he returned he was isolated in his office for a long time. I eventually went in to see him. I really did not know what to say, because Dick is such a generous man, and to have this happen to him and Anne was unbearable. And so I just sat there and started to cry. Dick was quiet. He kept smoking his pipe. And then he said, 'Sheelah, tell me about the transplant cases, tell me about the work.'"

Dick Lower made me laugh again when he told me, "After I left surgery, I had this nutty idea that I could run a cattle ranch. My manager at this ranch I had bought in Montana had announced he was leaving early in 1989, and so, after all the transplants and everything else that happened, I just took off. I spent most of the next seven years in Montana, looking after three hundred head of cattle on my own. I used to come in after a whole day out on the ranch, single-handedly looking after all these cattle, and I would try and eat these beans I had cooked. Boy, they would always smell delicious, but they were usually raw. I never left the place except to go to one of Norm's functions. It was my way of starting my life all over again."

I had always loved the way Shumway ended his short speech at a banquet held to celebrate his achievements when he retired from his post as Stanford's chief of surgery in 1993. Embarrassed by the adulation, Shumway kept his reply brief, and, in finding a way out of the spotlight, he said, "I would like all of you to meet my good friend and codefendant in heart transplantation, Dr. Richard Lower. Dr. Lower would you please stand up so that this audience may see a respectable landowner and cattle rancher? Thank you very much."

"Yeah," Lower said, laughing, "Norm never liked much attention. And he never really got his head around the charms of Montana or a cattle ranch either. He just likes hanging around Stanford, watching his old transplant program bloom while he flirts with the secretaries. They all love him up there—except the deans. They still remember what a hard time he gave them. He's some guy, Norm, and still funnier and sharper at eighty-one than anyone I've ever met. He's the king."

Lower paused thoughtfully. And then he looked up and said, "You *gotta* spend time with Shumway. Leave it to me. . . ."

The king wore baggy trousers and sneakers. He was deceptively shy but strangely enthusiastic. For a reluctant interviewee, Norman Shumway talked and laughed like we had climbed right back inside one of Sparky's old vans and slipped out for a little spin round the transplant block. The reserve finally fell away completely when, for our amusement, as if we were closing in on the corner of Clay and Webster, where he and Dick Lower used to "beguile the tedium" by switching hearts between dogs, we sat down and looked at a little homespun booklet Shumway had made for his lab boys as a Christmas present in 1962.

Charting the lab's first four years, *The Stanford Cardiac Surgical Team, 1958–1962* featured newspaper clippings, photographs, and pen portraits of all the key figures in the development of heart transplantation, in both the San Francisco and Stanford laboratories—Shumway, Lower, Ed Hurley, Eugene Dong, Ray Stofer, and technicians like Don Toy and Victor Villaluna. Shumway devoured the copy Dong had given me with chortling disbelief.

"Oh boy." He laughed, running his fingers lightly over some of the photos as if saying hello to his old friends. "I haven't seen this in thirty-odd years. This is terrific. Here we all are. Look at these gangsters."

Shumway pointed to a photograph titled *The Gang,* which had been taken inside the San Francisco laboratory where he and Lower had literally invented cardiac transplantation on a stainless-steel table. The accompanying text, written by Shumway, evoked the feel of the place and the spirit of the gang: "The high ceilings and dim lights of the narrow hallways gave abundant laboratory space in the old Lane building. As dark and dingy as the old lab was, it had a rather homely feeling. In the forty-one years of its existence it had undergone almost no changes. Instruments were boiled in the white pot on the gas burner in the far right-hand corner. The long black box at the left end of the workbench was a respirator. No one, except Don Toy, knew how to make it work. For years, medical students underwent surgical training in this laboratory. The stainless steel animal table in the left foreground was introduced by Ray Stofer. It was entirely out of place and technicians complained that it needed cleaning every day. Notice the well-fitting scrub clothes."

Shumway laughed a little harder. "I'd forgotten all about this. You know how I told you this building leaked? Well, I had an office in the corner, on the fifth floor, and when it rained you had to put a bucket on your desk to catch the water. It was hilarious. Can you see the blood splattered on the table legs? Ray Stofer, who was another ingenious guy, built this thing . . . You see this? Over here? That's where we boiled up the instruments. We didn't even have an autoclave. So we'd boil the instruments over there. Look at old Don Toy, the Chinese guy, who ran the lab. What an amazing character. This is how the whole damn thing started.

"Dick kept complaining about having a backache when we stood around that room for an hour or more—doing nothing while the heart cooled. We were involved in some interesting stuff with hypothermia back then. So I said to Dick, 'Why don't we just take out the dog's heart, and that'll take your mind off your back?' So we did it even though we had very primitive materials to work with—stuff that would have just been thrown out of the OR. But it was damn tricky sewing the same heart back into the same dog. And so Dick said, 'You know, if we take the heart from another dog we'll have more tissue to work with and we can bundle up the suture lines so they won't leak so badly'—otherwise they were like wet tissue paper. So, I said, 'Dick, that's some idea! Let's do it!' That's how the transplant from one dog to the other started."

Shumway was a master of the pithy and casual summary—just as he was expert in deflecting attention from himself. "Dick Lower," he would say softly, as if in awe of his friend's very name, "is the guru of cardiac transplantation." So determinedly self-effacing about his own work, Shumway was a charmingly relentless cheerleader for his gang. In celebrating Lower, Stinson, and Bruce Reitz, with whom he carried out the world's first successful heart-lung transplant in 1981, Shumway exalted a triumvirate that could equal any other trio of surgeons in the world.

In an even more endearing continuation of the pattern, his Stanford disciples were so shoe-shuffingly modest about their own exploits, it was as if he needed to bang the drum on their behalf. The contrast between Shumway and Barnard could not have been more stark. Yet just as you need to accept the rampant ego of Barnard if you want to discover his true worth, so you need to persevere and peel away Shumway's layers of reticence to finally grasp the essence of his achievements.

Shumway laughed wryly at his one professional setback. "It seemed cruel at the time. What is it they always say about being the first? We all know the first guy to get to the North Pole or the South Pole—or to step across the moon. It's just that second or third guy's name which is a little more elusive. I understand the whole drama of being the first, or not being the first. I've lived with it a few years now."

Shumway purposely didn't pause to allow further reflection. He was already veering back to Dick Lower. "You know, deep down, I always felt that Lower should have done the first, because he was the driving force behind all the experimental work. When Dick had that courtroom battle in the early seventies and transplant units were closing down around the world, I believed that even more strongly. The American College of Cardiology wanted to declare a moratorium on heart transplantation around 1970—the chairman of the Board of Trustees at Stanford called a meeting with the dean and university lawyers and they wanted to know why we shouldn't comply.

"And we just said, 'The idea of a moratorium and actually stopping our own transplant work would be ridiculous.' We already had patients who were surviving regularly for long periods of time, and I never had any doubt that we would win the battle. I had no concern that they could stop us—and that was precisely because of Dick's work in the lab. There's an old saying in experimental surgery, that anything you can do in a dog is much easier to do in a human. With the success Dick had with all our dog experiments, there was unequivocal evidence that it would work. And in the end, they all came around. It worked out fine."

Inevitably we drifted back to Chris Barnard. We flipped back and forth between their days in Minnesota and the madness of the first transplants. And in between, Shumway just shook his head as we contemplated those hot afternoons in Richmond when Barnard, silently, almost secretly, watched Lower at work in the lab. Yet I found Shumway most moving toward the end of our time together. Beyond the hurt and the concealed anger, I asked him about the tribute he had paid to Barnard in *The New York Times* a few days after his rival's death.

"Well," Shumway said, "I meant it, because, if only in one sense, he did make a hugely significant contribution to heart transplantation. What he did with brain death should never be forgotten. The fact that he chose to use a brain-dead donor brought this whole taboo subject out into the widest possible public arena. And so, in many ways, it was Chris Barnard who made the use of brain-dead victims for organ transplantation an acceptable concept. He paved the way on that issue—and, as we know, it became central to our whole early struggle in transplantation.

"Of course he and I didn't see much of each other. But I remember quite vividly the last time we met. It was June 2000, in Paris. He had this carcinoma of the nose, so his whole nose had been removed and grafts had been taken from his cheeks to build a new nose. Honest to God, I didn't even recognize him. I felt so sorry for him, because I knew what looking like that did to him."

Shumway, who had also suffered from skin cancer, rubbed a hand across his eighty-one-year-old face. "I didn't know it was him at first, but then I heard that voice. You could never miss his voice. So we chatted a bit, and it was okay, if a little stilted. But I just felt for him. I couldn't believe what had happened to him.

"In a way, I think he was a little sheepish. Maybe he was a little ashamed. I certainly thought so. Now that we're talking about it, let me tell you about the previous time we'd been together. I was with him at a conference in Spain, in about 1987, and it was pretty strange. I gave a little talk, and he gave a little talk, and then, in the middle of that, right up there on the podium, with me on the same stage, I thought he was going to break down. It was clear that he was deeply troubled. I didn't say anything to anyone then, but I understood. I remembered that his father was a minister back in South Africa, and so, deep down inside Chris Barnard, I think a sense of being righteous and fair had been inculcated."

"Do you think that's what haunted him?" I asked.

"Exactly," Shumway murmured. "Exactly . . ."

On the last morning of my final trip to Stanford, in the winter of 2004, I sat next to Shumway at the weekly conference of the hospital's transplant unit. Shumway and I were near the back of the circular gathering of surgeons, cardiologists, and transplant coordinators. We slurped our coffee and tucked into the spread that had been laid out by the Stanford catering crew for a seven-o'clock Friday-morning meeting.

"Oh yeah," Shumway said through a mouthful of pastry, "this one's real tasty. How's that muffin?"

"Beautiful," I confirmed, thrilled that my less-than-svelte body had been built on a diet that clearly did not disturb the world's most renowned cardiac surgeon.

We sat and listened as a roomful of doctors each took a turn to detail the mostly successful progress of their respective cardiac-transplant patients. The presentations were smooth yet passionate, concise yet emphatic, and I thought of Adrian Kantrowitz every time another mention was made of the balloon pump keeping a patient alive. And I could not help but think of how far transplantation had come in the forty-five years since Shumway and Lower had begun their work in that dark and leaky building in San Francisco. I also thought of Chris Barnard and his own contributions to transplantation. But mostly I thought of Shumway, as, in sidelong glances, I watched an eighty-one-year-old man listen attentively to the culmination of his life's work. He had forgotten the pastries and muffins as, discreetly and sagely, he listened to the younger people who had followed him.

When I went to see him in his office a few hours later, to say goodbye, Shumway jumped up with alacrity. "Aren't they great?" he said of all his Stanford surgeons and cardiologists. "Aren't they terrific?"

Norman Shumway died of cancer on February 10, 2006, the day after he turned eighty-three. Two years earlier, we spoke one last time about the journey he and his colleagues had taken—and specifically about the race to transplant the first human heart. "Maybe it was a blessing that we weren't the first," Shumway said as we walked slowly out of his office. "We had enough trouble anyway dealing with the press and all that hoo-hah. Boy, we had plenty of trouble. So maybe, in the end, it all worked out for the best."

Shumway paused, and then, with a little laugh, he stretched out his hand. "Yeah," he said, "I think it worked out just fine."

NOTES AND SOURCES

In addition to identifying the primary sources for the historical material in the previous pages, I have included below some background information on specific surgeons or incidents related to the book. This is obviously not meant to be read as a definitive series of notes on the early history of cardiac transplantation, but rather as a personal choice of facts, vignettes, and memories that, I hope, add a broader context to the preceding chapters.

Prologue: Into the Void

The depiction of Adrian Kantrowitz's preparations to transplant the world's first human heart on June 29, 1966, is based primarily on original research obtained during extensive interviews with the surgeon himself—as well as with Jordan Haller, his chief of thoracic surgery at Maimonides Hospital in Brooklyn, and William Neches, who was then a pediatric intern responsible for the care of the anencephalic donor infant. I also made extensive use of the case notes preserved by Neches and Kantrowitz. This attempted transplant is recalled briefly in two medical papers: A. Kantrowitz, "Moment in History: America's first human heart transplantation—The concept, the planning and the furor" (*ASAIO Journal* 44:4, July–August 1998, pp 244–52), and A. Kantrowitz et al., "Transplantation of the heart in an infant and an adult" (*American Journal of Cardiology* 22:782, 1968).

Rhoda and Richard Senz spoke to me in moving detail about the son they never saw—Ralph Senz was meant to be the donor patient in the world's first human heart transplant.

The references to Aristotle and Ovid come directly from an interview with Kantrowitz. Aristotle's quote, from 350 B.C., is also cited in *The Healing Heart: An Illustrated History of Cardiology* and *King of Hearts: The True Story of the Maverick Who Pioneered Open Heart Surgery*, G. Wayne Miller's fine biography of Walt Lillehei. Miller's book also mentions the Ovid quote, as does Louisa Young's *The Book of the Heart*.

Kantrowitz's memory of Theodore Billroth is from one of our interviews, and the Viennese surgeon's quote is confirmed by Miller and in Jon Palfreman's documentary series for Nova, *Pioneers of Surgery* (program two: "Into the Heart").

An initial allusion to Kantrowitz's years of transplant research with puppies is based on a reading of numerous medical papers, including Y. Kondo, F. Gradel, and A. Kantrowitz, "Heart homotransplantation in puppies: Long survival without immunosuppressive therapy" (*Circulation* 31 and 32 [Supp I]: 181, 1965); Y. Kondo, F. Gradel, and A. Kantrowitz, "Homotransplantation of the heart in puppies under profound hypothermia—Long survival without immunosuppressive treatment" (*Annals of Surgery* 162:837, 1965); and Y. Kondo et al., "Fate of orthotopic canine heart transplants" (*Journal of Cardiovascular Surgery* 8: 155, 1967).

Legislation surrounding the "definition of death"—so crucial to the outcome of the race to transplant the first human heart—is explored in more detail in later chapters. For the purposes of the prologue, I relied largely on my personal interviews with Kantrowitz, Richard Lower, Norman Shumway, and Marius Barnard. This issue is also considered in Tony Stark's book and four-part BBC television series about the history of organ transplantation, *Knife to the Heart*.

The number of heart transplants carried out annually, in the United States and globally, was supplied by Sharon Hunt, chief cardiologist at Stanford Medical Center.

Chapter One. On the Brink

In the archive section at the Groote Schuur Transplant Museum in Cape Town there is a copy of an undated letter Chris Barnard wrote to Walt Lillehei in which he candidly discusses hearing a South African Broadcasting Corporation radio report end with the words "heart transplant" and "Stanford Medical Center." He admits in vivid detail that he was convinced he had the lost the race to Norman Shumway. His despair is echoed by the memories of his first wife, Louwtjie, whose additional descriptions of his black suit and her car come from interviews she gave to the South African magazine *Scope* (December 29, 1967) and the Afrikaans newspaper *Beeld* (June 1970).

Her own book, *Heartbreak* (out of print), provides further background material, as do my interviews with Marius Barnard and Peggy Jordaan, who were both amusing on Chris's smoking habits. The specific moment when Barnard misheard the radio report about Stanford was also confirmed by François Hitchcock, then a young registrar at Groote Schuur Hospital, in Chris Logan's biography of Barnard, *Celebrity Surgeon*. Hitchcock remembers being phoned by Barnard and asked whether he had heard the full radio report; he supplies the quotation "You'd better go out and find a donor *now!*"

The strangest, and most cruelly misleading, myth to surround the first human heart transplant centers on the "involvement" of Hamilton Naki in Barnard's team. In late 2002 a couple of ambitious South African filmmakers began to peddle a bogus story that Naki had actually led the team of surgeons who excised the heart of Louis Washkansky in December 1967. It was claimed that only the existence of apartheid had kept this "fact" secret. Naki himself allowed the myth to grow—through either irresponsibility on his part or, more likely, his encroaching senility.

The apocryphal tale took full flight on April 25, 2003, when *The Guardian* in London printed an interview with Naki that fleshed out the saga with some imaginative flourishes. It was claimed that Naki worked tirelessly, and ceaselessly, during a "bloody forty-six hour marathon" in the OR—when the first transplant actually took just over four hours to complete. The article implied further that Naki had "taught" Barnard the art of cardiac surgery. I remember speaking that same day to Marius Barnard in Hermanus, and he was suitably contemptuous—claiming that the story was typical of the "rubbish" that had engulfed the first transplant. He urged me to ignore it and not to even challenge its astonishing lack of veracity. Marius, however, was emphatic in his praise of Naki's excellent technical and surgical skills as a laboratory technician and the key role he played as a member of their team.

In the ensuing years I heard talk of plans for a Hollywood feature film about Naki's "starring role" in the first transplant. It was more pleasing to read that he had, rightly, been awarded an honorary doctorate from the University of Cape Town on June 20, 2003—an appropriate acknowledgment of the great research work he had done over the years. It was also a reminder that, if not for apartheid, Naki would have certainly become a surgeon in his own right.

The misrepresentation of his true role in the transplant story reached its nadir with the obituaries that followed his death on May 29, 2005. Publications as esteemed as *The New York Times* and *The Economist* in London rehashed the myth they had first read in *The Guardian*. They eventually had to retract their obituaries and print dutiful apologies. In an editor's note in *The New York Times* on August 27, 2005, it was conceded that "an obituary on June 11 about Hamilton Naki, a black employee of the University of Cape Town, described him as having worked behind the scenes in 1967 to assist Dr. Christiaan N. Barnard in the first human heart transplant. In recent weeks, British news reports have challenged this description. Further reporting in South Africa by The New York Times has discounted many details of the original account, which was based largely on earlier published reports. The Times should have attributed the account in the obituary more specifically, and should have made further efforts to verify it independently before publication. The Times should also have corrected its account more quickly after the initial questions were raised."

Michael Wines, writing that same day in the paper, suggested that "there are few tales in the annals of medicine to rival the recent obituaries of Hamilton Naki, hailed as the unschooled and penniless black laborer who in 1967 secretly helped Dr. Christiaan N. Barnard perform the world's first heart transplant operation. Barred by apartheid from sharing the global acclaim for Dr. Barnard's feat, he won it only in death. The New York Times said Mr. Naki's skills were so esteemed that medical authorities 'quietly looked the other way' despite his black skin. The Spanish newspaper El País called him 'el héroe clandestino.' In an editorial, The Sydney Morning Herald wrote, 'Most of us are so blessed by relative privilege that the story of Hamilton Naki seems like an outrageous fiction.'

"Alas, it is. Much of it, anyway. This much is true: Mr. Naki, who was said to be 78 when he died in a black township in Cape Town, was a skilled self-taught surgeon, versed in the argot and techniques of transplants despite leaving school at 14. He was held in great regard by Dr. Barnard and other white colleagues at the University of Cape Town, where he worked for Dr. Barnard at the time of the historic transplant.

"But he did not extract the heart used in the transplant, given to Louis Washkansky, a 55-year-old diabetic, as many accounts had it. At the time, Mr. Naki was not even in Groote Schuur Hospital in Cape Town, where the surgery took place, according to former colleagues. His considerable surgical skills were limited to experimental work on pigs and dogs, and even his greatest admirers say he would not have been allowed to work on humans.

"Also, he was not a poor gardener at the university, as his obituaries reported, but a top-level laboratory assistant, paid a commensurate salary. He did not die penniless, either. How he became accepted by The Times and much of the global media as a world-class transplant surgeon in gardener's clothing is not at all clear. Some say Mr. Naki amplified his story, confusing myth and reality in his dotage. Others say an account in the British newspaper The Guardian of his pioneering role, which apparently went unchallenged for at least two years, seemed too authentic to require further checking."

The Economist had already responded contritely a month before. In a July 14 retraction headlined "How an Inspiring Life Became Distorted by Politics," the magazine suggested that Naki "changed" his story of not even being at the hospital at the time of the first transplant "not simply because of the confusion of old age—but because of pressure from those around him. Mr Naki was already a hero, as a man of scant education who had trained himself to carry out extremely difficult transplants on animals. He was also a martyr to apartheid: a man debarred from the proper exercise of his skills, and even from fair pay, by an iniquitous regime. (Christiaan Barnard admitted that 'given the opportunity,' Mr Naki would have been 'a better surgeon than me.') For both reasons, his role was gradually embellished in post-apartheid, black-ruled South Africa. By the end, he himself came to believe it.

"The process was assisted by hints from Barnard that Mr Naki had helped him in ways that were not fully known, and by the fact that, under apartheid, any such help on white human subjects would have had to be secret anyway. In the end, a story took shape that looked so plausible to the outside world that not only ourselves, but the *Lancet,* the *British Medical Journal* and many others accepted it. Yet the same story appeared so ridiculous to the University of Cape Town, staff say, that they did not trouble to deny it.

"To report this misapprehension is doubly sad, apart from our own regret at being caught up in it. It is sad that the shadow of apartheid is still so long in South Africa that blacks and whites can tell the same narrative in quite different ways, each suspecting the motives of the other. And it is especially tragic that it should have involved Mr Naki, a man considered 'wonderful' by both sides, black and white, and whose life should still be seen as an inspiration."

The November 21, 1967, story on preparations for a transplant at Groote Schuur comes from the front page of that day's final edition of the *Cape Times.*

My brief references here to Barnard's arthritis and his time at the University of Minnesota are amplified in later chapters—and stem directly from interviews with his daughter, Deirdre Visser, and Marius Barnard, Shumway, and Christian Cabrol, as well as from descriptions in his evocative and now out-of-print autobiography, *One Life,* cowritten with Curtis Bill Pepper and published in 1970.

Background material on his early family life and on research in the dog lab was provided by Marius Barnard, with direct quotations from Chris Barnard found in *One Life.* Barnard also writes in *One Life* about his patient's mood that Saturday afternoon—and those anecdotes were supplemented by firsthand accounts from Arnie Washkansky and Hettie Berman in my interviews with them in Cape Town.

The Stanford section is based on my interviews with Norman Shumway, Ed Stinson, Dick Lower, and Christian Cabrol, and supplemented by accounts of this time found at the Medical Center archive in Palo Alto. The page-long interview Shumway gave to the *Journal of the American Medical Association* (*JAMA*) was published on November 20, 1967.

This chapter's final section, relating to preparations for the first transplant at Maimonides Hospital (which changed its name to Maimonides Medical Center in 1968), stems from detailed interviews with Adrian Kantrowitz, Jordan Haller, and Bill Neches, and from my access to extensive archives maintained by Adrian and Jean Kantrowitz. The May 1966 operation on Louise Ceraso was discussed by Kantrowitz and supplemented by the account he gave to Allen B. Wiesse in his oral history *Heart to Heart: The Twentieth-Century Battle Against Cardiac Disease.* The New York Times reported the Ceraso case on May 21, 23, 24, 25, 26, 29, and 30, 1966.

I also consulted Stark's *Knife to the Heart,* both the book and television documentary, which feature interviews with Kantrowitz and Anna Scudero. The operation on Jamie Scudero is recounted in more clinical terms in A. Kantrowitz, "Moment in History: America's first human heart transplantation—The concept, the planning and the furor" (*ASAIO Journal* 44:4, July–August 1998, pp. 244–52), and A. Kantrowitz et al., "Transplantation of the heart in an infant and an adult" (*American Journal of Cardiology* 22:782, 1968).

Chapter Two. Out of the Cold

These detailed descriptions of Norman Shumway and Dick Lower's groundbreaking work in San Francisco are based on my interviews with the two surgeons. I also relied on their seminal transplant papers, including N. E. Shumway and R. R. Lower, "Topical cardiac hypothermia for extended periods of anoxic arrest" (*Surgical Forum* 1959; 10:563), and R. R. Lower and N. E. Shumway, "Studies on orthotopic homotransplantation of the canine heart" (*Surgical Forum* 1960; 11:18).

A more visual record, complete with Shumway's own handwritten notes, was given to me by their research colleague, Eugene Dong, M.D., whose extensive archive includes a photocopied pamphlet titled *The Stanford Cardiac Surgical Team, 1958–1962.* This informal but revealing journal was sent out to individual team members as a Christmas present by Shumway in 1962.

Apart from interviewing Gene Dong on three separate occasions, I particularly admired his written account of this time, "A Heart Transplant Narrative: The Earliest Years," which is featured in Paul Terasaki's *History of Transplantation: Thirty-five Recollections.*

The anecdote about a New York reporter comparing Minneapolis and St. Paul to Siberia comes from the website of St. Paul's Winter Carnival.

The bulk of material in this chapter relating to Minnesota and the work of John Lewis and Walt Lillehei emerged during my interviews with Shumway, Vince Gott, and Christian Cabrol, and was supplemented by the wealth of intricate detail in

G. Wayne Miller's *King of Hearts.* Shumway was especially incisive in his contributions and insights into Lewis, and those views were endorsed by Cabrol. Gott, meanwhile, highlighted the relentlessly witty banter Shumway and Lewis shared on their ward rounds.

The earliest hypothermia experiments carried out by Wilfred Bigelow were discussed in all these interviews, and by Miller, and illuminated further by footage in Jon Palfreman's documentary series for Nova, *Pioneers of Surgery,* as well as by Health Care's documentary series *Great Moments in Heart Surgery,* with particular reference to their second program, "It Must Have Been the Severe Climate in Minnesota." The title comes from a quip of Shumway's.

For additional context it should be pointed out that Bigelow had worked briefly under Alfred Blalock at Johns Hopkins Hospital in Baltimore, where he became preoccupied with the limitations of Blalock's famous "blue-baby" operation. The Blalock shunt could do no more than temporarily alleviate the cyanotic side affects of tetralogy of Fallot. Only the seemingly impossible fantasy of surgery inside the actual heart might eventually cure the tetralogy. Bigelow became obsessed with finding a method to work inside the opened chambers. The memory of the Canadian groundhogs returned to him one night while he lay in bed in Baltimore: What would happen if the entire body of a dog, and eventually a human, was cooled to the point of near hibernation? By the time he returned to Toronto, Bigelow was ready to experiment.

In April 1950, at the American Surgical Association's annual convention, at the Broadmoor Hotel in Colorado Springs, Bigelow presented his findings. Lewis and Lillehei sat captivated in an audience churning with skepticism. They were among the few to immediately understand the significance of Bigelow's breakthrough. Miller reveals that at the same convention Lillehei made a startling debut by presenting a paper that deftly outlined a way to induce chronic heart failure in dogs. He connected an artery to a vein, automatically increasing the flow of blood to the heart. Under the intense strain of having to pump harder and faster, the canine hearts failed within less than a month. Lillehei could then begin work on finding out how best to restore the damaged hearts. It was a technique as perfectly simple as his sharp suit, alligator shoes, grinning good looks, and Buick convertible were brilliantly gaudy.

Jordan Haller has remarked that even earlier work in hypothermia had been carried out by Temple Fay, a neurosurgeon in Philadelphia in the 1930s, who packed patients in ice to permit surgery and healing. According to Haller, Hugh Rosomoff used similar techniques—also while working as a neurosurgeon in the 1930s.

Miller writes in detail about both John Gibbon and Clarence Dennis, and more personal insights into Dennis were offered to me by Shumway and Gott. Adrian and Jean Kantrowitz also came to know Dennis extremely well after he moved from

Minnesota to New York. Notes on Gibbon come from detailed lectures on his work by both Shumway and Gott, as well as his friend Dwight Harken's biography, *To Mend the Heart—The Dramatic Story of Cardiac Surgery and Its Pioneers*. Additional visual material comes from the Nova documentary.

The first successful open-heart operation carried out by Lewis is covered in detail in *King of Hearts*, and discussed in interviews by Shumway and Gott. The two men's firsthand accounts of Lillehei's cross-circulation experiments were invaluable to me. A definitive portrayal of this period in Lillehei's life is supplied by Miller—who also writes about the DeWall oxygenator.

As an aside, soon after he arrived in Minnesota, Shumway became an intern with the aim of qualifying for a neurosurgical residency. His first medical paper bore a neurosurgery bias—"Two Cases of Ruptured Intra-Abdominal Aneurysm Complicated by Neurological Findings." Written in conjunction with William Peyton, it was published in the *Journal of Surgery* in 1951. Although he and Owen Wangensteen (Minnesota's chief) maintained their distance from each other, the professor was magnanimous enough to try to help Shumway find a residency at the world's then premier establishment for brain surgeons. Wangensteen arranged for the Montreal Neurosurgical Institute to interview Shumway as he approached the end of his internship.

Willie Cone, who was then second only to Wilder Penfield, the chief at the Montreal Institute, met Shumway in Wangensteen's office. He was another short man and, in the style of Wangensteen, began to tilt himself back in his chair—presumably to help him study the taller Shumway at a more oblique angle. Poor old Willie Cone succeeded only in toppling backward before he somehow managed to right himself by using one of his hands to push himself up. His little feet hurtled through the air before they came crashing down on the ground. And so he sat, dazed and stunned, quivering in his chair, with an astonished Shumway staring straight back at him.

In that moment of wretched vulnerability, Cone terminated the interview by offering Shumway a residency on the spot. Shumway thought he should be thanking the bucking chair rather than the blushing neurosurgeon. His own mind, however, had already changed tack before Cone spun on his chair. At twenty-eight, Norman Shumway had for some time been having doubts about his previous immersion in the brain. He would stay, instead, in Minnesota and work with John Lewis and Walt Lillehei. He would give himself up, utterly and totally, to the heart.

Shumway's eventual move to California is based on his own memories—and those given to me by Dick Lower. During our interviews, both Lower and Ed Hurley offered some invaluable insights into their relationships with Shumway, Victor Richards, and Frank Gebode in San Francisco. Shumway and Lower provide the background to their meeting and subsequent use of hypothermia. Robert Frater, another distinguished cardiac surgeon, who worked with Barnard before leaving Cape Town for New York, offered informed insight into the work of Dennis Melrose. As Frater stresses, it was not potassium per se that caused the damage, but rather the extremely high concentration that Melrose initially used.

Lower and Shumway's work in July 1958 is articulated by the surgeons themselves, while my very basic explanation of the workings of the heart and lungs was aided by Lower, Professor David Wheatley (the head of cardiac surgery at the Glasgow Infirmary), and by Channel 4's simple but cogent documentary "Circulation," in its *Anatomy for Beginners* series.

The start of the U.S. space program, and the race against their Soviet rivals, is detailed on the NASA website.

Chapter Three. Colored Hearts

From the outset it should be reiterated that, although it is associated with the country's troubled racial history, the word "colored" is still used in postapartheid South Africa to describe a racial grouping who see themselves, through both culture and language, as being distinct from the black majority. It does not now carry the same undertow of racism as in America or Europe.

The buildup to the first open-heart operation in Africa was recalled in intricate detail for me by Carl Goosen, who worked both as Barnard's research assistant in the lab and in the OR as his perfusionist on that momentous night. My interview with Goosen shed a sharp light on Barnard's character, and on his anxiety before that operation. Bob Frater and Marius Barnard provided me with much valuable background on Chris Barnard, Walter Phillips, and Jannie Louw. In David Cooper's collection of personal impressions and oral histories, *Chris Barnard: By Those Who Know Him Best,* Jannie Louw provides his own distinctive memories of this period.

Lillehei's letter of advice to Barnard can still be found in the Groote Schuur Transplant Museum's archive. In Cooper's interview with Lillehei, the same point is made, Lillehei stressing that "[Barnard] followed my advice. I told him not to do a transposition, nor a Tetralogy (both difficult operations). I said, 'Do something simple.' He did a straightforward pulmonary stenosis—with recovery of the patient."

It should also be remembered that Barnard had made such an impression on Wangensteen during his research stint in Minnesota that the venerable chief tried to persuade him not to return to Cape Town. The young Afrikaans surgeon was tempted, as South Africa seemed increasingly remote to him. But he knew intuitively that he needed to return home. After a long pause Wangensteen casually suggested that

Barnard should find out how much he would need to ship a heart-lung machine across the ocean to Cape Town.

Within a day, an elated Barnard established that it would cost a thousand dollars to buy the parts for the machine and then send them to South Africa. Wangensteen laughed softly. They could do better than that. He phoned the National Institutes of Health in Washington. Wangensteen explained that Barnard, a young South African surgeon, needed $2,000 for a bypass machine and an annual grant of $2,000 for the next three years. Barnard was incredulous. Eight thousand dollars would change his life. With eight grand he could take on the world.

Wangesteen, apart from the occasional grunt, was silent as he listened to the man on the other end of the line. He eventually put down the old black phone with a click. He looked at Barnard and then he grinned. "You got it," he said.

Barnard's trepidation over using a heart-lung machine is detailed in *One Life*, from which his direct quotes in this chapter are taken.

The background material on Joan and Victor Pick is an amalgam of my interviews with Marius Barnard and Ozzie Ozinsky, Barnard's recollections in *One Life*, archive material at the Groote Schuur Transplant Museum, and articles in the *Cape Times*, dated July 29, 1958, February 20, 1968, and (in a piece published soon after Victor's death) July 4, 1969.

Marius Barnard spent hours during our interviews reliving his and Chris's youth in Beaufort West, and he was especially moving in detailing their father's life and work. While Chris's memories of their childhood also feature in *One Life*, I was touched more by hearing Marius recount those days so poetically. For example, with Chris's best friend, Michel Roussouw, the Barnard brothers discovered a kind of freedom in the only department store in town. Mortimer & Hill was managed by the Rossouws' father, and it gave them hours of fantasy and pleasure. While they enjoyed eyeing the girls at the perfume counter, they were thrilled most by the gramophone, which played songs from faraway places near the front section for men's clothing. Marius, in particular, was fascinated by a Hawaiian lullaby as he sang along in his quivering falsetto: "*I want to go back, to my little grass shack, in Kealakekua, Hawaii . . .*" Hawaii was about as far as you could get from the Karoo. The Afrikaans boys yearned for the palm trees, rolling breakers, and exotic life of a world that lay far beyond their own. On Saturday afternoons they went to the movies—after first visiting the Good Hope Café, where they'd buy a cream soda or an ice cream.

The race against Daantjie Rabie is relived in *One Life*, where Barnard's direct quotes are found, but Marius provided a far more detailed account of the prejudice his father faced as a minister in a "colored" church.

Barnard's extraordinary research in producing intestinal atresia in unborn puppies was explained to me fully by Marius, and it is discussed in *One Life*, as well as by
Louw and Cooper in the latter's *Chris Barnard: By Those Who Know Him Best*.

The anecdotes about Barnard's arrival in Minnesota are from *One Life*. Shumway,
Gott, Cabrol, and Frater provided me with a more balanced account of his work in
Minnesota, while Lillehei and John Perry also described their memories of him to
Cooper.

Shumway's relationship with Wangensteen is detailed in my interviews with the
surgeon himself, and is supported by the amused recollection of Vince Gott and
Christian Cabrol.

In *King of Hearts*, Miller recounts how Lillehei had first noticed a small lump, on
the left side of his upper jaw, in late 1949. David State, a surgeon who would eventually replace Adrian Kantrowitz at Maimonides almost twenty years later, had removed it on February 9, 1950. Although it was yet to be examined in the lab, State
thought it had the look of a benign tumor. Two months later, when he spoke at
Broadmoor, an exultant Lillehei was watched closely by Wangensteen. The Minnesota
chief had sent specimens of the excised lump to pathologists at three prestigious
medical centers—the Mayo Clinic, Columbia University, and the Sloan-Kettering
Institute. The diagnoses were unanimous and endorsed the findings in Minnesota,
which Wangensteen had kept secret. Lillehei had lymphosarcoma; and the cancer was
widening inside him. He was given, at best, five years.

Wangensteen chose not to tell his star surgeon for months. Lillehei, meanwhile,
assumed the lab's apparent silence merely confirmed State's cheerful assumptions in
the OR. It was only toward the end of May 1950 that Wangensteen called in his senior
resident and gave him the devastating news. Lillehei took no comfort from the fact
that, as a surgeon, Wangensteen specialized in the removal of ulcers and cancerous
growths. The chief's approach to cancer was built on his conviction that it should be
attacked mercilessly. If one part of the body was found to be diseased, Wangensteen
believed that the surrounding tissue should be similarly hacked away. He also adhered to a "second look" policy, which meant that he would reopen even those patients of his who seemed to have fully recovered, sometimes removing another chunk
of body "just to be safe." Even if that pessimistic reexamination uncovered no further
signs of cancer, Wangensteen would often indulge in a third, fourth, and, on one notorious occasion, even a "fifth look."

At the same time, he supported his favorite residents, Lillehei most of all, with
searing commitment. Wangensteen was thrilled that Lillehei and Lewis and Richard
Varco led the most glamorous and newsworthy operations. Miller, Gott, and Shumway

all analyzed this curious contradiction in character that would never have been adopted by any of the grander surgical chiefs on the East Coast, who typically reserved the most significant cases for themselves.

In the early 1930s, not long after Wangensteen had assumed control of Minnesota, he had been forced to reject the application for residency of a talented young surgeon by the name of Robert Gross. He did not have the money to take on Gross and so lost him to Harvard. In 1938, Gross made international headlines after carrying out the first successful elective closed-heart surgical procedure in which he closed an eight-year-old girl's patent ductus. She made a full recovery and Gross closed almost a thousand patent ducti in the ensuing decade. He had pulled back the shutters on the dawn of heart surgery.

The fear of losing another young giant, this time to death, explained Wangensteen's mystifying reluctance to inform Lillehei of his condition. It was almost as if Wangensteen hoped that his silence might wish away a cancer as lethal as lymphosarcoma. When he finally submitted to reality, Wangensteen told Lillehei they would have to cut, and cut again. Lillehei privately urged three of the six additional surgeons who would also take the knife to his neck and chest—Lewis, State, and Varco—to try to restrain Wangensteen's instinct to cleave away at him. On June 1, 1950, Lillehei's cancer was attacked. He lost nine pints of blood in a ten-and-a-half hour operation. Only constant transfusions kept him alive during the cutting—and, as mentioned in this chapter, Shumway donated a pint of his own blood in the successful battle to save Lillehei.

Gott, in our interviews at Johns Hopkins, corroborated Barnard's account in *One Life* of how they worked together for the first time—and that Barnard's fascination with the heart emerged while he watched Gott operate the heart-lung machine. The direct quotes from Barnard came from *One Life*.

Gott recalled and explained Gil Campbell's work with the dog lung, which is also described in *King of Hearts*.

Of the many striking stories Christian Cabrol told me about his time working alongside Shumway and Barnard in Minnesota, I especially enjoyed this memory of the Parisian surgeon. He explained how on a snowy Friday afternoon in Minneapolis in December 1956, he and his French Canadian colleague Émile Bertho set about transplanting the heart of a dog. This was eighteen months before Shumway and Lower began their historic cardiac transplant experiments. In a far corner of Walt Lillehei's lab, Bertho and Cabrol hovered over the animal on their table. It was just after five p.m. Work was winding down for the week.

Vince Gott, continuing his tests to help Lillehei remedy heart block by attaching an electrode to the wall of the heart, had encouraged Bertho and Cabrol in their trials of his new sheet oxygenator. A large mongrel had survived their experimental surgery. When Cabrol asked, in his stuttering English, what they were expected to do with the dog, he and Bertho were greeted by a shrug from the lab technician. They could do what they liked, the man said, knowing that the dog could not be returned to the pound.

Cabrol knew that he and his wife could not keep a pet. The garden of their rented home in Minneapolis had given them unexpected pleasure, especially after their apartment-bound life in Paris, but it was too small for a dog.

"*Ça va*," Bertho said as he tickled the dog around the ears. "*Nous ferons une greffe du coeur.*" (Okay, then we'll do a heart transplant.)

"*Comment?*" (A what?)

"*Une greffe du coeur, vous comprenez . . .*" (You know, a heart transplant . . .) Bertho said it as if it was a concept they encountered every other day.

Cabrol nodded. He was suddenly curious to see what it might be like to remove the heart from one dog and transplant it into another.

As they began the operation, Chris Barnard rushed into the lab. He was racing as usual, looking frantic as he searched for Herb Warden, one of Lillehei's most experienced surgeons, who was helping Barnard develop a cardiac prosthesis, an artificial aortic valve through which oxygenated blood could be pumped into the left ventricle. Enthralled by his experience with Gott, Lillehei, and their bubbler, Barnard had persuaded Wangensteen to allow him to abandon his work on the gullet and switch to the heart.

Hearing that Warden had left the lab, Barnard turned away abruptly from the French residents, unaware that they were about to remove the heart from a dog they had just put down by lethal injection. They would then replace it with the heart belonging to a canine corpse stretched out on an adjoining table. Cabrol thought it typical of Barnard. While he was acknowledged as a relentless worker and a bright operator, Barnard could appear aggressive and self-absorbed. The severe haircut, the big ears, and the harsh accent also did not do much to endear Barnard to Cabrol, a smart and witty Parisian.

Cabrol preferred Norm Shumway, the cleverest and funniest of all Minnesota's brilliant residents. You could relax with Shumway. He was the kind of man you could tell a joke to and be assured that he would reply with an even more amusing riposte. When Shumway sauntered into Lillehei's lab that afternoon, not long after Barnard had dashed out again, he was immediately interested in the work of the French doctors.

"Hey, Chris," he called out to Cabrol, "what are you guys doing?"

Cabrol laughed while Bertho shouted out: "A heart transplant!"

Shumway let slip a surprised whistle. "A heart transplant?"

"It is true, Norm!" Cabrol confirmed in his heavily accented English.

318   NOTES AND SOURCES

"Well, good luck with your heart transplant, boys," Shumway grinned as he headed back out to his pregnant wife, Mary Lou, and their two young children, four-year-old Sara and two-year-old Mike.

"See you Monday, Norm," Cabrol waved before he returned to help Bertho stitch a dead heart into the empty chest of their first dog. They were nearing the end of their bizarre exercise and would not make any futile attempt to restart the transplanted heart. It was enough for them to have completed the intriguing procedure.

They did not know it then, but just over a dozen years later Shumway, Barnard, and Cabrol would carry out five of the world's first nine human heart transplants. Emile Bertho, who had dreamed up that zany and quickly forgotten Friday-afternoon idea in Minnesota, would remain in relative obscurity as a surgeon in Canada.

Barnard's various love affairs in Minnesota are mentioned in his less impressive and ultimately tawdry sequel, *The Second Life*, and are detailed further in Logan's *Celebrity Surgeon*. Deirdre Visser remembered the family's brief time together in Minnesota during our interviews, and I also read Louwtjie Barnard's own account in *Heartbreak*.

Lillehei, in the Cooper collection, confirms Barnard's memory in *One Life* of losing a patient on the table when he inadvertently cut a hole in the young boy's heart.

Marius Barnard remembered his father's death in powerful detail during our interviews, while Chris wrote of the remarkable funeral scene in *One Life*.

The actual first open-heart operation in Africa was described for me in our interviews by Goosen and "Ozzie" Ozinsky, who worked as the anesthetist on all of Barnard's most famous operations. Barnard's reactions, both during and after operating, emerged in these interviews, which matched the account offered in *One Life*. The quotation about Joan Pick's heart being "as strong as an ox" when she died in 2002 comes from *Celebrity Surgeon*.

The extract from Hendrik Verwoerd's speech was printed in *Die Vaderland*, July 30, 1958.

Chapter Four. Sparky's Gang

My interviews with Norman Shumway and Dick Lower form the basis of this chapter— supplemented, again, by their medical publications listed in the notes to Chapter Two.

Adrian Kantrowitz told me about his visit to Moscow to meet Vladimir Demikhov—with further background material on Demikhov obtained from a variety of sources, including interviews with Kantrowitz, Shumway, Haller, Gott, and Wheatley, and Eric Pace's article (published soon after the Russian surgeon's death at the age of eighty-two) in *The New York Times* on November 25, 1998.

Jean Kantrowitz provided much of the information about her meeting her future husband—as well as their respective family backgrounds. Adrian's older brother, Arthur, was a key figure in his intellectual development. As Adrian remembers, they were both electronics wizards and there was nothing that intrigued him more than working on some crazy gadget he and Arthur had invented in their mother's kitchen or in a back room of the old house. One of their first projects saw them develop a bath that maintained a constant temperature so that they could germinate bacteria. The medically minded Adrian took charge of germ production, while his physics-mad brother engineered the makeshift laboratory.

War focused their minds. Arthur lost himself in the intricacies of his Ph.D., in the hope that he would soon be designing fighter aircraft, while Adrian agreed with his mother's contention that it would be safer to work as a doctor rather than risk conscription as an ordinary soldier. He preferred the simultaneously glamorous and sensible idea of saving lives to dying in battle.

Kantrowitz himself relived for me his war years and spoke in detail about both Dwight Harken and Charles Bailey. It is also striking that, like Shumway, Kantrowitz initially planned on a career in neurosurgery. He told me that the highlight of his brief internship at the Jewish Hospital of Brooklyn had been the six weeks he'd spent working under a famous neurosurgeon, Leo Davidoff, who had studied under Harvey Cushing, revered as the "father of brain surgery." A lowly intern, Kantrowitz had done little but push his right foot down on a surgical cautery whenever Davidoff, at the head of the table, gave the instruction to "cook." Apart from pressing his foot toward the floor for the correct number of seconds, Kantrowitz had merely watched as Davidoff, following the procedure he had learned from Cushing to open the cranium, used a small series of clamps to pin back the galea—the layer of fibrous tissue running from the front to the back of the skull. Fifteen to twenty little clamps would dangle from the table before Davidoff reached for a wrap of gauze to bunch them together.

Kantrowitz saw how he could easily improve on this unwieldy technique. At home, he placed an eight-inch length of latex tubing over the long thin blades of an ordinary Carmalt clamp. Working like an adjustable elastic rubber band, the clamp could hold six of the smaller devices in a neat bundle and keep them out of Davidoff's way during intracranial surgery.

Aware of professional protocol, Kantrowitz showed his device to the surgical resident, who, impressed by the simple practicality of the instrument, then presented it to Davidoff. Without acknowledging his junior intern, whose name he did not even know then, Davidoff began to use the clamp. Kantrowitz stood at the far end of the OR and almost shivered when he finally heard Davidoff say to the senior resident, "This is good. Tell him to write it up."

In the summer of 1944, Kantrowitz wrote a one-page paper, his first as a doctor, describing the clamp. As was the custom, he placed Leo Davidoff's name above his own before adding, in delighted italics, *"F. Adrian Kantrowitz, Department of Neurosurgery, The Jewish Hospital of Brooklyn, New York."* When the final draft was returned to Kantrowitz he was shocked to see that nothing had been changed—apart from the removal of his chief's name. Davidoff did not need another publication on his long list, and, fittingly, he wanted the credit for an instrument that would be used by neurosurgeons for the next fifty years to go to the inventor alone. Kantrowitz's son, Allen, a neurosurgeon, used the clamp in the course of his surgical work in the 1980s. This simple invention is explained in the above-mentioned medical paper, A. Kantrowitz, "A method of holding galea hemostats in craniotomies" (*Journal of Neurosurgery* 1:392, 1944).

During his last few weeks in Brooklyn, Kantrowitz worked as a second assistant to Davidoff. The surgeon now knew his name. He was still using the new clamp. "Give me a Kantrowitz!" Davidoff would bark. The intern was relieved that he had a mask to cover his helpless grin. He now wanted, more than ever, to be a surgeon himself. He wanted to be the next Davidoff, to be another inspiring neurosurgeon. His mother, Rose, would be in ecstasy if he became a brain surgeon.

However, by the time Kantrowitz got back to postwar New York, most residencies had been filled by young doctors returning home before him. Davidoff had also moved—to Montefiore in the Bronx—but he had not forgotten Kantrowitz.

"Still using your clamp," he said gruffly. "How was the war?"

Davidoff was not a warm man, but he liked Kantrowitz. As soon as Davidoff was prompted about the possibility of a residency he called in his secretary to remind him when next they had an opening for an aspiring neurosurgeon at Montefiore.

"In about three years," the secretary sighed sympathetically. Every hot young buck wanted to be a brain surgeon.

"Look," Davidoff said, "you don't have to have a Jesus Christ complex. You don't have to be a damn neurosurgeon. Be a surgeon . . . you'll get an opening, and then see what comes from that."

Davidoff was right. Kantrowitz was offered a junior residency at Mount Sinai and within another year he became a resident surgeon at Montefiore. He soon developed new interests apart from the brain. Stirred by Harken, he began to lose himself in cardiac dreams. He learned more about the daring pioneers of the heart.

Fifty years earlier, in 1896, a German surgeon, Ludwig Rehn, opened the pericardium of a twenty-year-old man who had just been stabbed. Seeing a clear incision in the wall of the heart, Rehn went fearlessly to work. "The wound was closed with three silk stitches," he wrote. "The pulse immediately improved." Rehn's patient, the first man to have his heart saved by a surgeon, made a full recovery.

A year later, typifying the ignorance that haunted work on the heart for so long, the revered British thoracic surgeon, Stephen Paget, clearly oblivious to Rehn's successful operation, claimed that "Surgery of the heart has probably reached the limits set by Nature to all surgery; no new method and no new discovery can overcome the natural difficulties that attend a wound of the heart. It is true that 'heart suture' has been vaguely proposed as a possible procedure, and has been done on animals, but I cannot find that it has ever been attempted in practice." The heart, as Paget and thousands of doctors before him had been told, lay outside the domain of medicine.

Harken told Kantrowitz the story of an even more reckless German doctor. Inspired by an image in a veterinary journal that showed a catheter entering the vein of a horse in order to obtain a blood sample, Werner Forssmann, a twenty-five-year-old surgical intern in Berlin, decided to try and reach a human heart in the same way. In an outrageous experiment that would eventually lead to the development of cardiac catheterization and angiography, Forssmann attempted the technique in the summer of 1929, on a hot Sunday afternoon at the Berlin City Hospital.

Forssmann used his own body for the dangerous trial. He persuaded a bewildered nurse to assist him. Forssmann slid a ureteral catheter into a vein in his arm and, standing behind a fluoroscope screen while the nurse held a trembling mirror, he watched himself guide the catheter toward the right atrium. With the nurse crying out for him to stop, Forssmann entered the chamber of his own heart. Though he felt a burning sensation in his chest, his heartbeat remained constant. The blurred image of the tube in his heart could be seen on the screen, but with the nurse on the verge of hysteria, he knew no one would believe what he had just proved—that the atrium could survive catheterization.

In a daze of resolve, Forssmann forced himself to walk. With the catheter still in his heart, he climbed two flights of stairs, finally reaching the X-ray area, where he could take the images that would show that he was not as crazy as so many of his colleagues believed. He was eventually discovered in his own room by Dr. Joseph Fischman, who described the chilling scene in a letter to Harken:

> I and a few others of the resident staff were alarmed by the news that Dr. Forssmann had committed suicide. Upon arrival in his room we found Dr. F lying on his bed, silent and pale, staring at the ceiling, his clothes and the bed linen spotted with blood. He refused to give any information. The idea of suicide appeared to be not too remote as Dr. F was a rather queer, peculiar person, lone and desolate, hardly ever mingling with his co-workers socially. One never knew whether he was thinking or mentally deficient. On closer investigation of the situation one found his condition medically satisfactory. There

were a few surgical instruments lying around and also a catheter—still inserted into his antecubital vein (whether left or right, I do not remember). This latter was removed and a dressing applied to the wound. Whether he inserted the catheter in order to quench his scientific thirst or [something] else, I never was able to find out. What I still remember vividly [is] that the catheter was in the vein at a length of at least two-and-a-half feet.

Kantrowitz was captivated by such conviction, just as he was by the compelling way Harken damned the use of the word "impossible." It was, according to him, without meaning. Harken was already chasing a surgical cure for mitral stenosis. He was pushed even harder by his fiercest rival, Charles Bailey. Soon after his return from the war, Harken had shared the stage at the American Association for Thoracic Surgery with Alfred Blalock and Helen Taussig, who had just published their seminal work on "blue babies." After a glittering presentation, Harken was buttonholed by Bailey, a brash young surgeon from Philadelphia.

"Hey, Dwight," Bailey sneered, "I hear you're working toward mitral surgery. Well, guess what? I'm gonna beat you."

Bailey regarded Kantrowitz as a kindred spirit. They came from a similar background. Although a gentile, he described himself as the son of "a Jewish mother type," in the sense that she had determined, even before he was born, that he would become a doctor. Bailey also claimed that he had chosen to become a heart surgeon when he was only twelve, in 1922, long before Harken even had the thought. He had watched his father coughing blood into a basin while his mother tried to comfort him. His father died soon afterward from mitral stenosis.

Bailey had conducted extensive research on the mitral valve, both during autopsy and in the animal lab, and had always been struck by the similarity of its structure to an old-fashioned girdle. A cowboy like Bailey possessed a certain charm that had made him familiar with more than a few girdles in his time. He had also, he revealed to Kantrowitz, sold ladies's underwear while he was an undergraduate. "I promise you," he chuckled darkly, "I know girdles."

I also read Harken's autobiography, written with Lael Wertenbaker, *To Mend the Heart—The Dramatic Story of Cardiac Surgery and Its Pioneers*. Bob Frater was a fount of valuable information on the full story behind the history of mitral commissurotomy. His public lecture on the subject is a masterly exercise.

Kantrowitz spoke to me in detail about his early work on the mitral valve in cats. His vivid memories were underpinned by an extensive archive of written and filmed material—which I saw at the Kantrowitz archives in their Detroit office. I also read his various papers on the subject of this research, most notably Adrian Kantrowitz and Arthur Kantrowitz, "Experimental artificial left heart to permit surgical exposure of mitral valve in cats" (*Proceedings of the Society for Experimental Biology and Medicine* 74:193, 1950); Kantrowitz, Adrian, E. S. Hurwitt, and Arthur Kantrowitz, "Experimental artificial left heart for exposure of the mitral area" (first presented at the Surgical Forum, American College of Surgeons, Boston, 1951); and A. Kantrowitz, E. S. Hurwitt, and A. Herskovitz, "A cinematographic study of the function of the mitral valve in situ" (*Surgical Forum* 2:204, 1952).

With regard to the invaluable role that Jean Kantrowitz played it is important to state that, in marrying Adrian, she did not set out with any objective that she might become his professional partner; in fact, the exact opposite, as she stresses, was true. She did not want to work directly with her husband, but she was happy to assist him, on an informal basis, by offering her own considerable professional experience in business and accounting. In later years, with three small children at home, she assisted his team in drawing up budgets and overseeing the administrative side of grant applications. She also obtained her second master's degree in public health at the University of Michigan in 1973. And then, in 1975, at the age of fifty-six, Jean did some outstanding work under her own name when she planned and organized a successful child and adolescent psychiatry program at Case Western Reserve University in Cleveland. Today, after sixty years of marriage, she and Adrian still work together at their company headquarters, L-VAD Technology, in Detroit.

In addition to highlighting the innovation of Kantrowitz's imaginative research into heart surgery, it should be noted that when he joined Maimonides Hospital just over five years later, in 1955, he was appointed as their full-time Director of Cardiovascular Surgery—even though heart surgery had yet to begin as a full-fledged clinical entity.

Shumway and Lower's historic dog transplant on December 23, 1959, was described to me by the surgeons, and supplemented by their already cited medical papers on the operation as well as the case material still held at Stanford Medical Center archives. Eugene Dong's arrival at Stanford is recalled in our interviews and in his essay published in Terasaki's *History of Transplantation,* and also during an interview with Shumway. Dong had received his degree in physiology and had done a modicum of research as an undergraduate at the University of California at Berkeley and for two summers as a medical student in the new Clinical Research Unit at the University of California at San Francisco. He chose a medical internship in 1959 rather than a surgical one at Bellevue Hospital, New York City, for the broader experience it offered—and because it would allow him to study with both the chief of medicine at the Columbia University Division at Bellevue, Dickinson Richards, and the chief of pulmonary service, Andre Cournand. Richards and Cournard had shared the 1956 Nobel Prize for Medicine with Forssmann.

Dong told me that when applying to Stanford he met first with Roy Cohn, the acting chairman of surgery there. Cohn had explained that it was unlikely there would be a spot for Dong. However, as the interview unfolded at a leisurely pace, it eventually emerged that Cohn and Dong's uncle had been poker-playing buddies as students at Stanford Medical School. That changed everything. Cohn immediately had an idea as to how he might help his old friend's twenty-six-year-old nephew. He told Dong that Norm Shumway was clearly the rising star at Stanford. If anyone could dream up an opening for a smart new resident it would be Shumway.

Chapter Five. Heads and Hearts

John F. Kennedy's speech is reported on January 3, 1960, in *The New York Times.*

The history of transplant surgery in the 1950s—including the work done by Richard Lawler and Joseph Murray—is covered in a variety of publications, of which Tony Stark's *Knife to the Heart* and René Kuss and Pierre Bourget's *An Illustrated History of Organ Transplantation* were the most immediately useful to me.

Shumway and Lower were too immersed in the heart to closely follow parallel work being done by the renal transplant specialists, but their own experiments were being increasingly noticed. Another of their 1960 lab stars was honored by the National Society of Medical Research after he had thrived all year with a transplanted mitral valve.

"A frisky four-year-old pointer named Sam, once destined for execution in a public dog pound, is the Research Dog Hero of 1960," the society's press release confirmed in early January 1961. "Recognition came to Sam for his role in an experiment, by Drs. Norman E. Shumway, Richard R. Lower and Raymond C. Stofer of the Stanford School of Medicine, said to hold major hope for Americans whose hearts have been damaged by rheumatic fever. Sam will receive a silver collar at a San Francisco Medical Society ceremony on January 10. The purpose of the transplant was to see whether some way could be devised to replace disease-damaged mitral valves of human patients. Usually such patients are victims of rheumatic fever whose mitral valves have become too hardened to function properly. . . . At present Sam is in vigorous good health. He is playful and likes to greet members of the research team by jumping up on them. Dr. Shumway, the senior surgeon in the group, says that "if the method continues to prove effective in laboratory animals, we may be able to perform a similar operation on a human patient within a year."

Lower was struck more by the reaction of the Thoracic Board to his description of Shumway's repair technique for the tetralogy of Fallot. The mortality rate of most tetralogy cases across America hovered between 25 and 30 percent. Yet Shumway had carried out forty-five tetralogies at Stanford and only lost a single patient. The examiner had not heard of Shumway's extraordinary record and so he leaned back in his chair and quizzed Lower. "All right, Doctor," he said, the condescension dripping from his voice after Lower had correctly answered all his earlier questions, "now tell me how you would repair a tetralogy of Fallot."

Lower began to explain how he would use topical hypothermia—rather than potassium or more conventional methods of slowing the circulation—to obtain a reasonably dry field, thus allowing him to accurately repair the defect. As he outlined the surgical steps he would then take, the incredulous examiner interrupted him to ask him where on earth he had dreamed up such an idea. Lower revealed that it was the method Shumway had been using at Stanford for the past two years. He detailed his chief's near flawless record; and knew he had passed his boards when the older doctor asked him to again describe Shumway's cooling so that he could scribble down notes for his own use the next time he stepped back into the operating room.

Lower told me the "Shumberg" story, and Spyros Andreopoulos, the former chief media officer at Stanford Medical Center, offered me rich material on the work and character of Shumway, Arthur Kornberg, and Joshua Lederberg.

A copy of Chris Barnard's letter to Walt Lillehei, in January 1960, is held at the Transplant Museum at Groote Schuur Hospital.

The Nelson Mandela quotes come from Anthony Sampson's definitive biography, *Mandela.*

John Terblanche, Raoul de Villiers, Carl Goosen, and David Wheatley all spoke to me about Barnard's two-headed dog transplant (inspired by Demikhov), while Jannie Louw recalls the incident in Cooper's collection.

The U.S. State Department quote on Sharpeville comes from *The New York Times,* March 22, 1960. Further background on the impact of the Sharpeville massacre is provided by an assortment of books, including Sampson's *Mandela,* Joseph Lelyveld's *Move Your Shadow,* Stephen Clingman's *Bram Fischer,* and Nigel Worden's *The Making of Modern South Africa.* Barnard's response is gleaned from letters in the Groote Schuur Archive, which also holds records of his letters outlining his visit to Moscow in 1960.

Barnard's memories of Sharon Jorgensen are included in *The Second Life,* while his quote about springtime in Minneapolis comes from *One Life.* Chris Logan interviews Jorgensen in *Celebrity Surgeon,* and Deirdre Visser, in our interviews, remembered her father first suffering from arthritis in Minnesota. His encounter with the little girl watching him cling to the black rail was recorded in *One Life.* Louwtjie Barnard recalled her treatment for his arthritis, while Raoul de Villiers remembered Barnard's own stories of him drinking vodka over breakfast with Demikhov.

The details surrounding Shumway and Lower's lecture at the Clearwater Hotel were recounted by the surgeons themselves. I used selected quotes relating to their findings from the paper they presented that morning: "Studies on Orthotopic Homo-transplantation of the Canine Heart." Eugene Dong also reveals that, apart from the brief report in the *San Francisco Examiner* on October 11, 1960, their findings were mentioned at a lecture delivered later that week at the Surgical Forum by Watts Webb, who would carry out the first human lung transplant with James Hardy in Missis-sippi in 1963.

Both the BBC television documentary *Space Race* and the NASA website confirm the basic details of the Yuri Gagarin and Alan Shepard flights. The Victor Cohn arti-cle, "1970: Your Fantastic Future," is held at the Stanford Medical Center archive.

Adrian Kantrowitz detailed the case of Rose Cohen in our interviews. I also read two of his medical papers that explore this breakthrough in more clinical terms: A. Kantrowitz et al., "The treatment of complete heart block with an implantable, controllable pacemaker" (*Surg. Gynecol. Obstet.* 115:415, 1962); and W. Dressler, S. Jonas, and A. Kantrowitz, "Observations in patients with implanted cardiac pace-maker: Clinical experience" (*American Heart Journal* 66:325, 1963).

Kantrowitz was not the first, however, to make the connection between the heart and electricity as a way of either regaining or controlling a beat. In 1899, two Swiss physiologists, F. Battelli and J. L. Prevost, had shocked the fibrillating hearts of dogs and proved that they reverted to a more normal rhythm. Claude Beck had applied electrical paddles to the exposed heart of a postoperative patient in Cleveland in 1947 and achieved the first successful human defibrillation. Eight years later, the Boston cardiologist Paul Zoll replicated the technique, with the significant distinction that he was able to use the paddles outside the body. He soon created a large and unwieldy external pacemaker to reproduce the electrical force of the paddles.

Zoll, who had worked with Harken during the historic removal of shrapnel from a soldier's heart in World War II, was able to halve the mortality rate for acute my-ocardial infarction to 15 percent. Kantrowitz was still disconcerted by the horren-dous impact Zoll's giant pacemakers had on their hapless patients. The machines would be strapped to the chest, and at the first sign of a block they would produce a jolt of electricity that would restart the heart—but also knock recipients off their hospital bed or slam them against a wall.

In Minnesota, Lillehei and Gott experimented with the idea of attaching a small electrode to the heart as a less damaging way to regulate a wavering beat. With Gott carrying out the bulk of the work on dogs, they soon demonstrated that third-degree heart block could be controlled with a charge as low as 2.2 volts, without causing any painful jolts or burnt skin. In late 1957, Lillehei employed Earl Bakken to make a

portable pacer. Bakken, a brilliant local electrician and TV repairman who had assisted Lillehei with some electronics problems during his earliest cross-circulation
work, used an old issue of *Popular Electronics* to help him build a basic metronome.
Driven by a nine-volt battery, Bakken's little box produced an electric pulse that, attached by a wire to the heart, could regulate a beat.

Early the following year, Ake Senning reported a successful long-term implantation
of a pacemaker in Sweden. William Chardack, at the University of Buffalo, soon replicated the achievement. And then, on April 14, 1958, Lillehei used the portable Bakken
box to help save a young girl seized by heart block on the operating table. The age of the
pacemaker had begun—and decades later, Bakken's tiny company, Medtronic, originally operating out of his garage, would grow into a multibillion-dollar corporation.

Kantrowitz, in our interviews, recalled his and Kondo's first transplant experiments,
and further insights were provided by interviews with Yuki Nosé and Raoul de Villiers.
I also read their seminal publications: Y. Kondo, F. Gradel, and A. Kantrowitz, "Heart
homotransplantation in puppies: Long survival without immunosuppressive therapy"
(*Circulation* 31 and 32 [Supp I]: 181, 1965); Y. Kondo, F. Gradel, and A. Kantrowitz,
"Homotransplantation of the heart in puppies under profound hypothermia—Long
survival without immunosuppressive treatment" (*Annals of Surgery* 162:837 1965);
and Y. Kondo et al., "Fate of orthotopic canine heart transplants" (*Journal of Cardiovascular Surgery* 8: 155, 1967).

Chapter Six. Changing Tack

The relevant issues of the *Palo Alto Times* are held by the Stanford Medical Center
archive.

Beyond mastering the surgical art of transplantation, and preparing for the ultimate battle against rejection, Shumway and Lower had already proved that it was
possible to store a heart in cold saline for at least seven hours without damaging the
organ. "This is the first time such experiments have been performed successfully," a
1964 Stanford Medical Center newsletter boasted, "although surgeons have been trying to develop a suitable technique for fifty years. A report on the new development
was presented on April 18, 1962, at the annual meeting of the American Thoracic
Society in St. Louis, Missouri."

After Hurley had delivered his lecture on their cooling technique, Lower then
provided further resonant proof of Stanford's progress in transplantation. He quietly
put to rest an earlier argument proposed by C. Rollins Hanlon and Vallee Willman,
two St. Louis pundits of cardiac physiology. Lower smiled politely when he addressed
their prediction, based on what he described as an "elegant and neurochemical the-

ory," that heart transplants would never work because of autonomic denervation. Producing his slides and statistical records of rigorous experimental trials, Lower noted that, "the dogs, however, fooled the experts by showing that prolonged survival was not at all a physiologic problem—but entirely immunologic."

Eugene Dong provided me with some detailed insight into the racism endured by Chinese-Americans in California. Dong had been born and raised in Salinas. The bulk of Chinese immigrants to California, most of whom arrived in the 1870s, worked initially on the farmlands surrounding Salinas. Some then set up laundry businesses on Main Street but were soon displaced by a new Public Health Ordinance Act that "banned the washing of laundry" on that very street.

In the early 1930s, Dong's father set up the first Chinese-run pharmacy in California outside of those already operating in San Francisco's Chinatown. The Alien Land Act of 1913, barring the purchase of land by Chinese immigrants, had been repealed; and yet there were still stores along Salinas's Main Street that would not serve Chinese customers. His father, the first of ten children, and originally a herbalist before he became a pharmacist, returned to college and trained as a physician in the 1940s. Dong also had four uncles who'd graduated as physicians. They had come a long way from the laundry shops of Main Street.

Ed Hurley's battle with autotransplantation was relived in graphic detail in my interviews with Dong, Shumway, and Hurley himself. Dong also writes about some of these experiments in his recollection published in the Terasaki collection.

With regard to Dong's own crucial role in transplant history, it should be noted that he wrote grant requests formulating research ideas, backed by the data needed to convince the necessary review committees. More than anyone else at Stanford, he was able to articulate a research vision that others in positions of authority could appreciate as valid for funding purposes. Dong also raised private organization grants from local heart associations.

In the early 1960s Dick Lower left Stanford briefly for further training in lung surgery and for a while was not involved in much transplant research. Shumway's clinical work, meanwhile, consumed large chunks of his time. And so, from the winter of 1962 through the spring of 1964, Dong set about acquiring sufficient equipment and personnel to carry out Stanford's transplant research projects. He completed the denervated physiology experiments with Ed Hurley and published the results in 1964. Dong told me in our interviews of "the Eureka moment" when he discovered a method for monitoring heart rejection and administering medications on an "as needed" basis. As he told me: "I was starting from a blank slate, since no prior heart transplants had been followed by Dick for a long period of time with any monitoring equipment or chemical studies. Dick operated clinically on a number of transplanted animals, and I monitored as many of the physical and electrical attributes of the heart as the equipment of the times permitted. Then one stares at the data and looks for patterns. Once you could see a potential pattern, you would formulate an experiment to test that hypothesis."

Ed Stinson's arrival at Stanford is remembered by Lower and Stinson in our interviews.

Adrian and Jean Kantrowitz recalled the details of the National Heart and Lung Institute grant. Raoul and Suegnet de Villiers were interviewed in person. Their memories, in conjunction with my interviews of Yuki Nosé and Kantrowitz, form the basis of my descriptions of their work together at Maimonides in the early 1960s. Kantrowitz's key transplant papers from this period have been cited previously.

The first Barnard section in this chapter is driven by my interviews with de Villiers, Frater, Ozinsky, and Rodney Hewitson. Frater was particularly helpful in recalling Barnard and John Kirklin, and in detailing the significance of both the University of Minnesota Hospital and the Mayo Clinic to the development of open-heart surgery. Unlike the squabbling medical schools of New York or Boston, or Paris and London, where bitter local rivalries reigned, there was a constant exchange of information between the open-heart centers in Minnesota. And if Lillehei could hardly have been more different from the conservative Kirklin, they were bound together by mutual respect. Their contrasting methods also complemented each other, with Lillehei's constant search for the new being followed by Kirklin's determination to systemize cardiac surgery. Lillehei's bold approach allowed him to take risks, while Kirklin tested those seemingly reckless techniques until he had refined them to a point of such practicality that they could be followed by any competent surgeon around the world.

Aware of the more stylized approach at the Mayo, Shumway was among those who began to refer to it as "charm school." The Minnesota gang of delinquents was proud to be tagged, in turn, by the Mayo clinicians as being part of a very different "reform school" mentality. Kirklin and Lillehei encouraged their residents to visit each other's respective schools of surgical etiquette and risk so that they could swap ideas and experiences.

Most of the Minnesota boys traveled across to the Mayo late on Saturday mornings after Lillehei and Wangensteen's Mortality and Morbidity Conferences. As Lillehei did not operate on a Saturday, those early-morning meetings allowed an assortment of residents and surgeons to gather together in an attempt to assess their progress over the previous week. Personalities as contrasting as Lillehei and Varco, Shumway and Barnard, Gott and Cabrol shared that small space for a few hours every Saturday.

Barnard would then often drive over to Rochester to watch Kirklin at work. He was struck by another irony. One of the young University of Cape Town medical students he had tutored, while still a resident at Groote Schuur, had preceded his arrival in America. Frater, however, had followed his parents, who had both trained at the Mayo in the 1920s. They had also married each other in secret, since relationships between medical fellows at the Mayo were strictly forbidden. Frater himself arrived as a junior resident at the Mayo on October 1, 1955, almost three months before Barnard began working in Minnesota.

He understood the contradictions in Barnard's character, for Frater had observed them years before in Cape Town. He knew of Barnard's extraordinary work on tubercular meningitis and intestinal atresia, and he had always admired the flair and daring of the resident he had trailed down the corridors of Groote Schuur. Frater was an English-speaking South African and Barnard an Afrikaner, but they shared something more than just cardiac surgery whenever they met in Rochester. They were both still pulled toward their own country, with Barnard insisting that they would have so much more opportunity in South Africa than America. He was already dreaming of setting up Africa's first open-heart center on his return.

Frater recognized that, like every heart surgeon both before and after him, Barnard carried a small graveyard in his head. It was full of patients he had lost. The graveyards of Kirklin and Lillehei, especially Lillehei, were far bigger and more densely populated. Death comes most to those surgeons who try to be first. Perhaps this accounted for Kirklin's austere character. He was as tense as he was introspective, as driven as he was careful. Kirklin, as far as Frater could tell, had to do everything by the numbers. Whenever they went into the OR, Kirklin would have already written down in excruciating detail every step of the planned operation, and learned each by heart. If the stress of surgery became too much for Kirklin, he would walk away from the table toward a basin in a far corner. He would plunge his gloves, red with blood, into warm salty water and lower his head. Frater and the others would raise an eye at one another but wait silently for their chief to recover. And then back Kirklin would come. He would set to work again and do the most brilliant and complex surgery, slowly and deliberately.

Frater is also central to the discovery that Barnard had been offered a post at the Albert Einstein College of Medicine in 1962. This is confirmed further by Jordan Haller, who worked under Robert H. Goetz as his chief resident at Albert Einstein. Goetz had previously been one of Barnard's professors in Cape Town. When Barnard visited New York for further discussions, he joined one of the ward rounds in the company of Goetz, Chief of Surgery David State (who also came from Minnesota),

Haller, and various cardiologists. Haller remembers Barnard lamenting the fact that in South Africa "the blacks want to take over the country." His reactionary views riled his New York colleagues.

Barnard, of course, finally rejected the opportunity to move to Albert Einstein— he understood that he could dominate the cardiac terrain in his own country in a way that would be impossible in America. He also intuitively realized that, diverted by so much racial legislation, South Africa's lawmakers and judges allowed their doctors to work in an unfettered medical environment. Fittingly, the politically liberal Frater was finally offered, and accepted, the job at Albert Einstein—after he had been recommended by Barnard.

Barnard's immersion in his daughter's waterskiing rise is recounted by Deirdre herself, both in our interviews and in her lovely memoir *Fat, Fame, and Life with Father*. All the quotes from Barnard first appeared in *One Life*, while the chapter ends with a short extract from the Deirdre Visser book.

Chapter Seven. *Mississippi Gambling*

James Hardy's autobiography, *The Academic Surgeon*, provides the detailed list of his daily tasks—which is featured on the dust jacket of that book. Much of the background to his 1964 transplant of a chimpanzee heart comes from his autobiography and from the interviews he gave to Tony Stark in both the book and TV series *Knife to the Heart*. I also interviewed Marius Barnard, Adrian Kantrowitz, and Dick Lower about Hardy's work and read *The New York Times*'s coverage of that doomed transplant attempt.

Insight into Willem Kolff was obtained from my interviews with Adrian and Jean Kantrowitz, archival material provided by Shelley McKellar of ASAIO (the American Society for Artificial Internal Organs), the Willem Kolff Society, and Allen B. Wiesse's detailed interview with Kolff in *Heart to Heart*.

With reference to the January 1964 conference in New York, I quote from Lower and Shumway's paper "Special Problems in Transplantation of the Heart"—and asked both men, and Kantrowitz, for their memories.

The Nelson Mandela quote comes from his autobiography, *Long Walk to Freedom*, while Terblanche and Marius Barnard both discussed the impact of the Hardy attempt on Chris Barnard.

Bob Frater's comments on Barnard's intuitive brilliance are taken from his contribution to David Cooper's collection and from our subsequent interview.

John Terblanche spoke to me about his early transplant work with Barnard at

Groote Schuur, and Deirdre Visser provided further waterskiing references in this chapter. She also writes about these particular episodes in her memoir, while the direct quotes from her father were first printed in *One Life*.

The descriptions of David Hume are based on my interviews with Dick Lower and Carl Goosen, who had moved from Cape Town to Virginia, and also on H. M. Lee's essay on transplant work at MCV in Terasaki's *History of Transplantation*. Lower and Shumway both discussed with me the approaches Hume made to each of them, and the direct quotes were provided by Shumway.

Chapter Eight. The Prince

In our interviews, Kantrowitz discussed his work in left ventricular assist devices and compared his 1966 invention to that of Michael DeBakey's innovation. I also read the *New York Times* coverage of DeBakey's operation (from April 22–26, 1966), his fear of curbs on animal research (May 17, 1966), and the failure of his second attempt with the death of a patient called Walter L. McCans (May 21, 1966). I followed *New York Times* reports of the operation carried out by Kantrowitz on Louise Ceraso in May 1966 (see the list of dates in the notes to Chapter 1).

The description of the fated attempt to transplant the heart of Ralph Senz into the chest of Miller Stevenson is based on my personal interviews with Kantrowitz, Jordan Haller, William Neches, and Rhoda and Richard Senz. Kantrowitz and Neches also opened their archives to allow full access to their notes, correspondences, and case reports.

Chapter Nine. The Steal

Haller, Neches and, in particular, Ronald Hamaty allowed me to interview them at length about the subsequent attempt to use Baby Smith of Pittsburgh as a donor in a transplant to save Miller Stevenson.

Background information on Denton Cooley and Michael DeBakey came from my interview of Cooley in 2003, supplemented by Thomas Thompson's book *Hearts*, which documents the bitter rivalry between the Houston surgeons. The quote about DeBakey being "the handsomest son of a bitch to ever pick up a scalpel" comes from Thompson.

I interviewed Marius Barnard in detail about his work with DeBakey and Cooley, and he is the source for the direct quotes surrounding his spiky repartee with both surgeons. He also described his September 1966 trip to Virginia to see his brother.

Barnard's description of Cooley's dazzling skills as a surgeon first appeared in *One Life*, while the direct quotes from both Chris and Deirdre about him "dropping" her come from a copy of a 1986 London *Sunday Times* magazine profile that is kept at the Transplant Museum at Groote Schuur.

Tom Starzl told Tony Stark of Barnard's visit, which is also recounted in *One Life*.

My interview with Carl Goosen provided much of the background to the description of his move from Cape Town to Richmond, and he supplied the direct quote of Barnard on their first meeting in Virginia.

Memories of David Hume are supplied again by Lower, Shumway, Goosen, and H. M. Lee, while Barnard himself writes of their baboon experiment in *One Life* and supplies the direct quotes.

Carl Goosen and Richard Lower both describe Barnard watching the Richmond dog transplants in vivid detail. The direct quotes are recorded by Goosen. Donald Ross, whom I contacted personally in London, supplies the direct quote, "Christ, Donny, I'm going to do it."

The disaster of *Apollo 1* is recorded on the NASA website and in *New York Times* reports in the period January 28–30, 1967.

On May 18, 1967, the *Los Angeles Times* published an interview with Shumway in an article headlined "Full Transplant Near."

It is important to note that, from 1966 at Stanford, Eugene Dong carried out the bulk of research on the physiology of denervated hearts and artificial hearts and long-term cold storage of hearts with his own grants. Dong administered the experimental laboratory, hired staff, chose the research projects, and maintained all grants and communications with the granting agencies. Dong also mentioned his lab relationship with Bruce Reitz, who carried out the world's first successful heart-lung transplant at Stanford in 1981. As a young man, Reitz needed a senior thesis for graduation from Yale Medical School and, after contacting Shumway, was referred to Dong, under whom he completed his successful research.

Dong has pointed out further that while Shumway was hard at work in the OR, research in the mid-to-late 1960s continued at Stanford under his direction. He formulated and articulated the Stanford program to the federal government, thus ensuring the continued development of cardiac transplantation at Stanford. The inspiration of Shumway was always fundamental to this program, but the value of Dong's research contribution—particularly his data analysis—should not be underestimated, for it was vital in helping to raise money for still deeper research.

Lower told me during our interviews about his near transplant in 1966—foiled only by ABO blood incompatibility—and of the "reverse Hardy" he carried out, transplanting the heart of a human cadaver into a baboon on May 28, 1967.

Marius Barnard described their earliest attempts at cardiac transplantation in the research laboratories at Groote Schuur. He and Ozinsky also discussed with me the

Edith Black kidney transplant, while the direct quotes surrounding this operation come from *One Life*.

Jordan Haller's memory of attending, with Kantrowitz, Shumway's lecture at the American College of Surgeons in Chicago on October 5, 1967, was recounted during one of our interviews. I also read Harold M. Schmeck's article on the conference in *The New York Times* of October 7, 1967.

Chapter Ten. The Wait

Marius Barnard, Bob Frater, Raoul de Villiers, and Rodney Hewitson all spoke to me in detail about the qualities of Val Schrire and his working relationship with Chris Barnard. Marius was particularly useful in highlighting Schrire's caution as the buildup to the first transplant intensified. The direct quotes at the outset of this chapter are from *One Life*.

Background on Louis Washkansky was provided during my interviews with some of his surviving relatives in Cape Town—most notably Arnie Washkansky and Hettie Berman, while Harry and Sybil Washkansky also added to my understanding of the world's first heart transplant patient. Both *One Life* and Peter Hawthorne's *The Transplanted Heart* (published shortly after the first transplant but out of print now for almost twenty-five years) offer additional insights into Washkansky, but the quoted conversation between surgeon and patient come from Barnard's first autobiography.

Ann Washkansky was a much more timid and anxious personality than her husband—and, again, her family offered valuable insights into her character during our interviews. I also took note of the interview she gave to Tony Stark for the BBC's *Knife to the Heart*.

Ed Stinson, Norman Shumway, and Spyros Andreopoulos all shared with me their memories of their possible first recipient, and Andreopoulos described the gathering media interest in the transplant story. The letters quoted—between him and Harry Nelson of the *Los Angeles Times*—are still housed in the Stanford Medical Center archive.

Adrian Kantrowitz relived the tense prelude to Jamie Scudero's transplant, and both Kantrowitz and Bill Neches shared their respective archive materials on this case with me. Neches and Jordan Haller were also interviewed about this period as the hunt for a donor intensified.

Marius Barnard, Rodney Hewitson, and Ozzie Ozinsky were interviewed about the potential "colored" donor for Washkansky, and Chris Barnard records his own memories and the direct quotes in *One Life*.

Shumway told me in an interview about the impossibility of using a Chinese donor—and the sign on his door was remembered by Stinson, transplant coordinators Pat Gamberg and Joan Miller, and, of course, Shumway himself.

The drama of the accident that rendered Denise Darvall brain-dead was remembered by her father and brother in *One Life*. Ann Washkansky added her memory of coincidentally passing the scene of the accident in *Knife to the Heart*.

Marius Barnard, Hewitson, Ozinsky, Cecil Moss (the assistant anesthetist), Peggy Jordaan (the chief OR nurse), and Dene Friedmann (then a young perfusionist on Barnard's team) were all interviewed at length about the buildup to that first transplant and the operation itself, while the direct quotes come from *One Life*. Marius Barnard provides the key revelation—kept secret for almost forty years—that he persuaded his brother to stop Denise Darvall's heart with a concentrated dose of potassium so that they could proceed with the transplant and give Washkansky the best possible chance of survival. I also studied the commemorative *South African Medical Journal* of December 30, 1967, as the entire edition was given over to Barnard and his team's clinical account. Countless newspapers and magazines in December 1967 provided their own accounts of arguably the twentieth century's most famous medical feat.

Chapter Eleven. Fame and Heartbreak

Marius Barnard and Rodney Hewitson offered their own memories of the immediate aftermath to Denise Darvall's heart starting to beat inside Louis Washkansky's chest, and Marius spoke especially eloquently of his brother's sheer exhaustion in the hospital tearoom. He also told me about monitoring Chris's racing pulse.

The *Sunday Times* (Johannesburg) report on John Vorster's palpitating heart at Ellis Park was printed on December 3, 1967.

Arnie Washkansky and Hettie Berman remember the family being contacted by Barnard, and Raoul de Villiers relived for me his feelings of compassion for Kantrowitz and Shumway when he met his exultant fellow Afrikaner that morning. The quotes come from that interview.

Adrian Kantrowitz recalled his own reaction in one of our interviews, while the mood in the Stanford cafeteria was evoked for me by Ed Stinson.

All the newspaper quotes in this chapter were sourced directly from actual editions at the British Library's newspaper archive in Colindale.

The quoted conversation between Barnard and Washkansky comes from *One Life*, while Peter Hawthorne captures the banter between the surgeon and the reporters in *The Transplanted Heart*. Marius Barnard, however, was a key source for me with his personal recollections of this extraordinary time. He provides the quotes about Chris's smoking "other people's" cigarettes and his brother's love of the limelight.

Chapter Twelve. The Man with the Golden Hands

Apart from Adrian Kantrowitz, Bill Neches was my main source for the background to the world's second heart transplant. Neches and Kantrowitz shared their archive material with me. Jordan Haller also revisited the operation from his own bank of memories, while I watched Tony Stark's interviews with Anna Scudero in *Knife to the Heart*. The operation is detailed in clinical terms in A. Kantrowitz, "Moment in history: America's first human heart transplantation—The concept, the planning and the furor" (*ASAIO Journal* 44:4, July–August 1998, pp. 244–52), and in Kantrowitz et al., "Transplantation of the heart in an infant and an adult" (*American Journal of Cardiology* 22:782, 1968).

I heard the South African Broadcasting Corporation interview between Bossie Bosman and Louis Washkansky at Arnie Washkanky's house in Cape Town thirty-five years after it was first recorded.

Barnard's description of listening to the news on his car radio on December 8, 1967, comes from *One Life*, while the newspaper quotes are held at the Transplant Museum in Cape Town.

Barnard recalls the decline of Washkansky in *One Life*, but vivid memories were voiced by Ozinsky, Marius Barnard, Arnie Washkansky, and Hettie Berman.

Chapter Thirteen. Death and America

Marius Barnard recalled the Washkansky autopsy and the selection of Philip Blaiberg as their next transplant patient, an account borne out by his brother's descriptions in *The Second Life*.

Donald Longmore and Adrian Kantrowitz were quoted in *The Star* (Johannesburg) on December 19, 1967.

Memories of Washkansky's funeral come from my interviews with Arnie Washkansky, Hettie Berman, and Marius Barnard, who, of course, was a pallbearer.

The quotes from Barnard, reliving his journey to Washington and his trepidation before appearing on American television alongside Kantrowitz and DeBakey, are from *The Second Life*.

I watched a recording of *Face the Nation* at the Library of Congress in Washington, D.C., and interviewed Kantrowitz about his memories of that night. The quoted newspaper cuttings are all held at the British Museum's Newspaper Archive. Memories of Barnard and Lillehei in New York are from *The Second Life* and from Cooper's interview with Lillehei in his collection *Chris Barnard: By Those Who Know Him Best*. I read G. Wayne Miller's account of this time in *King of Hearts*—and also spoke to Kantrowitz about the visit of Lillehei and Barnard to his lab.

The Louwtjie Barnard quote comes from the *Cape Times*, December 27, 1967, while the Reuters report was quoted in the *Cape Argus* on December 27, 1967. The article from *Die Vaderland* was printed that same day. Lillehei's memory of accompanying Barnard to meet Pik Botha, then the South African consul in New York, appears in Cooper's book. *The Star*'s report on Barnard's appearance on NBC and its account of his meeting John Lindsay, the mayor of New York, were both published on December 28, 1967. The *New York Post* quote is from that same date.

Chris Barnard writes about Louwtjie's response to his increasing fame in *The Second Life*, where he also remembers his bruising encounter with Harold M. Schmeck—Barnard supplies the direct quotes used here. I read Schmeck's account of their meeting, as well as all his related heart-transplant coverage from December 4, 1967, to January 31, 1968, in the *New York Times*.

I interviewed Lower and Shumway about the December 28, 1967, meeting at Chicago O'Hare Airport and read the report of this informal conference printed in *JAMA* on January 15, 1968 (Volume 203, Number 3).

Barnard provides his own downbeat description of meeting President Lyndon Johnson in *The Second Life*, and I read this in conjunction with the copious press coverage given to their meeting in both American and South African newspapers on December 30, 1967.

I interviewed Marius Barnard, Rodney Hewitson, Ozzie Ozinsky, and Peggy Jordaan about the second heart transplant in Cape Town, when Philip Blaiberg received the heart of Clive Haupt. I was also granted access to the medical notes relating to Blaiberg and the nursing report on Haupt when he was admitted to Groote Schuur. *The Second Life* covers the Blaiberg transplant, while Raymond Hoffenberg provided an illuminating account of his involvement in assessing the neurological condition, against an oppressive political backdrop, in the *British Medical Journal* (December 2001). I interviewed Marius Barnard about Hoffenberg's role, and his political situation at Groote Schuur, and also followed reports on his banning order and subsequent exile in the South African press from November 1967 to January 1968.

The quotes from Alfred Snyders, Haupt's brother-in-law, are from the *Cape Argus*, January 2, 1968. The same newspaper carried the front-page story about Blaiberg being "thirsty" the following day, while also reporting the quotes from both the *Daily Sketch* and *The Guardian*. The *Cape Argus*'s report on Haupt's funeral was printed on January 6, 1968.

Chapter Fourteen. The Trial

Ed Stinson and Norman Shumway were my primary sources for the background and subsequent description of the first transplant at Stanford on January 6, 1968. I also made extensive use of the archive at Stanford Medical Center. The quotes from Bill and Virginia White were printed in *The New York Times* and the *Los Angeles Times* on January 8, 1968.

The quoted exchange between Shumway and reporters is from a fully transcribed copy of the press conference on file at the Stanford Medical Center archive. My interviews with Ed Stinson, however, provided the bulk of material about the battle to save Mike Kasperak's life.

A copy of the cable Kantrowitz sent to Shumway has been kept on record at the L-VAD office in Detroit. I was also given access to the notes from the various meetings held just before the second transplant at Maimonides. Kantrowitz, Haller, and Neches spoke to me in detail about the operation, as well as about the donor and recipient patient. I also read the "Schedule of Performance of Heart Transplant" and "Protocol for Adult Human Cardiac Transplantation" documents drawn up by Kantrowitz and his team, as well as the necropsy reports on Louis Block and Helen Krouch. The newspaper quotes come from *The New York Times,* the *Los Angeles Times,* and *The Star* (Johannesburg) on January 10 and 11, 1968. The report on the unmanned U.S. space flight is from *The New York Times* of January 11, 1968.

The quotes from Philip Blaiberg and his daughter, Jill, appeared, respectively, in the *Cape Times* of January 23, 1968, and the *Cape Argus* of January 20, 1968.

Chris Barnard writes of his desire to escape South Africa for Europe in *The Second Life,* from which comes the quote about being "a stallion locked up in a stable." He also writes in further detail of his European tour, and all the quotes in this section are from that book. I interviewed Marius Barnard at length about Blaiberg's recovery and his brother's European jaunt. I transcribed the quotes from a BBC copy of Chris Barnard's appearance on *Tomorrow's World* and read all the British national newspaper reports of his U.K. television debut and his subsequent brawl outside the Crazy Horse in Paris. The condemnation of Barnard in *Die Vaderland* appeared in an undated clipping held at the Transplant Museum archive in Cape Town.

Barnard's relationship with Gina Lollobrigida and his quote that "it's only polite to tip the postman" are documented in *The Second Life,* where he also writes about his preparations to travel to Stanford. The *Palo Alto Times* report on his visit appeared on February 29, 1968. I also interviewed Norman Shumway, Spyros Andreopoulos, and Eugene Dong about Barnard's awkward tour of Stanford.

I interviewed Richard Lower in detail about Barnard's performance at the Hilton in San Francisco on March 2, 1968, and read Barnard's own version of that extraordinary day. The threatened suicide of Louwtjie is mentioned in *The Second Life*, from which Barnard's direct quotes are taken. Barnard's unpublished notes about this incident, seemingly intended for his biography, contain a fuller account and are held at the Transplant Museum archive. Walter Sullivan's report on the conference was printed in *The New York Times* on March 3, 1968. Dick Lower remembered the hostile reaction Barnard received after his speech—and the few words he and Barnard shared together after Lower offered his hand.

The transplant fever that gripped the world was a subject I covered in lengthy interviews with numerous cardiac surgeons, including Norman Shumway, Dick Lower, Marius Barnard, Denton Cooley, Christian Cabrol, Jordan Haller, and Vince Gott. Haller's updated paper "Heart Transplantation in Man: Compilation of Cases II," written with Marcel Cerruti, provided me with the necessary list of transplants during this period.

Cooley himself told me about his cable to Barnard and both Tony Stark's BBC documentary *Knife to the Heart* and Thomas Thompson's *Hearts* offered summaries of this period with particular emphasis on Cooley's work. The quote from Jim Nora is from *Knife to the Heart*. The Stanford Medical Center archive confirmed the number of transplants in 1968 and 1969.

Haller, after leaving Maimonides Hospital himself soon after Kantrowitz's departure, also worked under Cooley. He reveals that "Cooley's organization with three rooms at that time was remarkable—heart surgery on an assembly line! But the key point is that Cooley actually *did* these cases. Others opened and closed chests but he did the 'money part' [i.e., the actual surgery]. He later expanded to ten rooms and averaged about thirty-two cases a day. His total cardiac operations is over 100,000 and the most in a twenty-four hour period is, I believe, forty! I had the privilege of working in his department and was responsible for one of the three rooms. I saw Denton Cooley save lives that no one else could."

Adrian Kantrowitz discussed and explained his balloon-pump work and I read his various papers which cover this key aspect of his medical legacy. With regard to the joint clinical trial he instigated I made a particularly close reading of A. Kantrowitz et al., "Initial clinical experience with intraaortic balloon pumping in cardiogenic shock" (*JAMA*, 203:113, 1968); also the follow-up data in "Letters: Intraaortic balloon pumping" (*JAMA* 203: 998, 1968). Kantrowitz himself recalled his departure from Maimonides in our various interviews, which were supplemented by my interviews with Haller and Neches, as well as his success with the Haskell Shanks case in August 1971.

The breakdown of Chris and Louwtjie Barnard's marriage is covered in her book *Heartbreak,* while the Gina Lollobrigida affair is explored more fully in Chris Logan's *Celebrity Surgeon.* For the purposes of this book I relied mostly on my interviews with Marius Barnard and Deirdre Visser. Marius also documented their transplant work at Groote Schuur through May 1971, and at the British Newspaper Library I read much of the extensive South African coverage of all six transplants from December 1967 and studied the relevant files at the Transplant Museum archive.

Shumway, Ed Stinson, Bruce Reitz, Phil Oyer, Bill Baumgartner, Sharon Hunt, Joan Miller, Pat Gamberg, and Spyros Andreopoulos were all interviewed about Stanford's transplant program in the 1970s. Eugene Dong was again a central figure during this period, as he set up the grant that enabled the medical center to employ specially trained postdoctoral fellows to care for transplant patients, rather than rely on residents rotating through general training. Dong also employed full-time transplant coordinators (who came from the nursing staff) to monitor the clinical care of transplant patients and to assist in the gathering of clinical data. He initiated a transplant data sheet on which the multiple parameters of post-transplant follow-up could be shared by all—surgeons, cardiologists, and immunologists.

When the first desktop computers became available, Dong and Oyer wrote a program that kept track of their clinical data and allowed it be analyzed on demand, which allowed them to trace statistical trends in survival with different treatment protocols. The program was distributed to a number of centers around the world for standardized data-gathering long before the Internet made such availability an easy matter. The grant paid for the salaries of researchers in other departments, such as cardiologists, statisticians, social workers, and psychiatrists.

The death of Bruce Tucker and Lower's transplant of his heart of May 26, 1968, was recalled in close detail for me by the surgeon. Lower was also my main source for the subsequent court case, and I read closely the legal essay printed in the *San Diego Law Review,* March 1975 (vol. 12, no. 2). This paper, "But When Did He Die? Tucker *v.* Lower and the Brain-Death Concept," was given to me by Lower himself. An undated copy of the *National Observer* article "When Does Life End: Heart Can Beat After Death, Jury Says" is held at the Stanford Medical Center archive. Finally, I also interviewed Norm Shumway to hear his reaction to the charge laid against his close friend and chief collaborator in cardiac transplantation.

Epilogue: Acceptance

All direct quotes in the Epilogue are taken from my interviews with Peggy Jordaan, Deirdre Visser, Marius Barnard, Adrian Kantrowitz, Richard Lower, Sheelah Katz,

Eugene Dong, and Norman Shumway. The Chris Barnard quote in support of Nationalist politician Connie Mulder comes from a South African Broadcasting Corporation recording of February 19, 1978—a transcript of which I read at the Transplant Museum archive. On his death in September 2001, however, Barnard was praised by Nelson Mandela as one of South Africa's "main achievers" who "has also done very well in expressing his opinion" on apartheid.

I read the list and individual citations given to the world's leading cardiac surgeons at the Henry Ford International Symposium in October 1975 at the Kantrowitz archive in Detroit; the names of Barnard and Walt Lillehei are conspicuous by their absence.

Marius Barnard provided me with all the necessary documentation surrounding the use of "piggyback" hearts, as well as his brother's quote that "growing old is humanity's greatest tragedy." I also interviewed Marius about Chris's various marriages and his disastrous role as an exponent of Glycel. Marius showed me the quote in which his brother compared himself to the Elephant Man.

The direct quotes relating to Chris Barnard's guilty reaction to the suicide of his son, Andre, are from *The Second Life.*

Quotes from Claude Guthrie's letter to Alexis Carrel lamenting their "newspaper fame" appear in various Shumway lectures housed at the Stanford Medical Center archive. Further background on Carrel comes from television interviews with Merrill Chase, who worked with the Nobel Prize–winning French surgeon in New York, on the BBC's *Knife to the Heart*—and also from Dwight H. Harken's autobiography, written with Lael Wertenbaker, *To Mend the Heart: The Dramatic Story of Cardiac Surgery and Its Pioneers.*

Ed Stinson's quote comes from his celebration of Shumway's work, which is housed at the Stanford Medical Center, while notes relating to *The Stanford Cardiac Surgical Team, 1958–1962* are included in the source material relating to Chapter 2.

The Friday-morning meetings at Stanford's transplant unit had been instigated almost thirty years before by Eugene Dong.

After his generous reading of this text, and in particular the brief section set at Stanford, Shumway sent me the following reminder: "One further note—in 1990 I persuaded a young faculty member, Dr. Vaughan Starnes, to look into the possibility of living pulmonary lobe transplants. Dr. Starnes went on to become Chairman of Cardiovascular Surgery at the University of Southern California and has now a remarkable series of patients surviving lobar transplants of the lung." Shumway died shortly after writing that note about one of his many protégés.

Shumway's tribute to Chris Barnard's role in the history of cardiac transplantation is quoted in Lawrence K. Altman's September 3, 2001, obituary of Barnard in *The*

New York Times. He quotes Shumway as saying that Barnard's first transplant "made the use of brain-dead victims acceptable for organ transplantation . . . [and] without Dr. Barnard's initial use of the brain-dead patient we would not have gone ahead. It was a monumental advance, more societal perhaps than medical, because it applied to all organ transplants."

By contrast, in a South African television documentary made for the M-Net channel shortly before his death, Barnard strikes a different note. He suggests that American surgeons were "particularly bitter because a certain doctor by the name of Norman Shumway was not the first to do the transplant—why he should have been the first I don't know." He argues that Shumway had published all his work in medical journals long before 1967—so making it part of the public domain. Barnard's distinctive voice then trails away in defiance: "I give Shumway a lot of credit . . . I learnt quite a lot from him."

ACKNOWLEDGMENTS

This book could not have been written without the generous and patient involvement of four cardiac surgeons—Adrian Kantrowitz, Richard Lower, Norman Shumway, and Marius Barnard. They endured my repeated interviews and more deluded questions with a grace and good humor I did not always deserve. So to them, first of all, I say thank you.

I contacted Adrian and Jean Kantrowitz in 2002, and the way they immediately invited me to meet them set the tone for the rest of my research. Over the years I became a frequent visitor to Detroit, and I am indebted to Adrian for all the detailed and engaging interviews, and to Jean for opening their archive of historical material. During the many lunches we shared downstairs at River Place, not to mention in countless e-mails and telephone conversations, Jean was unfailingly enthusiastic and meticulously exact as she deepened my understanding of a vast subject. And when it came to the final days of writing, both she and Adrian spent many hours ensuring that every last query was given detailed concentration. I'd also like to acknowledge the work done on my behalf by the support staff at L-VAD Technology, especially Beverly Stella.

My days with Richard Lower and his wife, Anne, in Richmond, Virginia, were among the most special while I did research. His wry but miraculously clear descriptions of his early research with Norm Shumway were invaluable; and of course it was Dick who finally persuaded his old friend to meet me. I owe him a lot—as I do Anne for her close reading of an early draft, which she corrected with such grammatical precision that she is now in danger of being asked to repeat the favor on all future books of mine.

Understanding his reluctance to be interviewed, I greatly valued my time with Norm Shumway at Stanford. He turned out to be even smarter and wittier than everyone had promised—and he made me laugh, whether he was talking about dogs hearts or golf courses, the unexplored genius of Lower the cattle rancher or the contrasting tedium of publicity.

Marius Barnard was consistently kind and understanding about my work on this book. And he and his wife, Inez, were always good to me, whether in Hermanus or London. I look forward to the publication of his book—a project that means a great deal to both of us.

Many other cardiac surgeons were extraordinarily benevolent with their time and interest in this book, and I'd like to thank especially my fellow South Africans Bob Frater and David Wheatley for reading the medical descriptions and correcting my more embarrassing errors. Any mistakes remaining are my own. Bob became a good friend and a source of striking insights into anything and everything from the mitral valve to the character of the archetypal surgeon. David Wheatley, meanwhile, was the first surgeon I ever interviewed—at the Glasgow Infirmary in April 2002—and he remained someone I could always contact in moments of confusion or incomprehension.

Basil Lazarides, my old school friend from Germiston, now an esteemed anesthetist, read the manuscript at an early stage and did much to help me clarify some of the medical aspects. He also proved, once more, that the oldest friendships do not wither—despite the passing years and a six-thousand-mile distance between us.

Jordan Haller was another surgeon who always acted more like a friend than an interviewee—and I shall never forget the way he and his wife, Carna, looked after me in Pittsburgh while teaching me a thing or two about cardiac history and opera. It was through Jordan that I came to meet William Neches—and a morning in Bill's office, with Jordan at his side, opened a new door to all the work they had done alongside Adrian Kantrowitz at Maimonides. They were forever ready to answer yet another question.

Similarly, the brilliant Ed Stinson did much to guide me through the epic Stanford story with his renowned humility; his help to me was considerable. At

Stanford itself, Mary Burge was unwavering in her encouragement during some of the more difficult early stages of my research—and she also sent me a steady stream of great books she knew I would like. M. A. Malone was another Stanford ally, among many others, who went out of her way to make me feel at home. I acknowledge all the others at Stanford who helped me during my various visits: Spyros Andreopoulos, Marguerite Brown, Eugene Dong, Pat Gamberg, Sharon Hunt, Joan Miller, Phil Oyer, Liz Pope, Bruce Reitz, and Robert Robbins.

With regard to the South African section of this book, I thank Deirdre Visser for her warm and humane responses to my questions about her father, Christiaan Barnard—many of which she answered repeatedly. It was a treat to meet her in Cape Town. Many other South Africans allowed me to interview them at length about their memories of Christiaan Barnard, Louis Washkansky, and Adrian Kantrowitz or their own association with the first human heart transplant. The following contributed significantly to my research: Hetty Berman, Johan Brink, Raoul and Suegnet de Villiers, Dene Friedmann, Carl Goosen, Rodney Hewitson, Christine and Pat Heydenrych, Peggy Jordaan, Cecil Moss, "Ozzie" Ozinsky, Marion Summerfield, John Terblanche, Susan Vosloo, Arnold Washkansky, and Harry and Sybil Washkansky.

I am indebted to Rhoda and Richard Senz for allowing me to interview them about a particularly painful period in their lives. Rhoda's letter to me after she read a draft of this book will always mean a great deal to me. I thank both her and Richard.

The following surgeons also helped me at various stages of my research: Bill Baumgartner, Christian Cabrol, Denton Cooley, Vince Gott, Ronald Hamaty, Ed Hurley, Yuki Nosé, and John Wallwork. Many of the better stories in this book come from interviews with them.

Jonny Geller, my agent in London, proved again why he's the best in the business. His editorial input was vital during chaotic early versions of this book. Emma Parry, my New York agent, played a similarly deft role and was a constant source of support during both the research and the writing.

David Highfill did more than anyone to shape and improve the book. As my editor at Putnam in New York, he managed the trick of persuading me to rework whole chunks of narrative while making me think that I was already on the right path. And the moment when he subtly suggested that I concentrate on the medical milestones was a true turning point. In a seamless transition, Rachel Kahan saw the book through its final stages to publication.

In London, Tim Binding was one of the first to see the merit of this subject, and his unique eye for the telling overview always helped me. Rochelle Venables, once more, supplied a notably sharp line-edit, and was always there to answer yet another question from me. During the last few months, Andrew Gordon steered the book through to its UK publication.

My parents, Ian and Jess, were typically supportive, and their input was immeasurable. They listened and responded to my research stories by reliving their own memories of Barnard and the first heart transplant in 1967.

Finally, as always, my wife, Alison, is my first and last reader, my best pal, and my heart-opening accomplice through every twist and turn before, during, and after writing. It seems all the sweeter that, fourteen years after buying my first book, she should have lived through every word of the last four with me. Alison has the kind of verve and belief that make her the only person I know who would, in the interest of making this a better book, have helped me transplant a heart from one neighborhood dog to another in the backyard shed—had we not been too soft or liked the tail-wagging mutts so much. So thanks go, most of all, to Alison and to Isabella, Jack, and Emma—our small trio who drew red and purple hearts almost every day to remind me of the people in this book.

INDEX